Meningiomas

Jennifer Moliterno • Antonio Omuro
Editors

Meningiomas

Comprehensive Strategies for Management

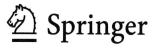 Springer

Editors
Jennifer Moliterno
Department of Neurosurgery
Yale School of Medicine
Yale New Haven Hospital
New Haven, CT
USA

Antonio Omuro
Department of Neurology
Yale School of Medicine
Yale New Haven Hospital
New Haven, CT
USA

ISBN 978-3-030-59557-9   ISBN 978-3-030-59558-6   (eBook)
https://doi.org/10.1007/978-3-030-59558-6

This Springer imprint is published by the registered company Springer Nature Switzerland AG
The registered company address is: Gewerbestrasse 11, 6330 Cham, Switzerland

We dedicate this book to all patients impacted by a meningioma diagnosis, and especially share our hope for more promising treatment with those who suffer from more aggressive ones.

Jennifer Moliterno
Antonio Omuro

Preface

Meningiomas are one of the most common types of brain tumors and frequently encountered by primary care physicians and brain tumor specialists alike. While these tumors are more often histologically benign (i.e., WHO Grade 1), approximately 15–20% can behave atypical (i.e., WHO Grade 2) or frankly malignant (i.e., WHO Grade 3). Some Grade 1 tumors may never become symptomatic and can be relatively simple to manage. However, for others, as they grow along certain locations of the dura and skull base, oftentimes invading the skull, they can become quite debilitating to patients based on their location, size, and mass effect on and/or involvement of critical neurovascular structures. Thus, for certain "*histologically benign*" tumors, their clinical behavior may be anything but benign. Tumor recurrence, seen more frequently with Grades 2 and 3 meningiomas, but also with Grade 1 tumors, can be difficult to predict and poses many challenges for treating physicians. When treatment is indicated, the first line modality is often surgical, but associated risks and morbidities can vary based on individual tumors. The use of radiation, more conventional or in the form of radiosurgery, can often be necessary, but similarly needs to be properly assessed and evaluated. While there is currently no standard or proven beneficial treatment with chemotherapy, clinical trials are underway. Thus, for a proportion of these seemingly simple and "benign" tumors, treatment can be quite complex, and paradigms, therefore, rely on a multidisciplinary clinical effort.

Recently, tremendous scientific advances have been made to better understand the molecular biology of meningiomas. Indeed, we now have a more in-depth understanding of the genetic alterations driving formation of these tumors, classifying them into molecular subgroups, with insight into why some transform into more malignant tumors and recur while others do not. More recent observations from translational research have underscored the difficulty with treatment of these tumors at the biological level and have identified specific genomic and pathological characteristics that suggest options for treatment. These findings can ultimately influence the management of meningiomas, both upfront and at the time of recurrence. To that end, precision medicine with care personalized to each individual is important, showing the most promise in the potential use of targeted drug therapies and clinical trials.

Given the prevalence and potential complexity of meningiomas, this text provides a comprehensive overview of the multidisciplinary management of meningiomas, organized by an overview, followed by evaluation and management considerations along a spectrum of benign to more malignant behavior. Its intent is to be highly informative and provide clarity for a wide audience of neurosurgeons, reconstructive surgeons, oncologists, neurologists, radiation oncologists, pathologists, radiologists, residents, and students who treat these patients and those who are training for a career in managing patients with these potentially challenging tumors.

New Haven, CT, USA   Jennifer Moliterno, MD
New Haven, CT, USA   Antonio Omuro, MD

Contents

Part III   Treatment Options for more aggressive meningiomas

Contributors

Ori Barzilai, MD Department of Neurosurgery, Memorial Sloan-Kettering Cancer Center, New York, NY, USA

Mark H. Bilsky, MD Department of Neurosurgery, Memorial Sloan-Kettering Cancer Center, New York, NY, USA

Priscilla K. Brastianos, MD Department of Medicine and Neurology, Massachusetts General Hospital/Harvard Medical School, Boston, MA, USA

Swathi Chidambaram, MD Department of Neurological Surgery, Weill Cornell Medicine, New York, NY, USA

Joseph N. Contessa, MD, PhD Department of Therapeutic Radiology, Yale School of Medicine, Yale New Haven Hospital, New Haven, CT, USA

Zachary A. Corbin, MD, MHS Department of Neurology, Yale School of Medicine, Yale New Haven Hospital, New Haven, CT, USA

William T. Couldwell, MD, PhD Department of Neurosurgery, Clinical Neurosciences Center, University of Utah, Salt Lake City, UT, USA

E. Zeynep Erson-Omay, MS, PhD Department of Neurosurgery, Yale School of Medicine, Yale New Haven Hospital, New Haven, CT, USA

Daniel M. Fountain, BSc MB BChir PGCME MRCS Manchester Centre for Clinical Neurosciences, Salford Royal NHS Foundation Trust, Salford, Manchester Greater Manchester, UK

Corey M. Gill, BS, BA Icahn School of Medicine at Mount Sinai, New York, NY, USA

Murat Gunel, MD, FACS, FAHA, FAANS Department of Neurosurgery, Yale School of Medicine, Yale New Haven Hospital, New Haven, CT, USA

Department of Neurosurgery, Yale New Haven Hospital, Tompkins Memorial Pavilion (TMP), New Haven, CT, USA

Christopher S. Hong, MD Department of Neurosurgery, Yale School of Medicine, Yale New Haven Hospital, New Haven, CT, USA

Anita Huttner, MD Department of Pathology, Yale School of Medicine, Yale New Haven Hospital, New Haven, CT, USA

Jana Ivanidze, MD, PhD Department of Radiology, Weill Cornell Medicine, New York, NY, USA

Michel Kalamarides, MD, PhD Department of Neurosurgery, Pitie-Salpetriere Hospital, AP-HP and Sorbonne Universite, Paris, France

Thomas J. Kaley, MD Department of Neurology, Memorial Sloan Kettering Cancer Center, New York, NY, USA

Sean S. Mahase, MD Department of Radiation Oncology, New York Presbyterian and Weill Cornell Medicine, New York, NY, USA

Declan McGuone, MB, BCh Department of Pathology, Yale School of Medicine, Yale New Haven Hospital, New Haven, CT, USA

Jennifer Moliterno, MD Yale New Haven Hospital and Smilow Cancer Hospital, New Haven, CT, USA

Yale Brain Tumor Center at Smilow Cancer Hospital, New Haven, CT, USA

Department of Neurosurgery, Yale School of Medicine, Yale New Haven Hospital, New Haven, CT, USA

S. Bulent Omay, MD Department of Neurosurgery, Yale School of Medicine, Yale New Haven Hospital, New Haven, CT, USA

Antonio Omuro, MD Yale New Haven Hospital and Smilow Cancer Hospital, New Haven, CT, USA

Yale Brain Tumor Center at Smilow Cancer Hospital, New Haven, CT, USA

Department of Neurology, Yale School of Medicine, Yale University, New Haven, CT, USA

Susan C. Pannullo, MD Department of Neurological Surgery, Weill Cornell Medicine, New York, NY, USA

Gabrielle W. Peters, MD Department of Radiation Oncology, Yale, New Haven, CT, USA

Matthieu Peyre, MD, PhD Department of Neurosurgery, Pitie-Salpetriere Hospital, AP-HP and Sorbonne Universite, Paris, France

Isabel P. Prado, MS Department of Neurology, Yale University, New Haven, CT, USA

Amol Raheja, MBBS, MCH Department of Neurosurgery, All India Institute of Medical Sciences, New Delhi, India

Ashley M. Roque, MD Department of Neuro-Oncology, Mount Sinai Hospital, New York, NY, USA

Diana A. Roth O'Brien, MD, MPH Department of Radiation Oncology, New York Presbyterian and Weill Cornell Medicine, New York, NY, USA

Robert J. Rothrock, MD Department of Neurosurgery and Radiation Oncology, Memorial Sloan-Kettering Cancer Center, New York, NY, USA

Thomas Santarius, MD, PhD, FRCS(SN) Department of Clinical Neurosciences, Cambridge University Hospitals NHS Foundation Trust, Cambridge, Cambridgeshire, UK

Theodore H. Schwartz, MD Department of Neurosurgery, Otolaryngology and Neuroscience, Weill Cornell Medicine, New York Presbyterian Hospital, New York, NY, USA

Yoshiya (Josh) Yamada, MD Department of Neurosurgery and Radiation Oncology, Memorial Sloan-Kettering Cancer Center, New York, NY, USA

Mark W. Youngblood, MD, PhD Department of Neurosurgery, Northwestern Memorial Hospital, Chicago, IL, USA

Amy Y. Zhao, BS Department of Neurosurgery, Yale School of Medicine, Yale New Haven Hospital, New Haven, CT, USA

Part I

Meningioma Basics

An Overview of Meningiomas

Michel Kalamarides and Matthieu Peyre

A Brief Historical Perspective on Meningiomas

While several historical examples of meningiomas have been retrospectively described under multiple designations (fonguous tumor of the dura mater, epithelioma, psammoma, dural sarcoma, and others) throughout centuries of medical literature, it was not until Harvey Cushing coined the term "meningioma" in 1922 that the knowledge of this tumor started to structure itself over detailed nomenclatures. Seminal work included the Cavendish lecture in 1922 and the publication of the monograph *Meningiomas, Their Classification, Regional Behaviour, Life History, and Surgical End Results* in 1938 by Cushing and Eisenhardt, which considered breakthroughs that defined the field for almost a century. The careful description of the clinical cases of meningiomas that Cushing operated on and the subsequent improvement of his surgical technique provided landmarks that led to the classification of meningiomas according to their site of origin. Based on early works under the tutelage of Cushing, Bailey and Bucy described the first definitive histological classification of meningiomas in 1931, which remained virtually unchanged until the early twenty-first century.

The field of meningioma surgery has witnessed several dramatic improvements since 1922, but our progress in the understanding of tumor biology and natural history remains astonishingly poor compared to the works of those pioneers. Quoting the words of H. Cushing during his Cavendish lecture in 1922: "There is today nothing in the whole realm of surgery more gratifying than the successful removal of a meningioma with subsequent perfect functional recovery, especially should a correct pathological diagnosis have been made. The difficulties are admittedly

M. Kalamarides (✉) · M. Peyre
Department of Neurosurgery, Pitie-Salpetriere Hospital, AP-HP and Sorbonne Universite, Paris, France
e-mail: michel.kalamarides@aphp.fr

© Springer Nature Switzerland AG 2020
J. Moliterno, A. Omuro (eds.), *Meningiomas*,
https://doi.org/10.1007/978-3-030-59558-6_1

great, sometimes insurmountable and though the disappointments still are many, another generation of neurological surgeons will unquestionably see them largely overcome." To date, while many of the aforementioned surgical difficulties have been indeed surmounted, nonsurgical therapies have remained elusive.

Demographics, Incidence, and Prevalence

Meningiomas are the most common primary brain tumor. Among the Central Brain Tumor Registry of the United States (CBTRUS) major histology-proven groupings, incidence rates were highest for tumors of the meninges, corresponding to 8.60 per 100,000 people [1]. Indeed, the most frequently reported histology overall was meningioma (37.1%), followed by tumors of the pituitary (16.5%) and glioblastoma (14.7%). Incidence rates of meningioma increase with age. In that registry, most meningiomas (79.8%) were described in the cerebral meninges and 4.2% in the spinal meninges, and approximately 15.2% did not have a specific meningeal site listed. Meningioma was most common in adults aged 65 years and older and remained very rare in children aged 0–14 years. The incidence of meningioma increased with age, with a dramatic increase after age 65 years. Even among the population age 85 years and older, these rates continued to increase.

Nonmalignant meningiomas overall were 2.16 times more common in females compared to males (Fig. 1.1). The female-to-male ratios were lowest in persons <20 years old, for whom incidence rates for males and females were approximately equal, and highest from 35 to 54, where incidence rates were three times

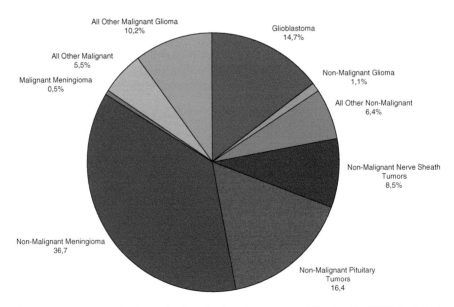

Fig. 1.1 Distribution of primary brain and other CNS tumors following CBTRUS Statistical Report [1]

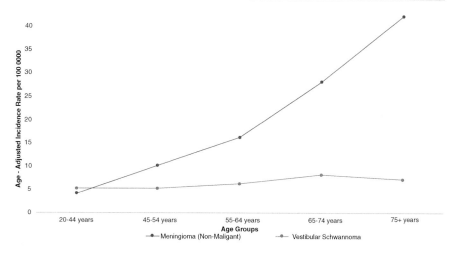

Fig. 1.2 Age-adjusted incidence rates of brain and other CNS tumors by selected histologies in patients more than 20 years old [1]

higher in females. One possible explanation is that WHO grades II and III are more frequent in males. Among the meningiomas with documented WHO grade, 80.6% were WHO grade I, 17.6% were WHO grade II, and 1.7% were WHO grade III. The prevalence of pathologically confirmed meningioma has been estimated to be approximately 97.5/100,000 in the United States, according to a 2010 CBTRUS report (Fig. 1.2).

It is noteworthy that a large number of meningiomas are asymptomatic and thus incidentally discovered during brain imaging performed for other reasons. Histology-based studies may therefore underestimate the true incidence of these tumors. In a study [2] of 2000 asymptomatic subjects (mean age, 63.3 years; range, 45.7–96.7), a brain MRI (1.5 T) without contrast enhancement was performed according to a standardized protocol. Meningiomas were recorded IN 0.9% of the population. Their size ranged from 5 to 60 mm in diameter, and their prevalence was 1.1% in women and 0.7% in men. The prevalence of meningiomas increased from 0.5% in 45- to 59-year-olds to 1.6% in persons 75 years of age or older.

Another source for analysis of the true incidence and prevalence of tumors is old autopsy series [3]. As the growth rate of meningiomas is typically slow, and most meningiomas remain asymptomatic throughout life, it was estimated that 50% of all meningiomas are discovered at autopsy. The prevalence of meningiomas found at autopsy in persons over 60 years of age is 3%, and the majority of the lesions are less than 1 cm in diameter.

Risk Factors

A number of genetic and environmental risk factors for the development of meningiomas have been identified, as summarized below.

Neurofibromatosis Type 2

Neurofibromatosis type 2 (NF2) is a rare genetic disorder (birth incidence 1/33,000) characterized by the development of multiple benign tumors of the nervous system. The hallmark of NF2 is the development of bilateral vestibular schwannomas [4]. Meningiomas are the second most frequent tumor type in NF2 and are found intra-cranially in 45% to 58% of patients. For those, the median number of meningiomas per patient was 3. The cumulative incidence of meningiomas was shown to be close to 80% by 70 years of age in a cohort of 411 patients with proven *NF2* mutation.

Other Genetic Risk Factors

Apart from NF2, other genetic risk factors for the development of meningiomas are rare. A subset of patients with *BAP1*-deficient rhabdoid meningiomas harbored germline *BAP1* mutations, indicating that rhabdoid meningiomas can be a harbinger of the *BAP1* cancer predisposition syndrome, which is associated with increased risk of uveal melanoma, cutaneous melanoma, malignant mesothelioma, renal cell carcinoma, cholangiocarcinoma, multiple non-melanoma skin cancers, and *BAP1*-inactivated nevi [5].

Two of the SWI/SNF chromatin remodeling complex subunits, *SMARCB1* [6] and *SMARCE1* [7], have been implicated in increased risk of meningiomas. Germline mutations of *SMARCB1* confer a risk of meningiomas as part of the schwannomatosis phenotype. More recently, loss-of-function mutations in *SMARCE1* were found to specifically predispose carriers to clear cell meningiomas. Another pathway implicated in meningiomas is the Sonic Hedgehog pathway. A nontruncating mutation in the Shh-Gli1 pathway gene, *SUFU*, was identified as the cause of multiple meningiomas in a single large Finnish family [8]. Finally, cranial hyperostosis and meningiomas are common in patients with Proteus syndrome, which is caused by a somatic activating mutation in *AKT1* c.49G > A. In a series of 29 patients with this syndrome, the most common intra-cranial tumor was meningioma, all co-localizing with cranial hyperostosis, and diagnosed at younger ages as compared to sporadic meningiomas and driven by the activation of the AKT/PI3K pathway [9].

Mutations of *CCM3/PDCD10* cause 10–15% of hereditary cerebral cavernous malformations. The phenotypic characterization of *CCM3*-mutated patients has been hampered by the limited number of patients harboring a mutation in this gene. In a series of 54 *CCM3*-mutated index patients, cerebral hemorrhage was the initial presentation in 72% of these patients. Multiple extra-axial, dural-based lesions were detected in seven unrelated patients [10]. These lesions were eventu-ally proven to be meningiomas in three patients who underwent surgical resection and histological examination. This multiple meningiomas phenotype is not associ-ated with a specific *CCM3* mutation. Hence, *CCM3* mutations are associated with a high risk of early-onset cerebral hemorrhage and with the presence of multiple meningiomas.

Radiation

The first report of an association between ionizing radiation and meningiomas was the Hiroshima study, which found an increased incidence of meningiomas linked to the distance from the center of the explosion [11]. Radiation-induced meningioma is a known late effect of cranial radiation therapy after childhood cerebral malignancy. In one recent study, the authors performed a screening brain MRI in asymptomatic survivors of childhood acute lymphoblastic leukemia treated with cranial radiation therapy ≥10 years previously [12]. The incidence of radiation-induced meningioma and outcomes of this group were compared with a historical cohort of survivors with the same exposure who underwent imaging only if symptoms were present. The study analyzed 176 patients, including 70 in the screening group and 106 unscreened. Screening MRI was performed a median of 25 years after radiation therapy and detected meningiomas in 15 (21.4%) patients. In the unscreened group, 17 patients (16.0%) had neurologic symptoms leading to an MRI with a median interval of 24 years after radiation therapy, 9 of whom (8.5%) were diagnosed with meningioma. There was no significant difference between screened and unscreened patients in the size of meningioma (mean diameter, 1.6 cm vs 2.6 cm; $P = 0.13$) and meningioma incidence (7.4% vs 4.0% at 25 years; $P = 0.19$). In a comprehensive review, the authors reviewed 251 cases of radiation-induced meningiomas [13]. The average age at onset for the primary lesion was 13.0 ± 13.5 years, and the average radiation dose delivered to this lesion was 38.8 ± 16.8 Gy. Secondary meningiomas could be divided into grades I (140), II (55), and III (10) tumors. Thirty patients (11.9%) had multiple lesions, and 46 (18.3%) had recurrent meningiomas. The latency period between radiotherapy for primary lesions and the onset of meningiomas was 22.9 ± 11.4 years. The latency period was shorter for patients with grade III meningioma and for those in the high-dose and intermediate-dose radiation groups who received systemic chemotherapy. Aggressive meningiomas and multiple meningiomas were more common in the high-dose and intermediate-dose groups than in the low-dose group. The 5-year and 10-year survival rates for all patients with meningioma were 77.7% and 66.1%, respectively. From a genomic standpoint, therapeutic radiation for childhood cancer typically drives structural aberrations of *NF2* in meningiomas [14, 15]. Further studies are needed to identify whether the observed predominant localization at the convexity is due to the axis of radiation, versus other biological reasons. Given the epigenetic and mutational similarity of sporadic meningioma of the convexity and radiation-induced meningiomas, the findings might potentially also point toward differential susceptibility for radiation-induced tumor formation, particularly by *NF2* mutations, in arachnoidal cells of the convexity compared to those of the skull base.

Hormonal Factors

Several observations indicate hormonal regulation of tumor growth including female predominance, frequent expression of progesterone receptors in approximately 70%

of meningiomas and epidemiological evidence of an association between meningioma and pregnancy [16], breast cancer, and exogenous hormone use. There is a modest increased risk of breast cancer among users of combined oral contraceptives and hormone replacement therapy. In contrast, several studies found no association between combined oral contraceptives and meningiomas, whereas several other studies did report an increased risk with hormone replacement therapy [17]. Several studies have also found an association between the use of synthetic progestins, including cyproterone acetate and megestrol acetate, and meningioma growth [18]. A recent study of meningiomas developing after long-term progestin therapy showed that they tended to be multiple and located at the skull base [19]. From a genetic point of view, a higher frequency of *PIK3CA* and *TRAF7* mutations and a lower frequency of *NF2*-mutated tumors were observed. This shift in mutational landscape indicates the vulnerability of certain meningeal cells and mutations to hormone-induced tumorigenesis. While the relationship between *PIK3CA* mutation frequency and hormone-related cancers such as breast and endometrial cancer is well-known, this hormonally induced mutational shift is a unique feature in molecular oncology.

Current Research Trends

Recent advances in the knowledge of tumor initiation of meningiomas, largely driven by advances in high-throughput gene sequencing, have led to the discovery of mutations that drive 80% of meningiomas, with two groups that are mutually exclusive. One group, mostly comprising skull base meningiomas, typically includes WHO grade I tumors with mutations in the *TRAF7* gene, in association with mutations in PI3K and SHH pathways genes. The other group consists of convexity meningiomas and that harbors *NF2* mutations. Remarkably, grade II and II meningiomas are much more common at the convexity with a predominance of *NF2* mutations. The multiple histological subtypes of meningiomas also seem to follow these mutation groups [20, 21]. Such advances in the understanding of the molecular biology of meningiomas will hopefully lead to a true histo-molecular associated with a topographic classification of those tumors in the next years that should aid in the clinical management of these patients.

The high incidence of meningiomas in autopsy series highlights that a high portion of those tumors remain asymptomatic throughout the individual life span. It is therefore of high importance to develop a heightened understanding of why and when meningiomas will escape their indolent clinical course to become symptomatic tumors. Advances in this field could lead to a more proactive clinical management of these tumors.

Similarly, another important focus of research is the characterization of the mechanisms underlying tumor progression to a more clinically and histologically aggressive behavior [22]. It is well-known that an aggressive behavior may be present from disease onset (de novo) or result from a malignant transformation from initially benign tumor [23]. It is possible that the progenitor cells of these meningiomas may differ, and intensive research efforts are being direct toward the identification of those, as well as the pathways involved in such striking shifts in biological behavior [24].

References

1. Ostrom QT, Gittleman H, Truitt G, Boscia A, Kruchko C, Barnholtz-Sloan JS. CBTRUS statistical report: primary brain and other central nervous system tumors diagnosed in the United States in 2011-2015. Neuro-Oncology. 2018;20(suppl_4):iv1–iv86.
2. Vernooij MW, Ikram MA, Tanghe HL, Vincent AJ, Hofman A, Krestin GP, et al. Incidental findings on brain MRI in the general population. N Engl J Med. 2007;357(18):1821–8.
3. Nakasu S, Hirano A, Shimura T, Llena JF. Incidental meningiomas in autopsy study. Surg Neurol. 1987;27(4):319–22.
4. Goutagny S, Bah AB, Henin D, Parfait B, Grayeli AB, Sterkers O, Kalamarides M. Long term of 287 meningiomas in neurofibromatosis type 2 patients: clinical, radiological, and molecular features. Neuro-Oncology. 2012;14(8):1090–6.
5. Shankar GM, Abedalthagafi M, Vaubel RA, Merrill PH, Nayyar N, Gill CM, et al. Germline and somatic BAP1 mutations in high-grade rhabdoid meningiomas. Neuro-Oncology. 2017;19(4):535–45.
6. Christiaans I, Kenter SB, Brink HC, van Os TA, Baas F, van den Munckhof P, et al. Germline SMARCB1 mutation and somatic NF2 mutations in familial multiple meningiomas. J Med Genet. 2011;48(2):93–7.
7. Smith MJ, O'Sullivan J, Bhaskar SS, Hadfield KD, Poke G, Caird J, et al. Loss-of-function mutations in SMARCE1 cause an inherited disorder of multiple spinal meningiomas. Nat Genet. 2013;45(3):295–8.
8. Aavikko M, Li SP, Saarinen S, Alhopuro P, Kaasinen E, Morgunova E, et al. Loss of SUFU function in familial multiple meningioma. Am J Hum Genet. 2012;91(3):520–6.
9. Keppler-Noreuil KM, Baker EH, Sapp JC, Lindhurst MJ, Biesecker LG. Somatic AKT1 mutations cause meningiomas colocalizing with a characteristic pattern of cranial hyperostosis. Am J Med Genet A. 2016;170(10):2605–10.
10. Riant F, Bergametti F, Fournier HD, Chapon F, Michalak-Provost S, Cecillon M, et al. CCM3 mutations are associated with early-onset cerebral hemorrhage and multiple meningiomas. Mol Syndromol. 2013;4(4):165–72.
11. Shintani T, Hayakawa N, Hoshi M, Sumida M, Kurisu K, Oki S, et al. High incidence of meningiomas among Hiroshima atomic bomb survivors. J Radiat Res. 1999;40(1):49–57.
12. Co JL, Swain M, Murray LJ, Ahmed S, Laperriere NJ, Tsang DS, et al. Meningioma screening with MRI in childhood leukemia survivors treated with cranial radiation. Int J Radiat Oncol Biol Phys. 2019;104(3):640–3.
13. Yamanaka R, Hayano A, Kanayama T. Radiation-induced meningiomas: an exhaustive review of the literature. World Neurosurg. 2017;97:635–44.
14. Agnihotri S, Suppiah S, Tonge PD, Jalali S, Danesh A, Bruce JP, et al. Therapeutic radiation for childhood cancer drives structural aberrations of NF2 in meningiomas. Nat Commun. 2017;8(1):186.
15. Sahm F, Toprak UH, Hübschmann D, Kleinheinz K, Buchhalter I, Sill M, et al. Meningiomas induced by low-dose radiation carry structural variants of NF2 and a distinct mutational signature. Acta Neuropathol. 2017;134(1):155–8.
16. Lusis EA, Scheithauer BW, Yachnis AT, Fischer BR, Chicoine MR, Paulus W, Perry A. Meningiomas in pregnancy: a clinicopathologic study of 17 cases. Neurosurgery. 2012;71(5):951–61.

17. Claus EB, Black PM, Bondy ML, Calvocoressi L, Schildkraut JM, Wiemels JL, Wrensch M. Exogenous hormone use and meningioma risk: what do we tell our patients? Cancer. 2007;110(3):471–6.
18. Gazzeri R, Galarza M, Gazzeri G. Growth of a meningioma in a transsexual patient after estrogen-progestin therapy. N Engl J Med. 2007;357(23):2411–2.
19. Peyre M, Gaillard S, de Marcellus C, Giry M, Bielle F, Villa C, et al. Progestin-associated shift of meningioma mutational landscape. Ann Oncol. 2018;29(3):681–6.
20. Clark VE, Erson-Omay EZ, Serin A, Yin J, Cotney J, Ozduman K, et al. Genomic analysis of non-NF2 meningiomas reveals mutations in TRAF7, KLF4, AKT1, and SMO. Science. 2013;339(6123):1077–80.
21. Brastianos PK, Horowitz PM, Santagata S, Jones RT, McKenna A, Getz G, et al. Genomic sequencing of meningiomas identifies oncogenic SMO and AKT1 mutations. Nat Genet. 2013;45(3):285–9.
22. Harmancı AS, Youngblood MW, Clark VE, Coşkun S, Henegariu O, Duran D, et al. Integrated genomic analyses of de novo pathways underlying atypical meningiomas. Nat Commun. 2017;8:14433.
23. Peyre M, Gauchotte G, Giry M, Froehlich S, Pallud J, Graillon T, et al. De novo and secondary anaplastic meningiomas: a study of clinical and histomolecular prognostic factors. Neuro-Oncology. 2018;20(8):1113–21.
24. Sahm F, Schrimpf D, Stichel D, Jones DTW, Hielscher T, Schefzyk S, et al. DNA methylation-based classification and grading system for meningioma: a multicentre, retrospective analysis. Lancet Oncol. 2017;18(5):682–94.

Histopathology and Grading of Meningiomas

Declan McGuone and Anita Huttner

Meningiomas are one of the most common intracranial tumor types encountered by neuropathologists in routine surgical pathology practice. When neuropathologists receive a tissue biopsy from a patient with a meningioma, they typically follow the mandate of the World Health Organization (WHO) Classification of Tumors of the Central Nervous System (2016), to accurately classify and grade the tumor. Although meningiomas are usually benign and are often slow-growing tumors, they are notable for their striking histologic diversity, and many different microscopic subtypes have been described over the years. Relatively few of these distinct histologic patterns are clinically significant, and, in practice, the most commonly encountered subtypes are the meningothelial, fibrous, and transitional variants. In this chapter we will consider the fundamental principles of tumor grading as they apply to meningioma, discuss the major morphologic subtypes of meningioma currently recognized by the WHO, and review common immunohistochemical studies that may be utilized to facilitate a diagnosis of meningioma. The tremendous histologic diversity of meningiomas means that they occasionally mimic other tumor types, including several malignant tumors, and this can be diagnostically problematic in centers that lack a dedicated neuropathologist. In this chapter we will also consider some of the major differential diagnoses that occasionally masquerade as meningioma.

D. McGuone
Department of Pathology, Yale New Haven Hospital, New Haven, CT, USA
e-mail: declan.mcguone@yale.edu

A. Huttner (✉)
Department of Pathology, Yale School of Medicine, New Haven, CT, USA
e-mail: anita.huttner@yale.edu

© Springer Nature Switzerland AG 2020
J. Moliterno, A. Omuro (eds.), *Meningiomas*,
https://doi.org/10.1007/978-3-030-59558-6_2

Meningioma Histogenesis

Although meningiomas usually occur as dural-based masses along the craniospinal axis, their histologic features actually resemble arachnoid rather than dura mater. As a result, they share many histologic similarities with normal arachnoidal cells, particularly the arachnoid cap cell, and have a tendency to occur at locations where this cell type is found most frequently [1–3]. Moreover, most meningiomas have an immunohistochemical profile that is similar to normal arachnoid mater including a characteristic patchy staining pattern for epithelial membrane antigen (EMA). In some instances, meningiomas recapitulate the functional properties of normal arachnoidal cells including a tendency to form whorls similar to the normal wrapping function of arachnoidal cells at cerebrospinal fluid (CSF) barrier sites [4]. Occasionally meningiomas occur at atypical locations in which arachnoidal cap cells are found such as the choroid plexus stroma, and this is the presumed basis for the rare intraventricular meningioma. Meningiomas that lack a dural connection are referred to as primary extradural meningiomas, and these have a predilection for head and neck regions such as the sinuses, orbit, skull bone, and scalp, although other sites including the lungs, mediastinum, and liver are described [5–9].

Grading of Meningioma

The most reliable morphologic predictor for tumor recurrence is the WHO grade, and the grade of a meningioma also plays an important role in guiding therapeutic decisions. The principles of meningioma grading are well established and enable meningiomas to be grouped into three categories, based on the extent of progressively atypical features that are defined by microscopic criteria (See Table 2.1). The vast majority of meningiomas correspond histologically to WHO grade I and are

Table 2.1 Meningioma morphologic variants grouped according to WHO grade and biological behavior

WHO grade I	WHO grade II	WHO grade III
Meningiomas with low risk of recurrence or aggressive behavior	Meningiomas with increased risk of recurrence or aggressive behavior	Meningiomas with high risk of recurrence or aggressive behavior
Meningothelial meningioma	*Atypical* meningioma	*Anaplastic* meningioma
Fibroblastic meningioma	*Clear cell* meningioma	*Rhabdoid* meningioma
Transitional meningioma	*Chordoid* meningioma	*Papillary* meningioma
Psammomatous meningioma		
Angiomatous meningioma		
Microcystic meningioma		
Secretory meningioma		
Lymphoplasmacyte-rich meningioma		
Metaplastic meningioma		

clinically benign [10]. The risk of recurrence for a grade I meningioma is 7–25% [11]. Higher-grade meningiomas arise either de novo or by transformation of a preexisting lower-grade tumor. Based on the degree to which atypical microscopic features are present, the tumor is classified as either atypical (WHO grade II) or anaplastic (WHO grade III). The risk for recurrence increases with progressively increasing grade, and grade III meningiomas are associated with a markedly elevated risk for recurrence and overall shorter survival times [12]. Cellular proliferation, as assessed using the Ki67 proliferation index, correlates well with tumor grade and biologic behavior [13]. An elevated proliferative index (i.e., >4%) is associated with a similar recurrence rate to atypical meningioma, while a markedly elevated proliferative index of >20% has been associated with death rates comparable to those of anaplastic meningioma [14]. Although the Ki67 proliferative index is an important adjunct in evaluating meningiomas, it is not currently recognized as a formal component of the WHO grading scheme, partly due to significant interlaboratory differences in technique and interpretation. It is worth noting that the boundary points between histologic tumor grades are also somewhat arbitrary. The relatively subjective nature of some of the softer morphologic criteria introduces inter- and intra-observer variability, which is sometimes associated with inconsistent tumor grading within institutions [15]. A subset of patients with grade I meningioma have one or two atypical features but not brain invasion or increased mitotic activity, and in these patients, the risk of recurrence is increased compared to individuals with otherwise benign grade I meningiomas that have no atypical features at all [16]. In patients who undergo a large tumor resection, grading of the excision specimen can be further complicated by the fact that meningiomas usually do not exist in a pure histologic form and often show significant heterogeneity between different regions within the tumor. This means that accurate grading often requires considerable sampling of different areas to exclude regions that could behave in a more clinically aggressive fashion. Several variants of meningioma have distinctive microscopic patterns that are associated with a significantly increased risk of recurrence and are automatically classified as higher grade based on these appearances alone. Examples of higher-grade meningiomas with distinctive microscopic appearances include the rhabdoid and papillary subtypes described below [11]. Progesterone receptor (PR) expression is inversely associated with tumor grade, and most grade III meningiomas do not express PR; however, this test has limited clinical utility because a significant number of grade I and grade II meningiomas also show no PR expression [17, 18].

WHO Grade I (Benign) Meningiomas

Tumors corresponding to grade I meningioma are characterized by striking histologic diversity, with nine variants currently recognized in the WHO Classification of CNS Tumors (see Table 2.2). By definition grade I tumors lack microscopic criteria of higher-grade atypical or anaplastic (i.e., malignant) meningiomas (see Table 2.1). Grade I meningiomas are permitted to have up to two atypical cytologic features

Table 2.2 WHO 2016 grading criteria for meningiomas

WHO grade I	WHO grade II Atypical meningioma	WHO grade III Anaplastic meningioma

Low grade with
  Any predominant morphology, except for clear cell, chordoid, papillary, or rhabdoid
  Mitoses <4/10HPF
  Lacks criteria of atypical or anaplastic meningioma
	Intermediate grade with
	  Brain invasion on histology
	  Increased mitotic activity (Mitoses >4/10 HPF)
	Or *at least 3* of the following features:
	  Sheet-like growth
	  Small cells with high N/C ratio
	  Increased cellularity
	  Foci of spontaneous necrosis
	  Macronucleoli
		High grade with
		  Overtly aggressive phenotype with sarcoma-, carcinoma-like histology
		  Mitoses >20/10 HPF

HPF high-power fields, *N/C ratio* nuclear-to-cytoplasmic ratio

(but not brain invasion or increased mitotic activity) before being classified as a grade II tumor. Moreover, invasion of the bone or skeletal muscle does not influence tumor grade, and some grade I tumors will exhibit considerable permeation of the skull bone, including occasional extension into the subcutaneous tissues of the scalp, without a corresponding change in grade [19]. The main features of the nine grade I variants are discussed in the following section.

Meningothelial Meningioma This is one of the most common and classic variants of meningioma that consists of well-demarcated lobules of arachnoidal cells partly surrounded by thin collagenous septa. Inside the lobules the tumor cells typically have imperceptible cell borders and appear to form a multinucleated syncytium. The tumor cells contain bland nuclei that tend to be relatively uniform with open chromatin and often contain nuclear pseudoinclusions which are a characteristic finding in this variant (Fig. 2.1). Unlike the transitional and fibrous subtypes described below, whorls and psammoma bodies are not a prominent finding although they can be seen in some cases. This variant has a predilection for the anterior skull base.

Fibrous Meningioma This is another common and classic grade I variant that typically has elongated tumor cells with a spindled appearance and intervening collagenous fibers. Whorls and psammoma bodies are often present, and the tumor cells may exhibit the classic nuclear features of meningothelial meningioma, at least focally. These features are helpful in distinguishing a fibrous meningioma from other spindle cell tumors such as schwannomas and tumors that contain abundant collagen such as solitary fibrous tumor/hemangiopericytoma. Fibrous meningiomas tend to have a convexity distribution (Fig. 2.2).

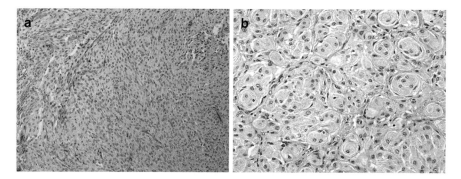

Fig. 2.1 (**a**) Meningothelial meningioma. Hematoxylin and eosin (H&E) stained section demonstrates a meningioma with lobular architecture, syncytium-like appearance due to ill-defined borders. (**b**) Variant with prominent whorl formation

Fig. 2.2 Fibrous meningioma with intersecting fascicles of spindled cells and variable collagen deposition (H&E stained section)

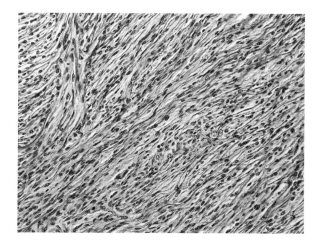

Transitional Meningioma   This is a common variant with microscopic features in transition between meningothelial and fibrous variants. The tumor often consists of meningothelial lobules with admixed fascicles of spindle cells, psammoma bodies, and whorls. Similar to the fibrous meningioma, these tumors tend to arise on the convexity dura.

Psammomatous Meningioma   Psammomatous meningiomas have a striking microscopic appearance and contain innumerable psammoma bodies which sometimes outnumber the tumor cells. In some cases, tumor cells can be difficult to identify due to the sheer abundance of psammoma bodies. Occasionally psammoma bodies coalesce and calcify or form metaplastic bone. These tumors classically occur in the thoracic spine of middle-aged women.

Fig. 2.3 Angiomatous meningioma. Composed of dense accumulation of numerous small blood vessels (H&E stained section)

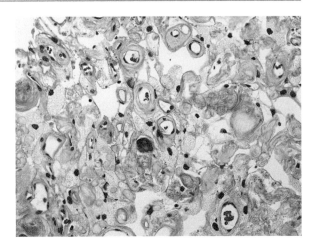

Angiomatous Meningioma This is a vascular variant characterized by innumerable blood vessels that comprise most of the tumor. The blood vessels typically vary in size and caliber and are often hyalinized. This tumor can mimic a vascular malformation or hemangioblastoma. A classic finding is degenerative atypia of the tumor nuclei which is sometimes striking and does not indicate a higher grade. Angiomatous meningiomas are sometimes associated with considerable peritumoral brain edema (Fig. 2.3).

Microcystic Meningioma This uncommon variant is characterized by numerus microcystic spaces demarcated by tumor cell processes and sometimes contains macrocysts detectable on imaging [20]. As with angiomatous meningioma, hyalinized blood vessels and degenerative atypia may occur. Microcystic meningiomas are thought to arise from arachnoid trabecular cells, and the microcysts are vaguely reminiscent of small subarachnoid spaces.

Secretory Meningioma This variant shows focal epithelial differentiation and contains intercellular eosinophilic secretions known as pseudopsammoma bodies. These secretions are usually periodic acid-Schiff-positive and can occur singly or in small clusters, in a background of otherwise classic meningioma. Focal epithelial differentiation can be highlighted by labeling with antibodies for cytokeratin and carcinoembryonic antigen (CEA) [21]. Pseudopsammoma bodies also label strongly for CEA, and this variant may be associated with elevated circulating CEA levels. Peritumoral edema is sometimes striking [22] (Figs. 2.4 and 2.5).

Lymphoplasmacyte-Rich Meningioma This is an uncommon variant characterized by a preponderance of chronic inflammation that often obscures the meningothelial component. The major differential diagnostic considerations are a clonal lymphoproliferative disorder, pachymeningitis, and other systemic hematologic and autoimmune conditions [23].

Fig. 2.4 Psammomatous meningioma. Numerous psammoma bodies dominate the tumor (H&E stained section)

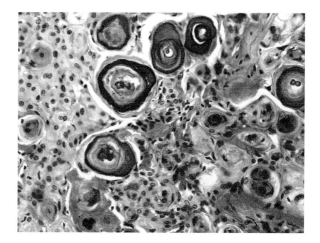

Fig. 2.5 Secretory meningioma shows gland-like spaces with brightly eosinophilic globules, also known as pseudopsammoma bodies (H&E stained section). These are PAS positive (not shown)

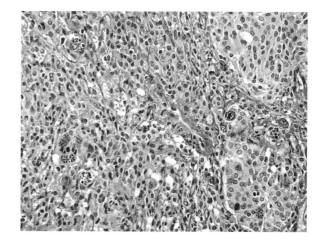

Metaplastic Meningioma This uncommon variant is characterized by focal or widespread mesenchymal differentiation that includes osseous, cartilaginous, lipomatous, myxoid, and/or xanthomatous tissue. Although the histologic appearances are striking, this variant has no known clinical significance.

WHO Grade II Meningiomas

Grade II meningiomas are a group of tumors characterized by a significantly increased risk of recurrence [11, 24]. Three entities are recognized in this group, the most common of which is the atypical meningioma, defined by the presence of atypical microscopic features (see Table 2.1). Two other grade II tumors, the clear cell and chordoid meningioma, are relatively uncommon and are defined by their distinctive microscopic appearances. Any previously mentioned grade I variant may also qualify for a diagnosis of atypical meningioma if microscopic criteria are met, even focally (see Table 2.1).

Atypical Meningioma The diagnosis of atypical meningioma is established by a mitotic count of greater than 4 mitotic figures per 10 high-power fields, evidence of brain invasion, and/or three or more microscopic criteria, including hypercellularity, small cell change, architectural sheeting, spontaneous necrosis, and macronucleoli (see Table 2.1). Despite the name, nuclear atypia is not a criterion for diagnosis. Moreover, nuclear atypia is not a reliable indicator of tumor grade because some grade I meningiomas such as the angiomatous and microcystic variants described above may also have considerable nuclear atypia. Only spontaneous tumor necrosis is scored, and correlation with clinical history is sometimes necessary to distinguish between embolization-induced necrosis and spontaneous necrosis [25]. Brain invasion is associated with a higher risk of recurrence and if present automatically indicates a grade II meningioma [26]. Demonstration of brain invasion requires confirmation of pial breach which is characterized by islands of meningioma cells completely surrounded by GFAP-positive brain parenchyma, often with reactive astrogliosis. Direct extension of a meningioma from the subarachnoid space along perivascular Virchow-Robin spaces, but without direct extension into the brain parenchyma, does not constitute invasion. Atypical meningiomas are more in common in males and tend to have a non-skull base location. The 5-year recurrence rate for atypical meningioma with gross total resection is significantly greater than grade I meningioma and has been estimated at up to 40% in some series [27] (Fig. 2.6).

Clear Cell Meningioma This rare meningioma variant has a predilection for the posterior fossa and spinal canal of younger patients and is recognized by its typical microscopic appearance. The tumor has a sheeting or patternless architecture and consists of polygonal cells with clear cytoplasm that are surrounded by interstitial and prominent perivascular collagen. This is a biologically aggressive tumor type, and frequent recurrence with occasional CSF seeding is described. *SMARCE1* mutations are described in familial and some sporadic cases, and loss of expression

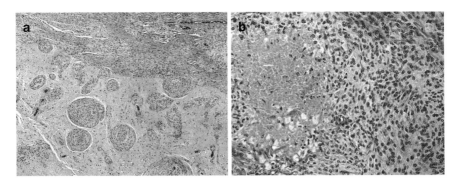

Fig. 2.6 Atypical meningioma. (**a**) H&E stained sections show brain invasion and (**b**) a focus of spontaneous necrosis

Fig. 2.7 Chordoid meningioma characterized by cords of epithelioid cells within a myxoid background (H&E stained section)

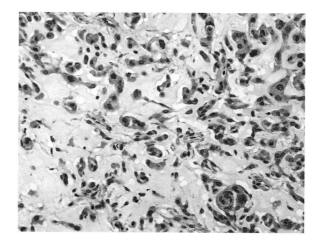

of SMARCE1 detected by immunohistochemistry may be a sensitive marker for clear cell meningioma [28].

Chordoid Meningioma These are rare tumors composed of nodules of vacuolated cells set in a myxoid stroma, with admixed regions of classic meningioma. The tumors histologically resemble chordoma. Psammoma calcifications are not common. In some instances, chronic inflammation and plasma cells are abundant, and rare cases are associated with Castleman disease and anemia (Fig. 2.7).

WHO Grade III (Malignant) Meningiomas

This is a group of malignant tumors characterized by markedly increased risk of recurrence and decreased overall survival when compared to other meningioma types. Three entities are recognized: anaplastic (malignant) meningioma, rhabdoid meningioma, and papillary meningioma.

Anaplastic (Malignant) Meningioma Anaplastic meningioma accounts for 1–3% of all meningiomas and is characterized by frankly anaplastic cytology that resembles undifferentiated carcinoma, melanoma, or sarcoma. Often the tumor is so poorly differentiated that it is difficult to discern the tumor as meningioma without additional immunohistochemical studies for confirmation. These tumors typically exhibit brisk mitotic activity (i.e., greater than 20 mitotic figures per 10 high-power fields), and atypical mitotic figures are usually found [29]. The Ki67 proliferative index is often markedly elevated, and tumor necrosis and brain invasion are frequent. Some anaplastic meningiomas also exhibit focal epithelial or mesenchymal differentiation, and this can sometimes pose additional diagnostic difficulties. In most instances a history of a prior meningioma at the same site, with immunohistochemical or genetic support, is required to establish the diagnosis (Fig. 2.8).

Rhabdoid Meningioma This is an uncommon high-grade variant characterized by tumor cells with eccentric nuclei, prominent nucleoli, and globular hyaline cytoplasmic material [30]. Most rhabdoid meningiomas have other overtly malignant features such as necrosis and brisk mitotic activity. Occasional grade I tumors have focal rhabdoid cytology without other malignant features, and this is acceptable as a minor component of those tumors, although closer clinical follow-up may be indicated. Unlike the rhabdoid cells of atypical teratoid/rhabdoid tumors of the posterior fossa of childhood, rhabdoid meningiomas retain expression of SMARCB1 (Fig. 2.9).

Papillary Meningioma This is a rare variant with a predominant papillary or perivascular pseudopapillary growth pattern comprising greater than 50% of the tumor. True papillary tumors have a classic cauliflower-like appearance; however, in most cases the appearance is actually pseudopapillary with tumor cells clinging to blood vessels that are separated by intervening clefts. Some papillary tumors exhibit focal rhabdoid features.

Fig. 2.8 Anaplastic (malignant) meningioma with high mitotic activity and markedly atypical cells (H&E stained section)

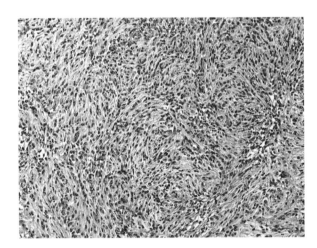

Fig. 2.9 Rhabdoid meningioma. Characterized by eccentrically displaced nuclei and prominent paranuclear eosinophilic globular inclusions (H&E stained section)

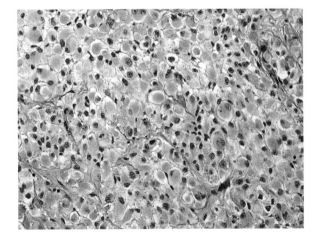

Other Meningioma Variants Acknowledged by the WHO   Several additional meningioma variants are acknowledged by the WHO although the clinical significance of these individual variants is currently unknown due to their overall rarity. Examples of these unusual variants include oncocytic, sclerosing, whorling-sclerosing, GFAP-expressing, granulofilamentous inclusion-bearing, rosette-forming, and mucinous meningiomas [4, 11, 31–34].

Meningioma Immunophenotype

The canonical confirmatory immunostain for meningioma is EMA, with most meningiomas having a characteristic wispy pattern of positive staining. Malignant tumors may show less intense EMA staining. Vimentin is expressed by all meningiomas, but as this protein is broadly expressed by many other cell types, it is of limited diagnostic utility. Somatostatin receptor 2A is expressed in most meningiomas and can be helpful in confirming arachnoidal lineage particularly in poorly differentiated tumors, although caution is required because this stain is also positive in many neuroendocrine neoplasms. GFAP is negative in meningioma cells but can be helpful in confirming brain tissue invasion by the tumor. Keratin stains are usually negative unless the meningioma shows focal epithelial differentiation, as in the secretory variant. Ki67 has an important role in evaluating cell proliferation, as discussed above.

Differential Diagnoses of Meningioma

Most meningiomas are slow-growing masses with characteristic imaging and clinical findings. In the majority of cases, a diagnosis is often clinically suspected before pathologic confirmation. In some instances, non-meningothelial tumors will present with unusual clinical or radiologic features or have a dural attachment, and this may pose a diagnostic challenge. Moreover, the histologic diversity of meningiomas can be problematic if the tumor is one of the rarer microscopic variants or if the tumor is of higher grade and poorly differentiated. Some of the more common differential diagnostic considerations are discussed below.

Non-meningothelial Mesenchymal Tumors

Non-meningothelial soft tissue tumors are a large and heterogeneous group of neoplasms ranging from benign to locally invasive or overtly malignant. They share similar histologic features with soft tissue tumors found at extracranial sites and are classified by cell lineage into adipocytic, vascular, fibroblastic, smooth muscle, skeletal muscle, nerve sheath, and undifferentiated types. The most common tumor belonging to this category is the solitary fibrous tumor/hemangiopericytoma, a tumor characterized by diffuse STAT6 nuclear expression [11]. This tumor typically has prominent staghorn-shaped blood vessels and either a solitary fibrous pattern comprising alternating hypercellular and hypocellular areas, bland spindled cells, and prominent collagen or a hemangiopericytoma pattern with high cellularity and prominent reticulin. These tumors typically express CD34 and lack EMA which facilitates their distinction from meningioma.

Metastatic Neoplasms

Dural-based metastatic neoplasms are sometimes confused for meningioma, particularly if the metastatic deposit is a solitary lesion, a primary origin for the tumor is not known, or there is no systemic disease. A diverse range of tumor types can exhibit dural metastases with tumors of the breast, prostate, lung, and other unusual locations such as uterus and gastrointestinal tract overrepresented in some series [35, 36]. Microscopic examination of the tumor typically reveals cytologic anaplasia with evidence of glandular or squamous differentiation, thereby confirming a diagnosis of metastatic carcinoma. Melanoma is often recognized by its brown cytoplasmic pigment and prominent nucleoli although non-pigmented variants of melanoma occur. Metastatic sarcomas typically have a spindled appearance and often require detailed immunohistochemical studies to differentiate them from anaplastic meningioma or other more common meningioma types. Occasionally clear cell and secretory meningiomas (see above) may resemble metastatic carcinoma, but these variants are readily distinguished from carcinoma by their distinct immunohistochemical profiles. In rare instances meningiomas can act as a receptor bed for metastatic tumor, and coexistent meningioma and metastatic carcinoma are occasionally described [37].

Other Differential Diagnoses

Specific variants of meningioma are also associated with specific differentials particular to the histologic features of that subtype. Examples include the microcystic meningioma which may resemble hemangioblastoma, angiomatous meningioma which can be confused for a vascular malformation, and the chordoid meningioma which can resemble a chordoma. The differential diagnosis of spindle cell tumors occurring at the cerebellopontine angle includes schwannoma and fibrous meningioma. The rare lymphoplasmacyte-rich meningioma raises several differentials including infectious and inflammatory etiologies, as well as low-grade lymphoma. In these diagnostically challenging cases, the histopathologic differential diagnosis is usually readily resolved by detailed immunohistochemical analysis of the tumor, careful clinicopathologic correlation, and ancillary studies.

References

1. Langford LA. Pathology of meningiomas. J Neuro-Oncol. 1996;29(3):217–21.
2. Kepes JJ. Presidential address: the histopathology of meningiomas. A reflection of origins and expected behavior? J Neuropathol Exp Neurol. 1986;45(2):95–107.

3. Cyril B, Courville KHA. The histogenesis of meningiomas: with particular reference to the origin of the 'meningothelial' variety. J Neuropathol Exp Neurol. 1942;1(3):337–43.
4. Perry A, Brat DJ. Practical surgical neuropathology: a diagnostic approach. Philadelphia: Churchill Livingstone/Elsevier; 2010.
5. Lang FF, Macdonald OK, Fuller GN, DeMonte F. Primary extradural meningiomas: a report on nine cases and review of the literature from the era of computerized tomography scanning. J Neurosurg. 2000;93(6):940–50.
6. Liu Y, Wang H, Shao H, Wang C. Primary extradural meningiomas in head: a report of 19 cases and review of literature. Int J Clin Exp Pathol. 2015;8(5):5624–32.
7. Bae SY, Kim HS, Jang HJ, et al. Primary pulmonary chordoid meningioma. Korean J Thorac Cardiovasc Surg. 2018;51(6):410–4.
8. Luo JZ, Zhan C, Ni X, Shi Y, Wang Q. Primary pulmonary meningioma mimicking lung metastatic tumor: a case report. J Cardiothorac Surg. 2018;13(1):99.
9. Zulpaite R, Jagelavicius Z, Mickys U, Janilionis R. Primary pulmonary meningioma with rhabdoid features. Int J Surg Pathol. 2019;27(4):457–63.
10. Alahmadi H, Croul SE. Pathology and genetics of meningiomas. Semin Diagn Pathol. 2011;28(4):314–24.
11. Louis DN. International Agency for Research on C, Deutsches Krebsforschungszentrum H, Organització Mundial de la S. WHO classification of tumours of the central nervous system. Lyon: International Agency for Research on Cancer; 2016.
12. Greenfield JG, Love S, Budka H, Ironside JW, Perry A. Greenfield's neuropathology. Boca Raton: CRC Press; 2015.
13. Mukhopadhyay M, Das C, Kumari M, Sen A, Mukhopadhyay B, Mukhopadhyay B. Spectrum of meningioma with special reference to prognostic utility of ER, PR and Ki67 expression. J Lab Physicians. 2017;9(4):308–13.
14. Perry A, Stafford SL, Scheithauer BW, Suman VJ, Lohse CM. The prognostic significance of MIB-1, p53, and DNA flow cytometry in completely resected primary meningiomas. Cancer. 1998;82(11):2262–9.
15. Willis J, Smith C, Ironside JW, Erridge S, Whittle IR, Everington D. The accuracy of meningioma grading: a 10-year retrospective audit. Neuropathol Appl Neurobiol. 2005;31(2):141–9.
16. Marciscano AE, Stemmer-Rachamimov AO, Niemierko A, et al. Benign meningiomas (WHO Grade I) with atypical histological features: correlation of histopathological features with clinical outcomes. J Neurosurg. 2016;124(1):106–14.
17. Perry A, Cai DX, Scheithauer BW, et al. Merlin, DAL-1, and progesterone receptor expression in clinicopathologic subsets of meningioma: a correlative immunohistochemical study of 175 cases. J Neuropathol Exp Neurol. 2000;59(10):872–9.
18. Roser F, Nakamura M, Bellinzona M, Rosahl SK, Ostertag H, Samii M. The prognostic value of progesterone receptor status in meningiomas. J Clin Pathol. 2004;57(10):1033–7.
19. Ironside JW. Diagnostic pathology of nervous system tumours. Edinburgh: Churchill Livingstone; 2002.
20. Paek SH, Kim SH, Chang KH, et al. Microcystic meningiomas: radiological characteristics of 16 cases. Acta Neurochir. 2005;147(9):965–72; discussion 972.
21. Colakoglu N, Demirtas E, Oktar N, Yuntem N, Islekel S, Ozdamar N. Secretory meningiomas. J Neuro-Oncol. 2003;62(3):233–41.
22. Buhl R, Hugo HH, Mehdorn HM. Brain oedema in secretory meningiomas. J Clin Neurosci. 2001;8(Suppl 1):19–21.
23. Bruno MC, Ginguene C, Santangelo M, et al. Lymphoplasmacyte rich meningioma. A case report and review of the literature. J Neurosurg Sci. 2004;48(3):117–24; discussion 124.
24. Champeaux C, Dunn L. World Health Organization grade II meningiomas. Acta Neurochir. 2016;158(5):921–9; discussion 929.
25. Ng HK, Poon WS, Goh K, Chan MS. Histopathology of post-embolized meningiomas. Am J Surg Pathol. 1996;20(10):1224–30.

26. Brokinkel B, Hess K, Mawrin C. Brain invasion in meningiomas-clinical considerations and impact of neuropathological evaluation: a systematic review. Neuro-Oncology. 2017;19(10):1298–307.
27. Perry A, Stafford SL, Scheithauer BW, Suman VJ, Lohse CM. Meningioma grading: an analysis of histologic parameters. Am J Surg Pathol. 1997;21(12):1455–65.
28. Tauziede-Espariat A, Parfait B, Besnard A, et al. Loss of SMARCE1 expression is a specific diagnostic marker of clear cell meningioma: a comprehensive immunophenotypical and molecular analysis. Brain Pathol (Zurich, Switzerland). 2018;28(4):466–74.
29. Perry A, Scheithauer BW, Stafford SL, Lohse CM, Wollan PC. "Malignancy" in meningiomas: a clinicopathologic study of 116 patients, with grading implications. Cancer. 1999;85(9):2046–56.
30. Perry A, Scheithauer BW, Stafford SL, Abell-Aleff PC, Meyer FB. "Rhabdoid" meningioma: an aggressive variant. Am J Surg Pathol. 1998;22(12):1482–90.
31. Roncaroli F, Riccioni L, Cerati M, et al. Oncocytic meningioma. Am J Surg Pathol. 1997;21(4):375–82.
32. Berho M, Suster S. Mucinous meningioma. Report of an unusual variant of meningioma that may mimic metastatic mucin-producing carcinoma. Am J Surg Pathol. 1994;18(1):100–6.
33. Elmaci I, Altinoz MA, Sav A, et al. Whorling-sclerosing meningioma. A review on the histological features of a rare tumor including an illustrative case. Clin Neurol Neurosurg. 2017;162:85–90.
34. Zheng J, Geng M, Shi Y, Jiang B, Tai Y, Jing H. Oncocytic meningioma: a case report and review of the literature. Surg Oncol. 2013;22(4):256–60.
35. Nayak L, Abrey LE, Iwamoto FM. Intracranial dural metastases. Cancer. 2009;115(9):1947–53.
36. Kleinschmidt-DeMasters BK. Dural metastases. A retrospective surgical and autopsy series. Arch Pathol Lab Med. 2001;125(7):880–7.
37. Sayegh ET, Burch EA, Henderson GA, Oh T, Bloch O, Parsa AT. Tumor-to-tumor metastasis: breast carcinoma to meningioma. J Clin Neurosci. 2015;22(2):268–74.

Radiographic Assessment of Meningiomas

3

Thomas J. Kaley

Introduction

The radiology of meningiomas at first may sound like a rather simple topic as they tend to have a very stereotypic appearance on traditional CT and MRI. However, as we delve further into the topic, it will become apparent that there are still many aspects for which further research is needed including accurate diagnostic imaging to differentiate meningiomas from other less common diagnosis, noninvasive measures of tumor grade, postoperative assessment to determine extent of resection, clinical trial assessment for both eligibility and determination of response to therapy (i.e., volumetric assessment), and utility of advanced imaging methods (PET scans, perfusion imaging, MR spectroscopy).

Standard Imaging Assessment of Meningioma

Meningiomas are most commonly first identified on either a CT or MRI scan. Occasionally these scans are performed for neurologic symptoms related to the meningioma, but more often they are performed for a reason completely unrelated, and the meningioma is found incidentally. One of the major limitations of standard imaging assessment with CT or MRI is the lack of validated, reliable, or definitive characteristics that can discriminate between the various subtypes and grade of meningioma. Having a way to particularly distinguish between a grade I and II meningioma would provide very valuable information in the initial assessment of a meningioma.

T. J. Kaley (✉)
Department of Neurology, Memorial Sloan Kettering Cancer Center, New York, NY, USA
e-mail: kaleyt@mskcc.org

© Springer Nature Switzerland AG 2020
J. Moliterno, A. Omuro (eds.), *Meningiomas*,
https://doi.org/10.1007/978-3-030-59558-6_3

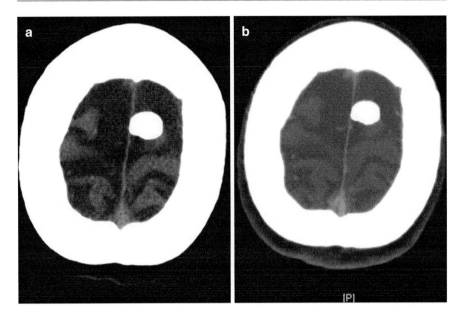

Fig. 3.1 Radiographic appearance of a calcified meningioma on CT without contrast (**a**) and post-contrast (**b**)

CT

When a meningioma is identified on a CT scan, it has a very characteristic appearance as demonstrated in Fig. 3.1. On noncontrast CT scans, meningiomas may appear as either hyperdense or isodense. The hyperdense appearance is found when meningiomas have calcified, and some postulate that this is a marker of a more indolent and lower-grade meningioma, with less growth potential for the future. On post-contrast CT images, meningiomas very brightly and homogenously enhance.

MRI

If a meningioma is found on CT scan, it should be followed by assessment with MRI except if there are contraindications to MRI. Contrast is necessary to best identify a meningioma. On contrast-enhanced T1-weighted images, a meningioma appears as a brightly and homogenously enhancing mass with, oftentimes, the classic "dural tail" which is simply a continuation of the meningioma into the dura (Fig. 3.2). FLAIR sequences are helpful to identify any peritumoral edema which is not typical for lower-grade or incidental meningiomas but may more likely be present in the WHO grade II and III meningiomas. The presence of peritumoral edema may influence the decision to treat a meningioma earlier. Although no clear

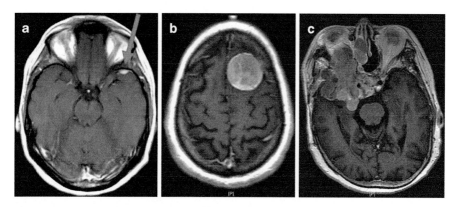

Fig. 3.2 Radiographic appearance of meningiomas on T1-weighted post-contrast MRI images: small incidental meningioma with dural tail (**a**), larger atypical meningioma (**b**), aggressive surgery and radiation refractory meningioma with irregular shape (**c**)

validated MRI criteria exist to serve as a biomarker which can distinguish between grades of meningioma, occasionally intratumoral necrosis may be visible which may suggest a higher-grade and more aggressive tumor.

Current Limitations of Standard Imaging

As discussed above, the major limitation of standard imaging is the inability of these techniques to distinguish between grades of meningioma which would have great utility in identifying patients who may need earlier intervention with surgery and/or radiation. Despite multiple attempts to investigate various imaging parameters, no clear criteria exist. The presence of peritumoral edema may suggest a higher-grade meningioma [1]. Although WHO grade III meningiomas tend to have substantial peritumoral edema, the more difficult challenge is differentiating a WHO grade II meningioma from a WHO grade I meningioma because the treatment decision may be different.

Standard imaging techniques also present a challenge for determining growth in meningioma to identify those that are progressing and in need of treatment as well as those currently on a therapy or in a clinical trial. Many meningiomas are amorphous or ameboid in shape, and standard 2D assessment is insufficient to accurately determine progression. This inaccuracy causes a major downstream problem for clinical trials and the accurate evaluation of new therapies.

Postsurgical assessment is another area where standard imaging falls a bit short. As described elsewhere in this book, surgical excision is graded according to Simpson grading. However, neither CT nor MRI is able to accurately determine Simpson grade. Instead, postsurgical imaging can at best utilize categories of gross total resection, subtotal resection, and biopsy. When evaluating therapies and prognosis, it is not clear that these MRI categories are sufficient.

Fig. 3.3 Hemangiopericytoma on T1-weighted
post-contrast MRI image
with similar appearance to
meningioma

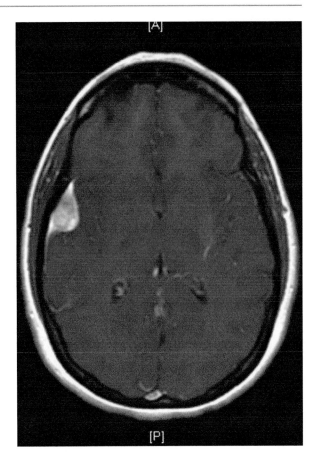

Lastly, standard imaging is inadequate at differentiating meningiomas from other dural diseases. For example, dural metastases from a systemic malignancy or indolent dural lymphomas may have a very similar appearance and are usually only distinguished by growth on subsequent scans and then histologic diagnosis via biopsy or resection. The other primary dural extra-axial tumor that may have a near identical radiographic appearance is a solitary fibrous tumor/hemangiopericytoma which may only be distinguished on histology as well, although these tumors tend to grow at a higher rate than meningiomas (Fig. 3.3). Advanced imaging techniques (discussed later) such as MR perfusion and spectroscopy may be helpful in differentiating meningioma from hemangiopericytoma [2].

Volumetric Analysis of Meningiomas

Accurate determination of growth in a meningioma is not only necessary for potential treatment decisions (i.e., the slow-growing meningioma where growth may not be evident over short intervals but only apparent on conventional analysis over longer periods of time) but is vital to the proper evaluation of new investigational therapies in order to accurately assess efficacy. Due to their irregular geometric shapes and variable growth rates, standard 2D assessment of meningiomas may be insufficient to accurately evaluate novel therapies. As most chemotherapies have proven ineffective in the treatment of meningioma, response criteria for trials are particularly challenging [3, 4]. The most consistent response criteria utilized in trials of the progression-free survival rate at 6 months (PFS6). However, the PFS6 rate is directly dependent on accurate diagnosis of progression which on 2D assessment is typically defined as ≥25% growth. One can easily visualize situations where a slow-growing tumor may consistently grow, yet not grow enough to measure as a 25% increase.

A 3D technique such as volumetric analysis provides a more accurate assessment of overall tumor burden and growth. The major limitation is that volumetric analysis is technically challenging and overall quite time-consuming. Additionally, there can be substantial interobserver variability (and even intraobserver variability). To date, there is no reliable computerized technology that can be readily utilized and available to deploy automated volumetric analysis. However, volumetric analysis may provide a more accurate and early assessment of tumor growth [5]. This early diagnosis would be particularly beneficial to patients who are receiving an ineffective therapy in both allowing them to switch therapies earlier, potentially avoid symptoms from further tumor growth, as well as avoid additional toxicity from a drug that is not providing benefit.

Advanced Imaging Techniques

Usually advanced ancillary imaging is not needed in the diagnosis of meningioma, but on occasion there may be limited value in the initial evaluation of a meningioma and trying to distinguish it from other entities. However, rarely is this necessary as usually there are only two circumstances: one, when there is the identification of a meningioma that necessitates treatment and surgical resection is pursued and therefore a definitive diagnosis is obtained via pathology, and, second, when there is a presumed meningioma identified on standard imaging that does not necessitate urgent intervention and early surveillance to identify growth can be pursued, and if there is growth, then again surgical resection is often sought for definitive diagnosis.

One area where advanced imaging would be particularly helpful is in the distinction between histologic grade and aggressivity. When a small meningioma is identified on imaging, if there was a noninvasive way of distinguishing a WHO grade II meningioma from a WHO grade I meningioma, there may be some value. However, again, this is typically made a moot point by utilizing a short interval surveillance follow-up image in order to determine treatment.

PET Imaging

Various PET tracers have been utilized for the diagnosis and management of meningiomas. Although rarely useful in the diagnostic accuracy of meningiomas, there may be certain circumstances where they may prove helpful in the future. In addition to the most common PET modalities described here, there are multiple other PET tracers under investigation.

Somatostatin receptors (SSTRs) are overexpressed in most, if not nearly all, meningiomas, and there are multiple different tracers designed to target the SSTR. Although PET scans using SSTRs may have high meningioma specificity, they are rarely needed. Historically there was interest in drugs to target the SSTR, although this has largely been found to be ineffective [6]. Even in these circumstances, given the ubiquity of SSTRs on meningiomas, these SSTR targeting PET scans do not provide a reliable biomarker for the very few patients who are possibly going to respond to therapy. Therefore, these scans are not considered standard in the management of meningioma currently, although may possibly play a role in the management in the future as research suggests they may be useful in identifying more aggressive or higher-grade tumors [7].

By far the most commonly available PET tracer at most institutions and facilities is FDG-PET, although its value is still quite limited. There are no reliable PET criteria as FDG avidity may vary with glucose metabolism which is not uniform across meningiomas, and it is unclear if FDG-PET can differentiate meningioma from other diagnostic considerations. For example, an FDG-avid meningioma may appear similar to a dural metastasis. There are two scenarios where an FDG-PET scan may be beneficial: first, in a previously radiated meningioma, FDG-PET may be helpful in the distinction between radiation necrosis and true tumor progression, and, second, if a treated meningioma (either with radiation or systemic therapy) converts from a hypometabolic tumor to a hypermetabolic tumor to suggest progression or vice versa and to suggest response to therapy.

MR Perfusion

MR perfusion (MRP) is a technique that attempts to quantify blood flow to a specific area on MRI. MRP has been valuable in the management of other brain tumor, in particular glioblastomas. However, its value in the management of meningiomas is not yet known.

Similar to PET imaging, the main investigation of MRP is as a technique to try to characterize meningiomas better at diagnosis with respect to grade and aggressivity, although the literature in this area is inconclusive and not yet validated as a reliable biomarker [8, 9]. Similarly, it is not clear if MRP can distinguish between various grades or alternate diagnoses (Fig. 3.4). In current practice though, the main utility of MRP is in the differentiation between true recurrence and radiation necrosis in the previously radiated meningioma, similar to FDG-PET scans.

Other Modalities

There of course are other imaging techniques which are under investigation in the evaluation and management of meningiomas. These include not only novel PET tracers but also other MR techniques such as MR spectroscopy and hyperpolarized MRI. In general, these investigational techniques, as with the more common ones

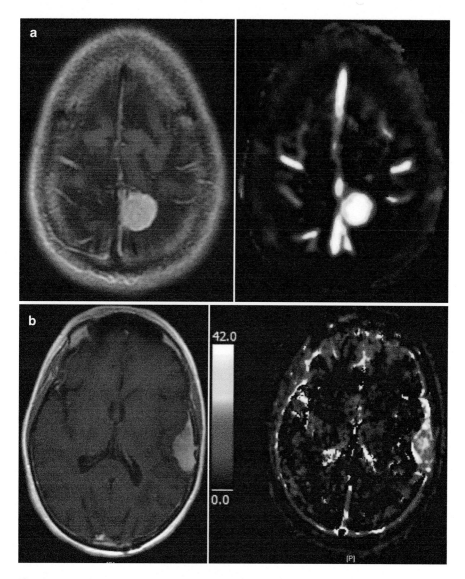

Fig. 3.4 MR perfusion imaging showing elevated plasma volume in an incidental meningioma (**a**), recurrent growing atypical meningioma (**b**), and hemangiopericytoma (**c**)

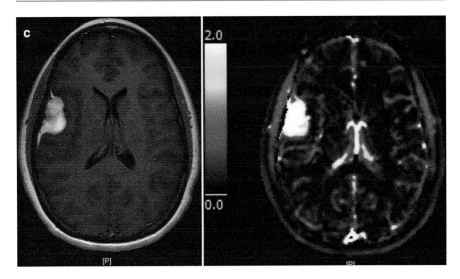

Fig. 3.4 (continued)

above, seek to identify a reliable noninvasive biomarker to identify tumor grade and aggressivity with the hopes of better identification of which patients would benefit from early intervention.

References

1. Ressel A, Fichte S, Brodhun M, Rosahl SK, Gerlach R. WHO grade of intracranial meningiomas differs with respect to patient's age, location, tumor size and peritumoral edema. J Neuro-Oncol. 2019;145(2):277–86.
2. Ohba S, Murayama K, Nishiyama Y, Adachi K, Yamada S, Abe M, et al. Clinical and radiographic features for differentiating solitary fibrous tumor/hemangiopericytoma from meningioma. World Neurosurg. 2019;130:e383–e92.
3. Huang RY, Bi WL, Weller M, Kaley T, Blakeley J, Dunn I, et al. Proposed response assessment and endpoints for meningioma clinical trials: report from the Response Assessment in Neuro-Oncology Working Group. Neuro-Oncology. 2019;21(1):26–36.
4. Kaley T, Barani I, Chamberlain M, McDermott M, Panageas K, Raizer J, et al. Historical benchmarks for medical therapy trials in surgery- and radiation-refractory meningioma: a RANO review. Neuro-Oncology. 2014;16(6):829–40.
5. Huang RY, Unadkat P, Bi WL, George E, Preusser M, McCracken JD, et al. Response assessment of meningioma: 1D, 2D, and volumetric criteria for treatment response and tumor progression. Neuro-Oncology. 2019;21(2):234–41.
6. Norden AD, Ligon KL, Hammond SN, Muzikansky A, Reardon DA, Kaley TJ, et al. Phase II study of monthly pasireotide LAR (SOM230C) for recurrent or progressive meningioma. Neurology. 2015;84(3):280–6.
7. Sommerauer M, Burkhardt JK, Frontzek K, Rushing E, Buck A, Krayenbuehl N, et al. 68Gallium-DOTATATE PET in meningioma: a reliable predictor of tumor growth rate? Neuro-Oncology. 2016;18(7):1021–7.

8. Chidambaram S, Pannullo SC, Roytman M, Pisapia DJ, Liechty B, Magge RS, et al. Dynamic contrast-enhanced magnetic resonance imaging perfusion characteristics in meningiomas treated with resection and adjuvant radiosurgery. Neurosurg Focus. 2019;46(6):E10.
9. Qiao XJ, Kim HG, Wang DJJ, Salamon N, Linetsky M, Sepahdari A, et al. Application of arterial spin labeling perfusion MRI to differentiate benign from malignant intracranial meningiomas. Eur J Radiol. 2017;97:31–6.

The Genomic Landscape of Meningiomas

4

Amy Y. Zhao, Mark W. Youngblood, E. Zeynep Erson-Omay, Jennifer Moliterno, and Murat Gunel

Introduction

Meningiomas are typically slow-growing tumors that arise from the meninges of the brain. These tumors accounted for 145,916 cases or 37.1% of all primary central nervous system tumors diagnosed in the United States between 2011 and 2015 [1]. When treatment is indicated, meningiomas are typically managed with

A. Y. Zhao
Department of Genetics, Yale University, New Haven, CT, USA
e-mail: amy.zhao@yale.edu

M. W. Youngblood
Department of Neurosurgery, Northwestern Memorial Hospital, Chicago, IL, USA
e-mail: mark.youngblood@northwestern.edu

E. Z. Erson-Omay
Department of Neurosurgery, Yale School of Medicine, Yale-New Haven Hospital, New Haven, CT, USA
e-mail: zeynep.erson@yale.edu

J. Moliterno
Yale New Haven Hospital and Smilow Cancer Hospital, New Haven, CT, USA

Yale Brain Tumor Center at Smilow Cancer Hospital, New Haven, CT, USA

Department of Neurosurgery, Yale School of Medicine, Yale University, New Haven, CT, USA

Department of Neurosurgical Oncology, Yale School of Medicine, New Haven, CT, USA
e-mail: jennifer.moliternogunel@yale.edu

M. Gunel (✉)
Department of Neurosurgery, Yale School of Medicine, Yale-New Haven Hospital, New Haven, CT, USA

Department of Neurosurgery, Yale-New Haven Hospital, Tompkins Memorial Pavilion (TMP), New Haven, CT, USA
e-mail: murat.gunel@yale.edu

© Springer Nature Switzerland AG 2020
J. Moliterno, A. Omuro (eds.), *Meningiomas*,
https://doi.org/10.1007/978-3-030-59558-6_4

Table 4.1 Percentage of low- vs high-grade meningioma patients showing progression-free survival at 2, 3, and 5 years of follow-up

	2 Year PFS (%)	3 Year PFS (%)	5 Year PFS (%)
Low-grade	94.12	91.88	88.46
High-grade	88.37	84.85	69.23

Internal unpublished data

neurosurgical resection and/or radiation therapy, as there is no effective, standardized medical treatment currently.

While the majority of meningiomas are often low grade (i.e., WHO Grade I), approximately 15–20% can be higher grade, with a more aggressive clinical course [2–8]. Higher Grade II and III meningiomas, with worse prognosis and higher recurrence rates compared to Grade I lesions (see Table 4.1), can arise de novo or progress from lower-grade meningiomas [8–10]. The specific molecular mechanisms that drive this difference in tumor grade are not completely clear. Thus, dissecting the molecular mechanisms underlying the formation and growth of meningiomas could prove to be fundamental in the management of these tumors, especially in recurrent and higher-grade ones.

As compared to other intracranial tumors – in particular gliomas – meningiomas harbor a smaller number of somatic mutations and large-scale chromosomal alterations [5–7]. Indeed, Grade I meningiomas have, on average, 7.2 somatic protein-altering variants, compared to glioblastomas, which typically harbor approximately 35.1 variants [11, 12]. This relatively low somatic mutational burden, along with mutually exclusive driver mutations, has led to the classification of meningiomas into distinct molecular subgroups [5–7, 13]. With the advent of next-generation sequencing, driver somatic mutations have been identified in over 80% of meningiomas [14], and these mutations have been shown to correlate well with clinical variables, including tumor grade, histology, location, and prognosis [14–16]. These findings can now help to guide the clinical decision-making for management of meningioma patients [14–17]. Consequently, subsequent research focusing on understanding the differing behavior of these distinct subgroups, including more aggressive meningiomas, has helped to guide precision clinical care. Further research is imperative both to determine the etiology of the remaining 20% of cases and to aid in determining additional molecular targets for treatments for these patients [14, 15].

In this chapter, we present a systemic review of the known genomic landscape of meningiomas with a focus on the results of next-generation sequencing studies. The clinical implications of these studies, as well as possible future directions of meningioma genomics research, will also be discussed.

Genomic Profile of Meningiomas

The meningioma driver genes, in which mutations have been proposed or shown to lead to tumor formation or growth, have recently been elucidated with the development of next-generation sequencing technologies. Mutations affecting these genes can be inherited (germline) and/or sporadic (somatic). While the inherited mutations are present in all of the patient's cells, the latter arise spontaneously in non-germ cells, at the level of the meningeal cells. Moreover, meningiomas harboring these germline or somatic mutations can be classified into differing molecular subtypes based on the affected genes. These different subtypes and their associated genes will be discussed in the following two sections.

Hereditary Meningioma Syndromes

Knudson's "two-hit" theory of cancer causation proposes that inactivating hits on both copies of a tumor suppressor gene is required for tumorigenesis. This hypothesis has been demonstrated in several cancers, such as retinoblastoma, colorectal cancer, Li-Fraumeni syndrome, and nervous system tumors, including gliomas and meningiomas [18]. Thus, meningioma-associated inherited syndromes often have germline mutations in one copy of tumor suppressor genes and require another damaging somatic alteration in the second allele to drive oncogenesis.

The first meningioma germline mutations were discovered through studies of these inherited syndromes, including Gorlin syndrome, Cowden syndrome, and neurofibromatosis type II [19–21]. Studying these syndromes has been particularly informative about meningioma pathogenesis. Gorlin syndrome, a rare inherited disease, causes basal cell carcinomas and has been associated with malignant meningiomas [22–24]. In particular, germline mutations in the Sonic Hedgehog (SHH) signaling pathway – often inactivating mutations in a copy of *Patched1* (*PTCH1*) coupled with somatic or copy number alterations in the second allele – are associated with meningiomas. Germline activating mutations in *PI3K* pathway components, such as *AKT Serine/Threonine Kinase 1* (*AKT1*) and *Phosphatidylinositol 3-Kinase* (*PI3KCA*), cause Cowden syndrome, which is characterized by multiple hamartomas and an increased risk for tumor formation, including meningiomas [25, 26]. Cowden syndrome has also been associated with loss of tumor suppressor *Phosphatase and tensin homolog* (*PTEN*), which represses the PI3K signaling pathway.

Neurofibromatosis II is an autosomal dominant disorder that affects approximately 1 in 33,000 individuals and presents with multiple meningiomas, bilateral vestibular schwannomas, and ependymomas [27, 28]. Initial linkage studies localized the causative gene to chromosome 22q12 [29, 30]. Subsequent molecular cloning showed the responsible gene to be *neurofibromatosis 2* (*NF2*) [31]. *NF2* encodes merlin protein, which is a member of the FERM family [32]. Merlin is involved in pathways that regulate cytoskeleton structure (Rac/Cdc42/PAK), protein synthesis (mTORC1), and cellular growth (Hippo, CRL4) and has an anti-mitogenic effect [33–38]. When merlin is depleted, cell growth is dysregulated and tumorigenesis occurs [39]. Moreover, neurofibromatosis type II syndrome patients' tumors tend to have chromosomal instability and can be more commonly higher grades [40]. In addition to *NF2*, inherited mutations in two of the SWI/SNF group of transcription factors – namely, *SWI/SNF-Related, Matrix-Associated, Actin-Dependent Regulator of Chromatin, Subfamily B, Member 1*, and *Subfamily E, Member 1* (*SMARCB1* and

SMARCE1, respectively) – can lead to familial meningiomas [41–43]. Interestingly, somatic mutations in the genes underlying these inherited disorders and the molecular pathways involved, especially *NF2,* are commonly observed in sporadic meningiomas, which will be discussed in the next section.

Common Variants in Meningioma Susceptibility

Single nucleotide polymorphisms (SNPs) are common substitutions at particular nucleotides, and tens of millions of SNPs have been identified in the human genome [44]. Genome-wide association studies (GWAS) attempt to identify SNPs that may be associated with a particular trait by comparing the allele frequencies of each SNP in individuals with the phenotype in question, against population-matched controls (i.e., people presumed not to have the phenotype) [45, 46].

By performing GWAS on 850 cases and 700 controls, Dobbins et al. found a meningioma susceptibility locus in *Myeloid/Lymphoid or Mixed-Lineage Leukemia 10 (MLLT10)* on chromosome 10p [47]. MLLT10 activates the Wnt signaling pathway [47]. This finding was substantiated specifically in females by Claus et al., who established 30% of meningiomas to demonstrate loss of heterozygosity on chromosome 10p [48]. It is important to note that the majority of participants in these studies were of European descent. For a more all-encompassing view of meningiomas, it would be relevant to include people with diverse ethnicities [47, 48].

Radiation-Induced Meningiomas

It has been shown that exposure to ionizing radiation, even with low doses, can increase the risk of meningioma [49]. Types of exposure can vary from dental x-ray radiation, radiotherapy for childhood tumors, to exposure to atomic explosions [49–51]. These meningiomas usually differ in their clinical presentation from sporadic meningiomas as they usually present as multiple or multifocal meningiomas and show increased rates of recurrence with higher proliferation indices [52, 53]. They are observed in a much younger population (range, 29.2–37.9 years of age) [51]. Twenty-three percent of high-dose radiation exposure-related meningiomas present as either atypical or malignant [54]. Consistent with this aggressive clinical course, these meningiomas show genomic instability caused by chromosomal copy number changes [55].

Sporadic Meningiomas

Unlike inherited syndromes where the mutations arise in the germline, de novo somatic mutations occur solely in cells that give rise to tumors and not in other tissues. Therefore, individual patients can serve as both a control and a case, such that tumor and normal samples from a patient can be compared to each other to identify somatic variants. Through many cytogenetic, molecular, and genetic studies, the genomic profile of sporadic meningiomas has been established [11, 56–59]. These studies revealed the genomic events underlying meningioma formation as well as the mechanisms causing their atypical transformation.

Somatic Mutations in Meningiomas

We and others have established the somatic mutational profile of sporadic meningiomas, identifying the molecular events in over 80% of Grade I tumors [11, 13–15, 56–59]. These studies, mainly with the use of whole-exome sequencing, revealed six genomic subgroups of meningiomas, based on driver mutations in *NF2*, *TNF Receptor-Associated Factor 7* (*TRAF7*), PI3K and Hedgehog (HH) pathway molecules, *Kruppel-Like Factor 4* (*KLF4*), and *RNA Polymerase II Subunit A* (*POLR2A*) [12–14] (Fig. 4.1). Importantly, these somatic mutations differed based on the anatomical origins of the spinal and intracranial tumors, along the convexity or skull base (Fig. 4.2) [16]. The remaining 20% sporadic meningiomas that do not harbor a coding somatic mutation in these established genes are currently classified under the "mutation unknown" category [13–16]. This section will describe these established molecular subcategories of sporadic meningiomas.

Among these subgroups, approximately 50% of sporadic meningiomas are due to loss of *NF2* [60–62]. Similar to the tumors of neurofibromatosis II patients, sporadic meningiomas also exhibit biallelic *NF2* loss, typically via an inactivating variant and concomitant loss of *NF2* locus on chromosome 22q [63]. Indeed, consistent with the human phenotype, mice with *cre*-induced biallelic loss of NF2 also develop meningiomas [64, 65]. *NF2* mutant meningiomas develop laterally in the skull base and posteriorly along the convexity, typically behind the coronal suture (Fig. 4.2) [16]. Histologically, there is a prevalence of fibrous and transitional tumor histology

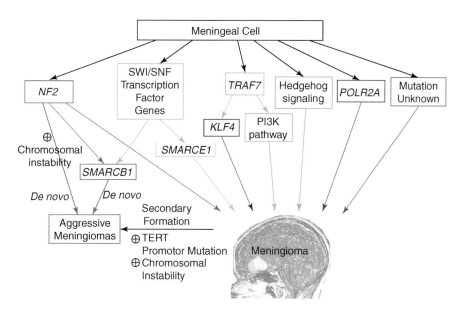

Fig. 4.1 Genomic subgroups of meningioma

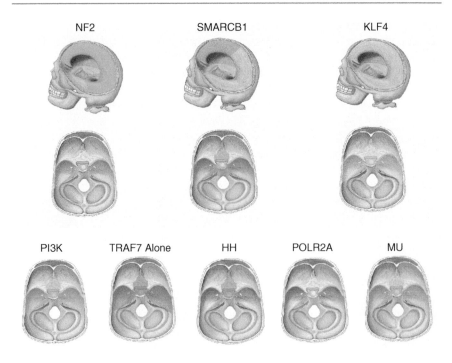

Fig. 4.2 Distinct molecular subtypes localize to different brain regions. (Reprinted from Young blood et al., (C) 2019, https://thejns.org/view/journals/j-neurosurg/aop/article-10.3171-2019.8. JNS191266/article-10.3171-2019.8.JNS191266.xml, with permission from Journal of Neurosurgery and AANS [16])

[15, 16]. While the predominantly convexity location should allow for less morbidity with treatment, *NF2* mutated meningiomas inherently confer more aggressive biological behavior with the potential for atypical transformation. Indeed, Harmanci et al. demonstrated that 75% atypical sporadic meningiomas harbor damaging mutations in *NF2* [59].

Recurrent somatic mutations that affect specific residues in *SMARCB1* are observed as co-mutations in a subset of *NF2* mutant meningiomas. As mentioned above, SMARCB1 is a member of the SWI/SNF group of transcriptional regulators [11, 42, 66, 67]. Indeed, damaging variants in *SMARCB1* almost always occur concurrently with *NF2* mutations and/or with loss of chromosome 22q, accounting for approximately 2.4% of WHO Grade I meningiomas [15, 41, 68]. Recurrent mutations in *SMARCB1* have been shown to lead to rhabdoid cancer [69]. However, somatic *SMARCB1* mutations in meningiomas are recurrent, almost always affecting the R386 residue. *SMARCB1/NF2* co-mutated meningiomas are significantly enriched in non-skull base regions and also seen in de novo atypical meningioma [16, 59]. Interestingly somatic *SMARCE1* mutations, in addition to the germline variants (see above), without co-occurring *NF2* mutations, have been identified in familial spinal clear cell and cranial clear cell meningiomas [43, 70, 71].

More recent studies have also identified somatic mutations in genes that have not been previously linked to neoplasia, including *TRAF7*, *KLF4*, and *POLR2A* [11, 13, 57, 59]. These non-*NF2* mutant meningiomas show a predilection for the junction of the anterior and middle cranial fossa, along the sphenoid wing, varying in terms of their laterality (Fig. 4.2) [16, 59]. Given the intimate association of these tumors with critical neurovascular structures, such as the optic nerve/chiasm and internal carotid artery bifurcation, these locations can be particularly relevant for treatment. Among these, TRAF7 is a linker protein between TNF receptors and cell survival pathways. It binds *MEKK3* to polyubiquinate and consequently degrade NF-kB factors *NEMO* and *p65* [72–74]. Somatic *TRAF7* mutations are identified in approximately 25% of WHO Grade I meningiomas [15, 72, 73]. Almost all of the meningioma-associated *TRAF7* mutations affect its WD40 repeat domain, which is the domain that interacts with MEKK3, leading to NF-kappaB activation [11, 73]. Mutations in this region may exert a dominant negative effect as the protein can no longer recognize binding substrates [14]. *TRAF7* mutant meningiomas are typically enriched in skull base lesions [16].

TRAF7 mutations almost always co-occur with either a recurrent $KLF4^{K409Q}$ mutation or PI3K pathway molecule mutations [57]. $TRAF7/KLF4^{K409Q}$ co-mutated meningiomas account for ~10% of WHO Grade I meningiomas [11, 14–16, 57]. *KLF4* is one of the four transcription factors (Yamanaka factors) that are sufficient for the transformation of somatic cells into induced pluripotent stem cells (iPSCs) [75]. It can act both as a tumor suppressor and as an oncogene, regulating both cellular apoptotic and proliferative pathways [76]. Previous work has suggested that *KLF4* may regulate the *PI3K* pathway through the *PDGF* receptor cascade [77–79], though this has yet to be demonstrated directly in meningiomas. The 409th residue of KLF4 lies in its zinc finger domain, which makes direct contact with DNA [57]. Disrupted DNA binding due to the *K409Q* mutation appears to lead to differential gene expression, ultimately leading to tumorigenesis [57]. Tumors with concurrent *TRAF7* and *KLF4* mutations have been associated with more lateral, non-midline anterior skull base locations and with secretory histology, which is known to cause peritumoral edema [16, 57]. This finding is significant as Grade I meningiomas typically do not have edema, which is associated with higher-grade tumors and can indicate significant brain involvement [80–82]. While surgical treatment of the meningioma is often required, this procedure can be associated with morbidity due to large intraoperative increases in intracranial pressure [82].

Another 10% of Grade I meningiomas and 30% of tumors confined to the skull base are caused by co-mutations in *TRAF7* and various molecules in the phosphoinositide 3-kinase/*AKT Serine/Threonine Kinase 1* (PI3K/AKT) pathway [11, 13, 56]. Among these co-mutations, a recurrent activating $AKT1^{E17K}$ mutation is the most common one [11, 14–16, 56, 83]. *AKT1* is involved in growth factor-induced survival by inhibiting apoptotic factors [84, 85]. The E17K mutation affects its pleckstrin domain, which then traps *AKT1* at the plasma membrane, leading to constitutive activation of the PI3K pathway [11, 14–16, 56, 83]. Similar to *TRAF7/KLF4* co-mutated meningiomas, PI3K pathway mutant tumors are enriched in anterior fossa skull base locations, with these tumors occurring more midline along the sphenoid wing and skull base (Fig. 4.2) [16]. Additionally, somatic *PIK3CA* activating and *PIK3R1* damaging mutations, both of which lead to subsequent PI3K pathway activation, have also been identified to be somatically in meningiomas [86–89].

Polymerase RNA II Subunit A (POLR2A) encodes RPB1, a member of the polymerase II complex, which is involved in the transcription of all mRNAs in eukaryotic cells [90]. Approximately 3% of meningiomas have recurrent mutations in *POLR2A*, and these are typically Grade I [11, 13–16]. Meningiomas are the only tumors known to harbor variants in this essential enzyme, which has been conserved through evolution [13]. Meningiomas with these mutations exhibit decreased expression of meningeal identity genes, including *Wnt Family Protein 6 (WNT6)*, *Zic Family Member 1 (ZIC1)*, and *Zic Family Member 4 (ZIC4)* [91, 92]. *POLR2A* mutated meningiomas are frequently present in the tuberculum sellae region with implications for clinical treatment as it can affect pituitary function (Fig. 4.2) [11, 13, 16, 56].

The Hedgehog (HH) pathway, which is physiologically associated with developmental patterning during embryogenesis and in stem cell and cell-cycle regulation in adults, is activated in another subgroup of meningiomas (6%) [11, 15, 56, 93]. Dysregulation in the HH pathway has been associated with several malignancies, including basal cell carcinoma, medulloblastoma, and pancreatic carcinoma, as well as Gorlin syndrome [93–97]. Ligands of the HH pathway – *Sonic Hedgehog (SHH)*, *Indian Hedgehog (IHH)*, and *Desert Hedgehog (DHH)* – bind to the receptor *Patched (PTCH)*, which then un-anchors the protein *Smoothened (SMO)* and allows it to increase transcription of HH-associated genes through downstream *Glioma-Associated Oncogene (GLI)* transcription factors [93, 98]. Typically, *GLI* transcription factors are anchored by *Suppressor of Fused (SUFU)* [93, 98]. Damaging variants in *SUFU* can lead to inherited cases of meningiomas, while activating mutations in *GLI* can lead to sporadic ones [11, 99]. Interestingly, the HH pathway is involved in midline patterning during embryogenesis, and most HH-mediated meningiomas occur at the midline, specifically along the olfactory groove or planum sphenoidale region [16, 100]. The majority of HH mutant meningiomas tend to be Grade I, and inherently slow-growing, often reaching considerable size before presenting clinically [16]. Tumors in this area can be difficult to surgically access, rendering potential precision medicine treatments, which are available for other tumors, for HH-driven meningiomas even more desirable.

Somatic Copy Number Variations in Meningiomas

Copy number variations (CNVs) are large-scale chromosomal number aberrations. In the context of neoplasia, CNVs can lead to either deletions of regions with tumor suppressors or amplification of oncogenes, thereby driving neoplasia [101].

The most frequently observed CNV event in meningiomas is the deletion or loss of heterozygosity of chromosome 22q, which harbors *NF2* and *SMARCB1*, among other genes [60]. Other frequently detected CNV events such as deletion of chromosomes 1p, 6q, 9p, 10, 13, and 14q, as well as chromosome 17p amplification, are associated with higher-grade meningiomas [60, 102–104]. Chromosome 1p harbors *Tumor Protein P73 (TP73)* and *Rho Guanine Nucleotide Exchange Factor 16*

(*ARHGEF16*) [102]. Loss of chromosome 1p is observed in a number of atypical cases and linked with tumor recurrence and progression. Specifically, chromosome 1p36 deletion has been suggested to predict shorter survival [102]. Deletion of chromosome 9p, containing tumor suppressors *Cyclin-Dependent Kinase Inhibitor 2A* and *2B* (*CDKN2A* and *CDKN2B*), which regulate the G1-S checkpoint, is a frequent event in cancer as in meningiomas [59, 105, 106].

Different chromosome number abnormalities are associated with certain histologic types of meningioma as well. For example, chromosome 2p loss is associated with choroid meningiomas, chromosome 5 polysomy is common in angiomatous meningiomas, and losses of chromosomes 1p, 6p, 14, and 22q are observed in anaplastic meningiomas [107–109]. In spinal meningiomas, amplification of chromosome 17q is observed in approximately 12% of cases [110].

Overall, a significant limitation of interpreting CNV studies is the difficulty in identifying specific tumor suppressor or oncogenes in regions of deletion and amplification, respectively, which highlights the importance of gene expression studies to establish possible driver mutations.

Somatic Noncoding Alterations in Meningiomas

In addition to somatic protein-coding variants, previous studies have suggested that alterations in noncoding regions may play a role in meningioma pathogenesis, including somatic noncoding variants and structural variants. Approximately 98.8% of the human genome is comprised of noncoding regions, and variants in these noncoding regions could lead to gene expression changes that underlie meningioma formation [111]. The advent of both long- and short-read whole-genome sequencing has allowed for observation of these noncoding pathogenic events.

Recent studies have demonstrated that noncoding variants near and genomic rearrangements involving *Neuronal Growth Regulator 1* (*NEGR1*) and SWI/SNF complex members are associated with meningiomas [56, 112, 113]. *NEGR1* is involved in CNS development, and mutations in this gene are associated with neuroblastoma [114, 115]. In addition, up to 5.5% of meningiomas may harbor *telomerase reverse transcriptase* (*TERT*) promoter mutations [116]. TERT maintains chromosomal length by maintaining telomere ends [82, 83], and mutations in the promoter (noncoding) region of *TERT* are markers for progression to malignancy in up to 90% of all cancers [117–121]. Meningioma patients with recurrent C228T and C250T mutations have a shorter time to progression, indicating these variants may be a strong prognostic indicator [122]. Promising results in cell culture studies have suggested that *TERT*-associated meningiomas may be responsive to ETS transcription factor inhibitor YK-4-270 [116].

Epigenetic Regulation/Deregulation in Meningiomas and Atypical Meningiomas

The aforementioned genomic findings explain the somatic variation in approximately 80% of meningioma cases [11, 15]. Epigenetic histone or DNA modifications can mediate gene expression changes via several different mechanisms, including methylation and acetylation. Gene silencing through DNA hypermethylation is observed commonly in tumors, including meningiomas [123–126]. These and other epigenetic modifications might be important in understanding the molecular landscape of the "mutation unknown" meningiomas.

Epigenetic regulation leads to modification of gene expression by remodeling the chromatin structure. Typically, tightly packed chromatin (heterochromatin) renders its corresponding genomic regions transcriptionally inactive, whereas its looser state (euchromatin) makes it transcriptionally active [127]. Histone modifications at specific histidine residues, such as acetylation and methylation, result in changes in chromatin accessibility and thus regulate the expression of genes [127]. Overexpression of oncogenes or under-expression of tumor suppressors can then lead to tumorigenesis.

Chromatin modifications and accessibility have been studied through many sequencing techniques, including chromatin immunoprecipitation (ChIP) followed by next-generation sequencing, specifically interrogating acetylation or trimethylation of the lysine 27 residue on histone 3 (H3K27) [128–134]. Interestingly, the epigenetic and genetic drivers for meningioma do not appear to have significant overlaps [135].

We have shown expression of the repressive H3K27me3 signal and a hypermethylated phenotype in de novo atypical meningiomas [59]. These meningiomas, which are mostly *NF2* mutant, become atypical through either genomic instability or co-mutations in *SMARCB1* [59]. Both of these groups show hypermethylation of the polycomb repressive complex 2 (PRC2) binding sites in human embryonic stem cells [59]. This phenocopies a more primitive cellular state with increased proliferation and decreased differentiation. Indeed, these atypical meningiomas exhibit upregulation of EZH2, the catalytic subunit of the PRC2 complex, as well as the E2F2 and FOXM1 transcriptional networks, suggesting novel therapeutic targets [59, 136, 137].

Matrix metalloproteinases (MMPs) facilitate tumor invasion by destabilizing the extracellular matrix [138]. TIMP3 covalently binds to and inhibits MMPs, thus preventing metastases [139]. Hypermethylation of TIMP3 is associated with lower TIMP3 and higher MMP expression, leading to higher-grade and/or metastatic meningiomas [30, 125]. Moreover, p14ARF – a protein product of *CDKN2A* – typically potentiates the effect of cell cycle controller TP53 through facilitating the degradation of MDM2 proto-oncogene [140]. Methylation of P14ARF thus increases P53 breakdown and leads to anaplastic meningiomas as well as other brain tumors [141, 142]. *N-myc downstream-regulated gene* 2 (NDRG2) is involved in cell growth and apoptosis pathways [143]. It is consistently hypermethylated and downregulated in Grade III meningiomas [144, 145]. Finally, *WNK Lysine Deficient Protein Kinase 2* (WNK2) is a potential cell growth suppressor as it inhibits colony formation when exogenously expressed and cell proliferation in vitro [146]. In particular, WNK2 inhibits MEK1, ERK1/2, and EGFR signaling [146]. In over 70% of Grade II and III meningiomas, WNK2 expression is decreased through excessive methylation at CpG islands [147]. Moreover, higher-grade meningiomas demonstrate neovascularization, which is the formation of new blood vessels within the tumor and can support the fast growth of cancer cells. In 54% of Grade III meningiomas and 30% of all meningiomas, hypermethylation of *Thrombospondin 1* (THBS1), an inhibitor of angiogenesis, may lead to neovascularization and tumor progression [148, 149].

Hypermethylation of conserved homeobox genes, *Proenkephalin* (PENK) and *Insulin-Like Growth Factor 2 mRNA-Binding Protein 1* (IGF2BP1), has been linked to the likelihood of recurrence [150]. Homeobox genes are involved in developmental patterning during embryogenesis, PENK may physically bind with p53 and RELA to modulate cellular apoptosis, and IGF2BP1 stabilizes the mRNA of c-myc oncogene and IGF2 [151–154]. Increased *IGF2BP1* promoter methylation is associated with Grade II/III meningiomas [153]. Conversely, global hypomethylation has also been reported in meningioma and is associated with atypical and malignant cases [135].

Importantly, epigenomic changes correlate with clinical behavior. Sahm et al. showed that these methylation patterns are better at predicting patients' prognosis than WHO grading of their lesions (Fig. 4.3) [123]. Interestingly, some WHO Grade III tumors have a benign methylation status, signaling better prognosis, while loss

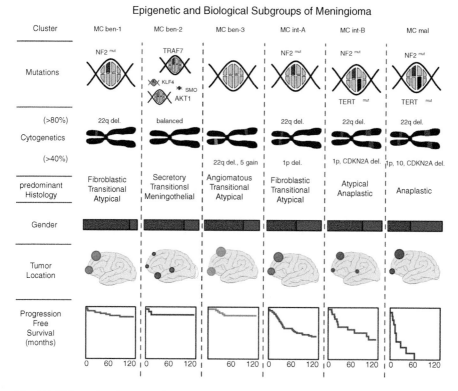

Fig. 4.3 Epigenetic subgroups of meningiomas. (Reprinted from Sahm et al., © 2017, with permission from Elsevier [123]

of suppressor histone marker, H3K27me3, is associated with poor prognosis [123, 155]. Among other cases, most non-*NF2* mutated tumors were found to fall into a single cluster with good prognosis, irrespective of grade (Fig. 4.2) [15, 123]. Two large and distinct subgroups of methylation patterns were observed, raising the possibility of distinct mechanisms or cells of origin [123]. Of note, previous reports suggest hierarchical clustering can only distinguish between Grade III and Grade I/II tumors but not between Grade I and Grade II tumors [123].

The aforementioned epigenetic modifications are related to methylation patterns. However, gene expression regulation through activating histone acetylation at the H3K27 residue also plays a role in meningioma development. Super-enhancer loci are enhancer-enriched regions with significant activating H3K27 acetylation patterns [11, 13, 14]. Several super-enhancers, some that are subtype specific and some that are enriched in all meningioma subtypes, were identified by our group [13]. Tumors with loss of *NF2* exhibited super-enhancer loci near Wnt pathway genes, including *secreted frizzled-related protein 2* (SFRP2), *naked cuticle homolog 1* (NKD1), and *disheveled-associated activator of morphogenesis 2* (DAAM2) [13, 14]. *POLR2A* has a differentially activated super-enhancer over *wingless-type MMTV integration site family, members 6 and 10 A* (*WNT6* and *WNT10A*) and loss of a super-enhancer near *Zic family member 1 and 4* (*ZIC1* and *ZIC4*) [13]. Interestingly, both ZIC and WNT signaling pathways are involved in meningeal differentiation and growth [13, 91, 92]. Finally, in *KLF4/TRAF7* co-mutated meningiomas, super-enhancer activity and expression are enriched in *grainyhead-like 3* (*GRHL3*), which codes for a transcription factor critical for neural tube development [13].

Clinical Correlates of Meningioma Genomics

As described in the previous sections, up to 80% of meningiomas fall into well-defined molecular subtypes based on mutations in driver genes [11, 13–15, 56–59]. These mutations strongly correlate with the patients' prognosis (through WHO grade predictions), as well as the tumor location and histology [16]. Cases with biallelic loss of *NF2* are enhanced in Grade II and III tumors [16]. On the other hand, *POLR2A* or *TRAF7/KLF4* tumors often present as low-grade lesions [16]. In terms of location, we were first to show that non-*NF2* meningiomas (i.e., *TRAF7*, *KLF4*, and *PI3K* mutants) localize to the skull base [13, 16]. *SMARCB1*, a regulator of the HH pathway, and HH mutated tumors (*SMO, SUFU, PRKAR1A*) often localize to the midline, where HH pathway is active during brain development [16, 92, 100]. *POLR2A* mutated lesions are found near the tuberculum sellae [11, 13, 56]. Histology is also related to tumor subtype: *NF2* mutated meningiomas are correlated with fibrous histology [15, 16], TRAF7/*KLF4*^{K409Q} with secretory [57], and *POLR2A/AKT1/SMO* with meningothelial [16].

In addition, gene expression studies are used to better understand and predict the prognosis of meningiomas [156]. Similarly, DNA methylation studies are leveraged to predict recurrence [157].

Precision Medicine for Meningiomas

In terms of treatment, meningiomas are typically managed by surgical resection and/or radiation. However, as discussed above, some meningiomas can arise in relatively higher-risk locations along the skull base, such as the *TRAF7*, *KLF4*, and *PI3K* subgroups, with the involvement of or close proximity to critical neurovascular structures [15, 16]. Other meningiomas (i.e., *NF2*) can occur in more favorable locations but are associated with higher grade and recurrence rates [15, 16]. How to treat residual tumors and those that recur and progress is of particular concern, not only in WHO Grade I tumors but also in higher-grade tumors [158]. Moreover, whether to treat residual tumor or wait for disease progression is another area of debate. Undeniably, there are limitations in terms of the current treatment strategies, as there are a finite number of times surgery and radiation can both be used and reused in any one patient. Also, radiation-induced meningiomas can occur, often presenting with multiple lesions, a more aggressive course, and a higher risk of recurrence [159, 160]. This is further complicated by the current lack of effective chemotherapy. Thus, finding an alternative way to medically manage these tumors is essential, and the low mutational burden and well-characterized genomic etiologies of meningiomas suggest that these tumors may respond well to specific drug-based treatments based on molecular profiling [15, 16]. For example, HH signaling pathway activation is well-described in cancer. There are targeted medications that exist for aberrant HH signaling, which have been repurposed for clinical trials in meningiomas [89]. More scientific investigation and clinical trials, like that for upregulated HH signaling, is imperative in meningiomas.

Conclusion and Future Directions

Recent scientific efforts have undeniably led to a significantly better understanding of the genetics and pathogenesis of meningiomas, both inherited and somatic, and have afforded insight into tumor progression. These studies have contributed hugely to identifying novel meningioma drivers – including *KLF4*, *TRAF7*, and *POLR2A*, which have not been previously associated with cancer – and to classifying the molecular subtypes of meningiomas, including up to 80% of all sporadic meningiomas. However, the downstream mechanisms for formation of these meningioma subtypes are still not well understood. Additionally, 20% of meningiomas do not harbor coding somatic mutations in one of the established meningioma driver genes. It is possible that these meningiomas harbor mutations in noncoding regions or have epigenetic abnormalities. With the advent of cheaper and more accurate next-generation sequencing, these questions may be answered and validated with functional studies. Thus, further genomic studies are merited, and with a better understanding of the molecular pathogenesis of meningiomas, targeted therapies and better patient outcomes will hopefully become a reality soon.

References

1. Ostrom QT, Gittleman H, Truitt G, Boscia A, Kruchko C, Barnholtz-Sloan JS. CBTRUS statistical report: primary brain and other central nervous system tumors diagnosed in the United States in 2011–2015. Neuro Oncol. 2018;20(suppl_4):iv1–86.
2. Dirks MS, Butman JA, Kim HJ, Wu T, Morgan K, Tran AP, et al. Long-term natural history of neurofibromatosis type 2–associated intracranial tumors. J Neurosurg. 2012;117(1):109–17.
3. Nakamura M, Roser F, Michel J, Jacobs C, Samii M. Volumetric analysis of the growth rate of incompletely resected intracranial meningiomas. Zentralbl Neurochir. 2005;66(01):17–23.
4. Jääskeläinen J, Haltia M, Laasonen E, Wahlström T, Valtonen S. The growth rate of intracranial meningiomas and its relation to histology. An analysis of 43 patients. Surg Neurol. 1985;24(2):165–72.
5. Choy W, Kim W, Nagasawa D, Stramotas S, Yew A, Gopen Q, et al. The molecular genetics and tumor pathogenesis of meningiomas and the future directions of meningioma treatments. Neurosurg Focus. 2011;30(5):E6.
6. Domingues PH, Teodósio C, Otero Á, Sousa P, Gonçalves JM, Nieto AB, et al. The protein expression profile of meningioma cells is associated with distinct cytogenetic tumour subgroups. Neuropathol App Neurobiol. 2015;41(3):319–32.
7. Smith MJ. Germline and somatic mutations in meningiomas. Cancer Genet. 2015;208(4):107–14.
8. Cahill KS, Claus EB. Treatment and survival of patients with nonmalignant intracranial meningioma: results from the Surveillance, Epidemiology, and End Results Program of the National Cancer Institute. J Neurosurg. 2011;115(2):259–67.
9. Al-Mefty O, Kadri PA, Pravdenkova S, Sawyer JR, Stangeby C, Husain M. Malignant progression in meningioma: documentation of a series and analysis of cytogenetic findings. J Neurosurg. 2004;101(2):210–8.
10. Nowak A, Dziedzic T, Krych P, Czernicki T, Kunert P, Marchel A. Benign versus atypical meningiomas: risk factors predicting recurrence. Neurol Neurochir Pol. 2015;49(1):1–10.
11. Clark VE, Erson-Omay EZ, Serin A, Yin J, Cotney J, Özduman K, et al. Genomic analysis of non-NF2 meningiomas reveals mutations in TRAF7, KLF4, AKT1, and SMO. Science. 2013;339(6123):1077–80.
12. Parsons DW, Jones S, Zhang X, Lin JC, Leary RJ, Angenendt P, et al. An integrated genomic analysis of human glioblastoma multiforme. Science. 2008;321(5897):1807–12.
13. Clark VE, Harmancı AS, Bai H, Youngblood MW, Lee TI, Baranoski JF, et al. Recurrent somatic mutations in POLR2A define a distinct subset of meningiomas. Nat Genet. 2016;48(10):1253.
14. Clark VE. Characterizing the genomic architecture and molecular mechanisms driving the formation of non-NF2 meningiomas. 2015. (Doctoral dissertation, Yale University).
15. Youngblood MW. Molecular features and translation applications of genomic alterations in meningioma. 2019. (Doctoral dissertation, Yale University).
16. Youngblood MW, Duran D, Montejo JD, Li C, Omay SB, Özduman K, et al. Correlations between genomic subgroup and clinical features in a cohort of over 3000 meningiomas. J Neurosurg. 2019;1(aop):1–10.
17. Gupta S, Bi WL, Dunn IF. Medical management of meningioma in the era of precision medicine. Neurosurg Focus. 2018;44(4):E3.
18. O'Connor C, Miko I. Developing the chromosome theory. Nat Educ. 2008;1(1):44.
19. Evans DR. Neurofibromatosis type 2 (NF2): a clinical and molecular review. Orphanet J Rare Dis. 2009;4(1):16.
20. Smith MJ, Beetz C, Williams SG, Bhaskar SS, O'Sullivan J, Anderson B, et al. Germline mutations in SUFU cause Gorlin syndrome–associated childhood medulloblastoma and redefine the risk associated with PTCH1 mutations. J Clin Oncol. 2014;32(36):4155–61.
21. Orloff MS, He X, Peterson C, Chen F, Chen JL, Mester JL, Eng C. Germline PIK3CA and AKT1 mutations in Cowden and Cowden-like syndromes. Am J Human Genet. 2013;92(1):76–80.

22. Lee CW, Tan TC. Meningioma associated with Gorlin's syndrome. J Clin Neurosci. 2014;21(2):349–50.
23. Albrecht S, Goodman JC, Rajagopolan S, Levy M, Cech DA, Cooley LD. Malignant meningioma in Gorlin's syndrome: cytogenetic and p53 gene analysis: case report. J Neurosurg. 1994;81(3):466–71.
24. Askaner G, Lei U, Bertelsen B, Venzo A, Wadt K. Novel SUFU frameshift variant leading to meningioma in three generations in a family with gorlin syndrome. Case Rep Genet. 2019;2019:9650184.
25. Yakubov E, Ghoochani A, Buslei R, Buchfelder M, Eyüpoglu IY, Savaskan N. Hidden association of Cowden syndrome, PTEN mutation and meningioma frequency. Onco Targets Ther. 2016;3(5–6):149.
26. Pain M, Darbinyan A, Fowkes M, Shrivastava R. Multiple meningiomas in a patient with cowden syndrome. J Neurol Surg Rep. 2016;77(03):e128–33.
27. Karajannis MA, Ferner RE. Neurofibromatosis-related tumors: emerging biology and therapies. Curr Opin Pediatr. 2015;27(1):26.
28. Ruttledge MH, Andermann AA, Phelan CM, Claudio JO, Han FY, Chretien N, et al. Type of mutation in the neurofibromatosis type 2 gene (NF2) frequently determines severity of disease. Am J Human Genet. 1996;59(2):331.
29. Peyrard M, Fransson I, Xie YG, et al. Characterization of a new member of the human beta-adaptin gene family from chromosome 22q12, a candidate meningioma gene. Hum Mol Genet. 1994;3:1393–9.
30. Barski D, Wolter M, Reifenberger G, et al. Hypermethylation and transcriptional downregulation of the TIMP3 gene is associated with allelic loss on 22q12. 3 and malignancy in meningiomas. Brain Pathol. 2010;20:623–31.
31. Rouleau GA, Seizinger BR, Wertelecki W, Haines JL, Superneau DW, Martuza RL, Gusella JF. Flanking markers bracket the neurofibromatosis type 2 (NF2) gene on chromosome 22. Am J Human Genet. 1990;46(2):323.
32. Trofatter JA, MacCollin MM, Rutter JL, Murrell JR, Duyao MP, Parry DM, et al. A novel moesin-, ezrin-, radixin-like gene is a candidate for the neurofibromatosis 2 tumor suppressor. Cell. 1993;72(5):791–800.
33. Zhou L, Ercolano E, Ammoun S, Schmid MC, Barczyk MA, Hanemann CO. Merlin-deficient human tumors show loss of contact inhibition and activation of Wnt/β-catenin signaling linked to the PDGFR/Src and Rac/PAK pathways. Neoplasia. 2011;13(12):1101–IN2.
34. Rong R, Tang X, Gutmann DH, Ye K. Neurofibromatosis 2 (NF2) tumor suppressor merlin inhibits phosphatidylinositol 3-kinase through binding to PIKE-L. Proc Natl Acad Sci U S A. 2004;101(52):18200–5.
35. Kissil JL, Wilker EW, Johnson KC, Eckman MS, Yaffe MB, Jacks T. Merlin, the product of the Nf2 tumor suppressor gene, is an inhibitor of the p21-activated kinase, Pak1. Mol Cell. 2003;12(4):841–9.
36. Thaxton C, Lopera J, Bott M, Baldwin ME, Kalidas P, Fernandez-Valle C. Phosphorylation of the NF2 tumor suppressor in Schwann cells is mediated by Cdc42-Pak and requires paxillin binding. Mol Cell Neurosci. 2007;34(2):231–42.
37. James MF, Han S, Polizzano C, Plotkin SR, Manning BD, Stemmer-Rachamimov AO, et al. NF2/merlin is a novel negative regulator of mTOR complex 1, and activation of mTORC1 is associated with meningioma and schwannoma growth. Mol Cell Biol. 2009;29(15):4250–61.
38. Hamaratoglu F, Willecke M, Kango-Singh M, Nolo R, Hyun E, Tao C, et al. The tumour-suppressor genes NF2/Merlin and Expanded act through Hippo signalling to regulate cell proliferation and apoptosis. Nat Cell Biol. 2006;8(1):27.
39. McClatchey AI, Giovannini M. Membrane organization and tumorigenesis—the NF2 tumor suppressor, Merlin. Genes Dev. 2005;19(19):2265–77.
40. Goutagny S, Yang HW, Zucman-Rossi J, Chan J, Dreyfuss JM, Park PJ, et al. Genomic profiling reveals alternative genetic pathways of meningioma malignant progression dependent on the underlying NF2 status. Clin Cancer Res. 2010;16(16):4155–64.

41. van den Munckhof P, Christiaans I, Kenter SB, Baas F, Hulsebos TJ. Germline SMARCB1 mutation predisposes to multiple meningiomas and schwannomas with preferential location of cranial meningiomas at the falx cerebri. Neurogenetics. 2012;13(1):1–7.
42. Christiaans I, Kenter SB, Brink HC, van Os TAM, Baas F, Van den Munckhof P, et al. Germline SMARCB1 mutation and somatic NF2 mutations in familial multiple meningiomas. J Med Genet. 2011;48(2):93–7.
43. Smith MJ, O'Sullivan J, Bhaskar SS, Hadfield KD, Poke G, Caird J, et al. Loss-of-function mutations in SMARCE1 cause an inherited disorder of multiple spinal meningiomas. Nat Genet. 2013;45(3):295.
44. Marth GT, Korf I, Yandell MD, Yeh RT, Gu Z, Zakeri H, et al. A general approach to single-nucleotide polymorphism discovery. Nat Genet. 1999;23(4):452.
45. Risch N, Merikangas K. The future of genetic studies of complex human diseases. Science. 1996;273(5281):1516–7.
46. Visscher PM, Brown MA, McCarthy MI, Yang J. Five years of GWAS discovery. Am J Hum Genet. 2012;90(1):7–24.
47. Dobbins SE, Broderick P, Melin B, Feychting M, Johansen C, Andersson U, et al. Common variation at 10p12. 31 near MLLT10 influences meningioma risk. Nat Genet. 2011;43(9):825.
48. Claus H, Calvocoressi L, Schildkraut J, Walsh K, Hansen H, Smirnov I, McCoy L, et al. Report from the meningioma consortium: confirmation of a meningioma risk locus at 10p12. Neuro-Oncology. 2016;18:103–3.
49. Ron E, Modan B, Boice JD Jr, Alfandary E, Stovall M, Chetrit A, Katz L. Tumors of the brain and nervous system after radiotherapy in childhood. N Engl J Med. 1988;319(16):1033–9. https://doi.org/10.1056/NEJM198810203191601.
50. Claus EB, Calvocoressi L, Bondy ML, Schildkraut JM, Wiemels JL, Wrensch M. Dental x-rays and risk of meningioma. Cancer. 2012;118(18):4530–7.
51. Umansky F, Shoshan Y, Rosenthal G, Fraifeld S, Spektor S. Radiation-induced meningioma. Neurosurg Focus. 2008;24(5):E7.
52. Louis DN, Scheithauer BW, Budka H, von Deimling A, Kepes J. Meningiomas. In: Kleihues P, Cavenee WK, editors. Pathology and genetics. Tumors of the nervous system: WHO classification of tumors. Lyon: IARC Press; 2000.
53. Kleihues P, Cavenee WK. World Health Organization classification of tumors. Pathology and genetics of tumors of the nervous system. Lyon: IARC Press; 2000.
54. Musa BS, Pople IK, Cummins BH. Intracranial meningiomas following irradiation-a growing problem? Br J Neurosurg. 1995;9(5):629–38.
55. Agnihotri S, Suppiah S, Tonge PD, Jalali S, Danesh A, Bruce JP, et al. Therapeutic radiation for childhood cancer drives structural aberrations of NF2 in meningiomas. Nat Commun. 2017;8(1):1–7.
56. Brastianos PK, Horowitz PM, Santagata S, Jones RT, McKenna A, Getz G, et al. Genomic sequencing of meningiomas identifies oncogenic SMO and AKT1 mutations. Nat Genet. 2013;45(3):285.
57. Reuss DE, Piro RM, Jones DT, Simon M, Ketter R, Kool M, Becker A, Sahm F, Pusch S, Meyer J, Hagenlocher C. Secretory meningiomas are defined by combined KLF4 K409Q and TRAF7 mutations. Acta Neuropathol. 2013;125(3):351–8.
58. Metzker ML. Sequencing technologies—the next generation. Nature Rev Genet. 2010;11(1):31–46.
59. Harmancı AS, Youngblood MW, Clark VE, Coşkun S, Henegariu O, Duran D, et al. Integrated genomic analyses of de novo pathways underlying atypical meningiomas. Nat Commun. 2017;8:14433.
60. Ueki K, Wen-Bin C, Narita Y, Asai A, Kirino T. Tight association of loss of merlin expression with loss of heterozygosity at chromosome 22q in sporadic meningiomas. Cancer Res. 1999;59(23):5995–8.
61. Ruttledge MH, Sarrazin J, Rangaratnam S, Phelan CM, Twist E, Merel P, et al. Evidence for the complete inactivation of the NF2 gene in the majority of sporadic meningiomas. Nat Genet. 1994;6(2):180.

62. Wellenreuther R, Kraus JA, Lenartz D, Menon AG, Schramm J, Louis DN, et al. Analysis of the neurofibromatosis 2 gene reveals molecular variants of meningioma. Am J Pathol. 1995;146(4):827.
63. Merel P, Hoang-Xuan K, Sanson M, Moreau-Aubry A, Bijlsma EK, Lazaro C, et al. Predominant occurrence of somatic mutations of the NF2 gene in meningiomas and schwannomas. Genes Chromosomes Cancer. 1995;13(3):211–6.
64. Kalamarides M, Niwa-Kawakita M, Leblois H, Abramowski V, Perricaudet M, Janin A, et al. Nf2 gene inactivation in arachnoidal cells is rate-limiting for meningioma development in the mouse. Genes Dev. 2002;16(9):1060–5.
65. Kalamarides M, Stemmer-Rachamimov AO, Niwa-Kawakita M, Chareyre F, Taranchon E, Han ZY, et al. Identification of a progenitor cell of origin capable of generating diverse meningioma histological subtypes. Oncogene. 2011;30(20):2333.
66. Rousseau G, Noguchi T, Bourdon V, Sobol H, Olschwang S. SMARCB1/INI1 germline mutations contribute to 10% of sporadic schwannomatosis. BMC Neurol. 2011;11(1):9.
67. Christiaans I, Kenter SB, Brink HC, van Os TA, Baas F, Van den Munckhof P, et al. Germline mutation of INI1/SMARCB1 in familial schwannomatosis. Am J Hum Genet. 2007;80(4):805–10.
68. Smith MJ, Wallace AJ, Bowers NL, Rustad CF, Woods CG, Leschziner GD, et al. Frequency of SMARCB1 mutations in familial and sporadic schwannomatosis. Neurogenetics. 2012;13(2):141–5.
69. Biegel JA, Zhou JY, Rorke LB, Stenstrom C, Wainwright LM, Fogelgren B. Germ-line and acquired mutations of INI1 in atypical teratoid and rhabdoid tumors. Cancer Res. 1999;59(1):74–9.
70. Smith MJ, Wallace AJ, Bennett C, Hasselblatt M, Elert-Dobkowska E, Evans LT, et al. Germline SMARCE1 mutations predispose to both spinal and cranial clear cell meningiomas. J Pathol. 2014;234(4):436–40.
71. Tauziede-Espariat A, Parfait B, Besnard A, Lacombe J, Pallud J, Tazi S, et al. Loss of SMARCE1 expression is a specific diagnostic marker of clear cell meningioma: a comprehensive immunophenotypical and molecular analysis. Brain Pathol. 2018;28(4):466–74.
72. Yang J, Lin Y, Guo Z, Cheng J, Huang J, Deng L, et al. The essential role of MEKK3 in TNF-induced NF-κB activation. Nat Immunol. 2001;2(7):620.
73. Bouwmeester T, Bauch A, Ruffner H, Angrand PO, Bergamini G, Croughton K, et al. A physical and functional map of the human TNF-α/NF-κB signal transduction pathway. Nat Cell Biol. 2004;6(2):97.
74. Zotti T, Uva A, Ferravante A, Vessichelli M, Scudiero I, Ceccarelli M, Vito P. TRAF7 protein promotes Lys-29-linked polyubiquitination of IκB kinase (IKKγ)/NF-κB essential modulator (NEMO) and p65/RelA protein and represses NF-κB activation. J Biol Chem. 2011;286(26):22924–33.
75. Takahashi K, Tanabe K, Ohnuki M, Narita M, Ichisaka T, Tomoda K, Yamanaka S. Induction of pluripotent stem cells from adult human fibroblasts by defined factors. Cell. 2007;131(5):861–72.
76. Yamanaka S, Takahashi K, Okita K, inventors; Kyoto University, assignee. Induced pluripotent stem cells produced with Oct3/4, Klf4 and Sox2. United States patent 8,278,104. 2012.
77. Rowland BD, Bernards R, Peeper DS. The KLF4 tumour suppressor is a transcriptional repressor of p53 that acts as a context-dependent oncogene. Nat Cell Biol. 2005;7(11):1074.
78. Chang YL, Zhou PJ, Wei L, Li W, Ji Z, Fang YX, Gao WQ. MicroRNA-7 inhibits the stemness of prostate cancer stem-like cells and tumorigenesis by repressing KLF4/PI3K/Akt/p21 pathway. Oncotarget. 2015;6(27):24017.
79. Zheng B, Han M, Bernier M, Zhang XH, Meng F, Miao SB, et al. Krüppel-like factor 4 inhibits proliferation by platelet-derived growth factor receptor β-mediated, not by retinoic acid receptor α-mediated, phosphatidylinositol 3-kinase and ERK signaling in vascular smooth muscle cells. J Biol Chem. 2009;284(34):22773–85.
80. Raslan A, Bhardwaj A. Medical management of cerebral edema. Neurosurg Focus. 2007;22(5):1–12.

81. Kaal EC, Vecht CJ. The management of brain edema in brain tumors. Curr Opin Oncol. 2004;16(6):593–600.

82. Regelsberger J, Hagel C, Emami P, Ries T, Heese O, Westphal M. Secretory meningiomas: a benign subgroup causing life-threatening complications. Neuro-Oncology. 2009;11(6):819–24.

83. Yesilöz Ü, Kirches E, Hartmann C, Scholz J, Kropf S, Sahm F, et al. Frequent AKT1 E17K mutations in skull base meningiomas are associated with mTOR and ERK1/2 activation and reduced time to tumor recurrence. Neuro-Oncology. 2017;19(8):1088–96.

84. Chen WS, Xu PZ, Gottlob K, Chen ML, Sokol K, Shiyanova T, et al. Growth retardation and increased apoptosis in mice with homozygous disruption of the Akt1 gene. Genes Dev. 2001;15(17):2203–8.

85. Kang JQ, Chong ZZ, Maiese K. Critical role for Akt1 in the modulation of apoptotic phosphatidylserine exposure and microglial activation. Mol Pharmacol. 2003;64(3):557–69.

86. El-Habr EA, Levidou G, Trigka EA, Sakalidou J, Piperi C, Chatziandreou I, et al. Complex interactions between the components of the PI3K/AKT/mTOR pathway, and with components of MAPK, JAK/STAT and Notch-1 pathways, indicate their involvement in meningioma development. Virchows Arch. 2014;465(4):473–85.

87. Bujko M, Kober P, Tysarowski A, Matyja E, Mandat T, Bonicki W, Siedlecki JA. EGFR, PIK3CA, KRAS and BRAF mutations in meningiomas. Oncol Lett. 2014;7(6):2019–22.

88. Pang JC, Chung NY, Chan NH, Poon WS, Thomas T, Ng HK. Rare mutation of PIK3CA in meningiomas. Acta Neuropathol. 2006;111(3):284–5.

89. Abedalthagafi M, Bi WL, Aizer AA, Merrill PH, Brewster R, Agarwalla PK, et al. Oncogenic PI3K mutations are as common as AKT1 and SMO mutations in meningioma. Neuro-Oncology. 2016;18(5):649–55.

90. Bernard G, Chouery E, Putorti ML, Tétreault M, Takanohashi A, Carosso G, et al. Mutations of POLR3A encoding a catalytic subunit of RNA polymerase Pol III cause a recessive hypomyelinating leukodystrophy. Am J Hum Genet. 2011;89(3):415–23.

91. Inoue T, Ogawa M, Mikoshiba K, Aruga J. Zic deficiency in the cortical marginal zone and meninges results in cortical lamination defects resembling those in type II lissencephaly. J Neurosci. 2008;28(18):4712–25.

92. Choe Y, Zarbalis KS, Pleasure SJ. Neural crest-derived mesenchymal cells require Wnt signaling for their development and drive invagination of the telencephalic midline. PLoS One. 2014;9(2):e86025.

93. di Magliano MP, Hebrok M. Hedgehog signalling in cancer formation and maintenance. Nat Rev Cancer. 2003;3(12):903.

94. Pastorino L, Ghiorzo P, Nasti S, Battistuzzi L, Cusano R, Marzocchi C, et al. Identification of a SUFU germline mutation in a family with Gorlin syndrome. Am J Med Genet Part A. 2009;149(7):1539–43.

95. Von Hoff DD, LoRusso PM, Rudin CM, Reddy JC, Yauch RL, Tibes R, et al. Inhibition of the hedgehog pathway in advanced basal-cell carcinoma. N Engl J Med. 2009;361(12):1164–72.

96. Berman DM, Karhadkar SS, Hallahan AR, Pritchard JI, Eberhart CG, Watkins DN, et al. Medulloblastoma growth inhibition by hedgehog pathway blockade. Science. 2002;297(5586):1559–61.

97. Thayer SP, di Magliano MP, Heiser PW, Nielsen CM, Roberts DJ, Lauwers GY, et al. Hedgehog is an early and late mediator of pancreatic cancer tumorigenesis. Nature. 2003;425(6960):851.

98. Rubin LL, de Sauvage FJ. Targeting the Hedgehog pathway in cancer. Nat Rev Drug Discov. 2006;5(12):1026.

99. Aavikko M, Li SP, Saarinen S, Alhopuro P, Kaasinen E, Morgunova E, et al. Loss of SUFU function in familial multiple meningioma. Am J Hum Genet. 2012;91(3):520–6.

100. Boetto J, Bielle F, Sanson M, Peyre M, Kalamarides M. SMO mutation status defines a distinct and frequent molecular subgroup in olfactory groove meningiomas. Neuro-Oncology. 2017;19(3):345–51.

101. Shlien A, Malkin D. Copy number variations and cancer. Genome Med. 2009;1(6):62.
102. Gabeau-Lacet D, Engler D, Gupta S, Scangas GA, Betensky RA, Barker FG, et al. Genomic profiling of atypical meningiomas associates gain of 1q with poor clinical outcome. J Neuropathol Exp Neurol. 2009;68(10):1155–65.
103. Carvalho LH, Smirnov I, Baia GS, Modrusan Z, Smith JS, Jun P, et al. Molecular signatures define two main classes of meningiomas. Mol Cancer. 2007;6(1):64.
104. Lee Y, Liu J, Patel S, Cloughesy T, Lai A, Farooqi H, et al. Genomic landscape of meningiomas. Brain Pathol. 2010;20(4):751–62.
105. Büschges R, Ichimura K, Weber RG, Reifenberger G, Collins VP. Allelic gain and amplification on the long arm of chromosome 17 in anaplastic meningiomas. Brain Pathol. 2002;12(2):145–53.
106. Schultz DC, Vanderveer L, Buetow KH, Boente MP, Ozols RF, Hamilton TC, Godwin AK. Characterization of chromosome 9 in human ovarian neoplasia identifies frequent genetic imbalance on 9q and rare alterations involving 9p, including CDKN2. Cancer Res. 1995;55(10):2150–7.
107. Sievers P, Stichel D, Hielscher T, Schrimpf D, Reinhardt A, Wefers AK, et al. Chordoid meningiomas can be sub-stratified into prognostically distinct DNA methylation classes and are enriched for heterozygous deletions of chromosomal arm 2p. Acta Neuropathol. 2018;136(6):975–8.
108. Abedalthagafi MS, Merrill PH, Bi WL, Jones RT, Listewnik ML, Ramkissoon SH, et al. Angiomatous meningiomas have a distinct genetic profile with multiple chromosomal polysomies including polysomy of chromosome 5. Oncotarget. 2014;5(21):10596.
109. Collord G, Tarpey P, Kurbatova N, Martincorena I, Moran S, Castro M, et al. An integrated genomic analysis of anaplastic meningioma identifies prognostic molecular signatures. Sci Rep. 2018;8(1):13537.
110. Amplifikasyonu G. Her-2/neu gene amplification in paraffin-embedded tissue sections of meningioma patients. Turk Neurosurg. 2009;19(2):135–8.
111. Esteller M. Non-coding RNAs in human disease. Nat Rev Genet. 2011;12(12):861.
112. Bi WL, Greenwald NF, Abedalthagafi M, Wala J, Gibson WJ, Agarwalla PK, et al. Genomic landscape of high-grade meningiomas. NPJ Genom Med. 2017;2(1):15.
113. Proctor DT, Patel Z, Lama S, Resch L, van Marle G, Sutherland GR. Identification of PD-L2, B7-H3 and CTLA-4 immune checkpoint proteins in genetic subtypes of meningioma. Onco Targets Ther. 2019;8(1):e1512943.
114. Kim H, Hwang JS, Lee B, Hong J, Lee S. Newly identified cancer-associated role of human neuronal growth regulator 1 (NEGR1). J Cancer. 2014;5(7):598.
115. Pischedda F, Szczurkowska J, Cirnaru MD, Giesert F, Vezzoli E, Ueffing M, et al. A cell surface biotinylation assay to reveal membrane-associated neuronal cues: Negr1 regulates dendritic arborization. Mol Cell Proteomics. 2014;13(3):733–48.
116. Spiegl-Kreinecker S, Lötsch D, Neumayer K, Kastler L, Gojo J, Pirker C, et al. TERT promoter mutations are associated with poor prognosis and cell immortalization in meningioma. Neuro-Oncology. 2018;20(12):1584–93.
117. Goutagny S, Nault JC, Mallet M, Henin D, Rossi JZ, Kalamarides M. High incidence of activating TERT promoter mutations in meningiomas undergoing malignant progression. Brain Pathol. 2014;24(2):184–9.
118. de Jesus BB, Blasco MA. Telomerase at the intersection of cancer and aging. Trends Genet. 2013;29(9):513–20.
119. Kong F, Zheng C, Xu D. Telomerase as a "stemness" enzyme. Sci China Life Sci. 2014;57(6):564–70.
120. Xu Y, Goldkorn A. Telomere and telomerase therapeutics in cancer. Genes. 2016;7(6):22.
121. Liu T, Yuan X, Xu D. Cancer-specific telomerase reverse transcriptase (TERT) promoter mutations: biological and clinical implications. Genes. 2016;7(7):38.
122. Horn S, Figl A, Rachakonda PS, Fischer C, Sucker A, Gast A, et al. TERT promoter mutations in familial and sporadic melanoma. Science. 2013;339(6122):959–61.

123. Sahm F, Schrimpf D, Stichel D, Jones DT, Hielscher T, Schefzyk S, et al. DNA methylation-based classification and grading system for meningioma: a multicentre, retrospective analysis. Lancet Oncol. 2017;18(5):682–94.
124. Gendreau JL, Chow KK, Sussman ES, Iyer A, Pendharkar AV, Ho AL. DNA methylation analysis for the treatment of meningiomas. J Vis Surg. 2017;3:178.
125. Liu Y, Pang JCS, Dong S, Mao B, Poon WS, Ng HK. Aberrant CpG island hypermethylation profile is associated with atypical and anaplastic meningiomas. Hum Pathol. 2005;36(4):416–25.
126. Gao F, Shi L, Russin J, Zeng L, Chang X, He S, et al. DNA methylation in the malignant transformation of meningiomas. PloS One. 2013;8(1):e54114.
127. Grewal SI, Moazed D. Heterochromatin and epigenetic control of gene expression. Science. 2003;301(5634):798–802.
128. Park PJ. ChIP–seq: advantages and challenges of a maturing technology. Nat Rev Genet. 2009;10(10):669.
129. Gavrilov A, Eivazova E, Pirozhkova I, Lipinski M, Razin S, Vassetzky Y. Chromatin immuno-precipitation assays. Totowa: Humana Press; 2009. Chromosome conformation capture (from 3C to 5C) and its ChIP-based modification; p. 171–188.
130. Mifsud B, Tavares-Cadete F, Young AN, Sugar R, Schoenfelder S, Ferreira L, Wingett SW, Andrews S, Grey W, Ewels PA, Herman B. Mapping long-range promoter contacts in human cells with high-resolution capture Hi-C. Nat Genet. 2015;47(6):598.
131. Buenrostro JD, Wu B, Chang HY, Greenleaf WJ. ATAC-seq: a method for assaying chromatin accessibility genome-wide. Curr Protoc Mol Biol. 2015;109(1):21–9.
132. Wang Z, Gerstein M, Snyder M. RNA-Seq: a revolutionary tool for transcriptomics. Nat Rev Genet. 2009;10(1):57.
133. Li G, Fullwood MJ, Xu H, Mulawadi FH, Velkov S, Vega V, Ariyaratne PN, Mohamed YB, Ooi HS, Tennakoon C, Wei CL. ChIA-PET tool for comprehensive chromatin interaction analysis with paired-end tag sequencing. Genome Biol. 2010;11(2):R22.
134. Hatada I, Hayashizaki Y, Hirotsune S, Komatsubara H, Mukai T. A genomic scanning method for higher organisms using restriction sites as landmarks. Proc Natl Acad Sci. 1991;88(21):9523–7.
135. He S, Pham MH, Pease M, Zada G, Giannotta SL, Wang K, Mack WJ. A review of epigenetic and gene expression alterations associated with intracranial meningiomas. Neurosurg Focus. 2013;35(6):E5.
136. Vasudevan HN, Braunstein SE, Phillips JJ, Pekmezci M, Tomlin BA, Wu A, et al. Comprehensive molecular profiling identifies FOXM1 as a key transcription factor for meningioma proliferation. Cell Rep. 2018;22(13):3672–83.
137. Paramasivam N, Hübschmann D, Toprak UH, Ishaque N, Neidert M, Schrimpf D, et al. Mutational patterns and regulatory networks in epigenetic subgroups of meningioma. Acta Neuropathol. 2019;138(2):295–308.
138. Coussens LM, Fingleton B, Matrisian LM. Matrix metalloproteinase inhibitors and cancer—trials and tribulations. Science. 2002;295(5564):2387–92.
139. Qi JH, Ebrahem Q, Moore N, Murphy G, Claesson-Welsh L, Bond M, Baker A, Anand-Apte B. A novel function for tissue inhibitor of metalloproteinases-3 (TIMP3): inhibition of angiogenesis by blockage of VEGF binding to VEGF receptor-2. Nat Med. 2003;9(4):407.
140. Zhang Y, Xiong Y, Yarbrough WG. ARF promotes MDM2 degradation and stabilizes p53: ARF-INK4a locus deletion impairs both the Rb and p53 tumor suppression pathways. Cell. 1998;92(6):725–34.
141. Yin D, Xie D, Hofmann WK, Miller CW, Black KL, Koeffler HP. Methylation, expression, and mutation analysis of the cell cycle control genes in human brain tumors. Oncogene. 2002;21(54):8372.
142. Boström J, Meyer-Puttlitz B, Wolter M, Blaschke B, Weber RG, Lichter P, et al. Alterations of the tumor suppressor genes CDKN2A (p16INK4a), p14ARF, CDKN2B (p15INK4b), and CDKN2C (p18INK4c) in atypical and anaplastic meningiomas. Am J Pathol. 2001;159(2):661–9.

143. Deng Y, Yao L, Chau L, Ng SS, Peng Y, Liu X, Au WS, Wang J, Li F, Ji S, Han H. N-Myc downstream-regulated gene 2 (NDRG2) inhibits glioblastoma cell proliferation. Int J Cancer. 2003;106(3):342–7.
144. Lusis EA, Watson MA, Chicoine MR, Lyman M, Roerig P, Reifenberger G, Gutmann DH, Perry A. Integrative genomic analysis identifies NDRG2 as a candidate tumor suppressor gene frequently inactivated in clinically aggressive meningioma. Cancer Res. 2005;65(16):7121–6.
145. Skiriute D, Tamasauskas S, Asmoniene V, Saferis V, Skauminas K, Deltuva V, Tamasauskas A. Tumor grade-related NDRG2 gene expression in primary and recurrent intracranial meningiomas. J Neuro Oncol. 2011;102(1):89–94.
146. Hong C, Moorefield KS, Jun P, Aldape KD, Kharbanda S, Phillips HS, Costello JF. Epigenome scans and cancer genome sequencing converge on WNK2, a kinase-independent suppressor of cell growth. Proc Natl Acad Sci. 2007;104(26):10974–9.
147. Jun P, Hong C, Lal A, Wong JM, McDermott MW, Bollen AW, et al. Epigenetic silencing of the kinase tumor suppressor WNK2 is tumor-type and tumor-grade specific. Neuro-Oncology. 2009;11(4):414–22.
148. Bello MJ, Amiñoso C, Lopez-Marin I, Arjona D, Gonzalez-Gomez P, Alonso ME, et al. DNA methylation of multiple promoter-associated CpG islands in meningiomas: relationship with the allelic status at 1p and 22q. Acta Neuropathol. 2004;108(5):413–21.
149. Panetti TS, Chen H, Misenheimer TM, Getzler SB, Mosher DF. Endothelial cell mitogenesis induced by LPA: inhibition by thrombospondin-1 and thrombospondin-2. J Lab Clin Med. 1997;129(2):208–16.
150. Kishida Y, Natsume A, Kondo Y, Takeuchi I, An B, Okamoto Y, Shinjo K, Saito K, Ando H, Ohka F, Sekido Y. Epigenetic subclassification of meningiomas based on genome-wide DNA methylation analyses. Carcinogenesis. 2011;33(2):436–41.
151. Di Vinci A, Brigati C, Casciano I, Banelli B, Borzì L, Forlani A, Ravetti GL, Allemanni G, et al. HOXA7, 9, and 10 are methylation targets associated with aggressive behavior in meningiomas. Transl Res. 2012;160(5):355–62.
152. Soshnikova N, Duboule D. Epigenetic regulation of Hox gene activation: the waltz of meth-yls. BioEssays. 2008;30(3):199–202.
153. McTavish N, Copeland LA, Saville MK, Perkins ND, Spruce BA. Proenkephalin assists stress-activated apoptosis through transcriptional repression of NF-κB-and p53-regulated gene targets. Cell Death Differ. 2007;14(9):1700.
154. Huang X, Zhang H, Guo X, Zhu Z, Cai H, Kong X. Insulin-like growth factor 2 mRNA-binding protein 1 (IGF2BP1) in cancer. J Hematol Oncol. 2018;11(1):88.
155. Katz LM, Hielscher T, Liechty B, Silverman J, Zagzag D, Sen R, Wu P, Golfinos JG, et al. Loss of histone H3K27me3 identifies a subset of meningiomas with increased risk of recurrence. Acta Neuropathol. 2018;135(6):955–63.
156. Olar A, Goodman LD, Wani KM, Boehling NS, Sharma DS, Mody RR, Gumin J, et al. A gene expression signature predicts recurrence-free survival in meningioma. Oncotarget. 2018;9(22):16087.
157. Nassiri F, Mamatjan Y, Suppiah S, Badhiwala JH, Mansouri S, Karimi S, Saarela O, et al. DNA methylation profiling to predict recurrence risk in meningioma: development and validation of a nomogram to optimize clinical management. Neuro-Oncology. 2019;21(7):901–10.
158. Peyre M, Zanello M, Mokhtari K, Boch AL, Capelle L, Carpentier A, et al. Patterns of relapse and growth kinetics of surgery-and radiation-refractory meningiomas. J Neuro Oncol. 2015;123(1):151–60.
159. Joachim T, Ram Z, Rappaport ZH, Simon M, Schramm J, Wiestler OD, von Deimling A. Comparative analysis of the NF2, TP53, PTEN, KRAS, NRAS and HRAS genes in sporadic and radiation-induced human meningiomas. Int J Cancer. 2001;94(2):218–21.
160. Shoshan Y, Chernova O, Jeun SS, Somerville RP, Israel Z, Barnett GH, Cowell JK. Radiation-induced meningioma: a distinct molecular genetic pattern? J Neuropathol Exp Neurol. 2000;59(7):614–20.

Part II

Initial Meningioma Management and Treatment Paradigms

The Initial Evaluation and Surveillance of Meningiomas

5

Isabel P. Prado and Zachary A. Corbin

Abbreviations

CNS   Central nervous system
DNA   Deoxyribonucleic acid
PET   Positron Emission Tomography
RNA   Ribonucleic acid
WHO   World Health Organization

Epidemiology

Meningiomas are the most common adult primary intracranial tumor, constituting over one-third of all primary central nervous system (CNS) tumors and over half of all nonmalignant CNS tumors in the United States [1]. Among specific histologic categories, meningioma incidence is the highest of CNS tumors, at 8.33 per 100,000 [1]. A projected 31,500 new meningioma cases in 2018 and 31,990 in 2019 is expected to contribute to a growing prevalence [1].

Prognostic Factors

The World Health Organization (WHO) classifies CNS tumors into grades based on aggressiveness. Meningiomas are divided into three grades: grade I, also called "benign," grade II or "atypical," and grade III or "anaplastic" [2]. Meningiomas present more frequently in women (60–70%), regardless of histopathological

I. P. Prado · Z. A. Corbin (✉)
Department of Neurology, Yale University, New Haven, CT, USA
e-mail: zachary.corbin@yale.edu

© Springer Nature Switzerland AG 2020
J. Moliterno, A. Omuro (eds.), *Meningiomas*,
https://doi.org/10.1007/978-3-030-59558-6_5

classification [3–5]. The age-adjusted incidence rates for males and females, respectively, are as follows: 3.68 per 100,000 and 8.56 per 100,000 for grade I, 0.26 per 100,000 and 0.30 per 100,000 for grade II, and 0.08 per 100,000 and 0.09 per 100,000 for grade III [6]. Meningioma incidence rises with age, with an incidence between 28.0 and 45.0 per 100,000 in adults over 65 [1]. These rates underestimate the true incidence and prevalence, for a large subset of meningioma patients have presumed diagnoses without pathological confirmation.

As suggested by the higher incidence among women, sex hormones may impact meningioma risk. Studies have examined the relationship between use of exogenous hormones, through oral contraceptives or hormone replacement therapy, and risk. The strongest association indicates hormone replacement therapy is a potential risk factor for meningioma, when adjusted for age [7, 8]. Other risk factors include environmental exposures and genetic syndromes. Ionizing radiation, often used for cancer treatment, has been linked to the development of meningiomas [9, 10]. Childhood cancer survivors who have been exposed to cranial radiation therapy therefore have an increased meningioma risk. Radiation-associated meningiomas, as compared to sporadic meningiomas, are more commonly high grade and multifocal [11]. The actuarial risks of developing a meningioma, 0.53% 5 years after cranial irradiation and 8.18% at 25 years, have since decreased with the modernization of radiotherapy [12]. Additionally, patients of the female sex, with earlier cancer diagnoses, or treated with higher radiation doses, are at particularly high risk for meningioma and subsequent neurologic morbidities, including seizures, sensory deficits, focal neurologic dysfunction, and severe headaches [13].

Perhaps the most extensively studied risk factors are those of genetic mutations. The association between meningiomas and the *NF2* gene may be causative in nature, as suggested by genetic syndrome studies. Mutations in the *NF2* tumor suppressor gene cause neurofibromatosis type 2, a familial tumor predisposition syndrome. A range of 50% to 76% of these patients develop at least one meningioma [2]. A range of 30% to 70% of sporadic meningiomas exhibit an inactive *NF2* gene [9]. Furthermore, the increasing rate of mutations among higher-grade meningiomas, 50–60% of grade I and up to 75% of grades II and III, suggests a correlation between *NF2* mutations and tumor progression [2, 14].

Patients with other genetic syndromes, including neurofibromatosis type 1, nevoid basal cell carcinoma, Li-Fraumeni syndrome, von Hippel-Lindau syndrome, and Cowden disease, have also been diagnosed with meningiomas, although the strength of these relationships is not thoroughly studied [9]. The most well-reported genetic mutation unassociated with a familial syndrome is that of the *TERT* promoter. This mutation has prognostic value for risk stratification because of its indication of both rapid recurrence and more aggressive tumor growth, regardless of WHO grade [11, 15]. Mutations in *SMO* and *AKT1* also correlate with an increased risk of recurrence, suggesting the need for tighter surveillance for these high-risk patients [16]. Epigenetic mechanisms that may describe meningioma pathogenesis include aberrant DNA methylation of homeobox genes and decreased levels of microRNAs, which are important for regulating posttranslational silencing and may contribute to higher risks of meningioma recurrence [17].

The role of genetics in the risk of recurrent meningioma continues to be considered for its prognostic importance. According to a study measuring several independent variables, mutations in chromosome 14, in addition to patient age and WHO grade, provided the best prognostic stratification to predict recurrence [18]. Ultimately, the histopathological characterization, as illustrated by WHO grade, remains the primary risk stratification tool for meningioma recurrence.

Pathogenesis

The cells of origin for meningiomas are proposed to be arachnoid cap or meningothelial cells [2]. These solitary tumors may be round or sheetlike and are typically well-demarcated. While most are intracranial and extra-axial, with broad dural attachments, meningiomas may also originate in the spinal cord. They range drastically in size, but the larger meningiomas often inwardly shift the underlying brain structures [9, 12]. The greatest predictor of tumor behavior is grade, as determined through certain histopathological characteristics.

Grading

The most recent update of the definitions for meningiomas was included in the WHO Classification of Tumors of the CNS, published in 2016 [19]. Meningioma grades are based on histopathological characteristics, including mitotic rate, cellular features of atypia, and local invasion, and define 81% of meningiomas as grade I; 18% as grade II, also called atypical; and 2% as grade III, also called anaplastic (Fig. 5.1) [1, 2]. Despite the small percentage of anaplastic meningiomas, nearly 300 patients receive a new diagnosis of this type of tumor every year [12]. Of note, intraoperative frozen section analysis of meningioma has many limitations [3]. WHO grade continues to be primarily determined from histopathological characteristics of tissue specimens.

Clinical Evaluation

Asymptomatic or incidentally discovered meningiomas comprise nearly 40% of all newly diagnosed meningiomas, as reported by international studies [20, 21]. The majority of tumors, however, trigger symptoms associated with their size and location. The most common single symptom is headache, resulting from increased intracranial pressure due to either space-occupying tumors or vasogenic cerebral edema [3, 9]. Seizures and focal neurological deficits are also prevalent among newly diagnosed meningioma patients. Other presenting symptoms tend to vary with location: hemispheric lesions may cause partial weakness or sensory loss, while skull base tumors can induce cranial nerve dysfunction, including vision loss [9].

Fig. 5.1 Proportion of meningiomas by WHO grade. (Data from the Central Brain Tumor Registry of the United States (CBTRUS) for meningioma with documented WHO grade. Data from Ostrom et al. [1])

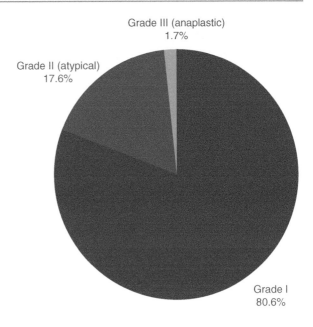

Imaging Studies

Brain imaging is one of the initial diagnostic screens for patients who present with neurological symptoms. In fact, the expanded use of diagnostic intracranial imaging has contributed to the high prevalence of asymptomatic, incidentally discovered meningiomas [9]. These imaging studies offer a noninvasive approach to characterize potential tumors and the associated structural or functional changes.

Magnetic resonance imaging (MRI) represents the optimal and likely most widely used imaging technique for newly diagnosed meningiomas. These tumors present radiographically as well-demarcated, globular, extra-axial masses, often connected to the dura mater [9, 11]. As compared to the cortex of normal brain, meningiomas are isointense-to-hypointense on T1 sequences and isointense-to-hyperintense on T2 sequences [9]. Tumors that are T2 hypointense are associated with harder consistency during surgery, a factor that can also be evaluated using a more advanced MRI technique known as diffusion tensor imaging (DTI) [9]. Most meningiomas do not display restricted diffusion, necrosis, or hemorrhage [9].

Meningiomas typically display strong, homogenous enhancement with gadolinium contrast. Blood vessels may display a "sunburst" appearance around the tumor due to vasculature leakage [9]. The dural tail, describing the broad dural attachment that is visible with contrast in T1-weighted images, most accurately represents reactive dural thickening rather than extension from the tumor [9]. Other MRI features include (1) more dural infiltration in cases of en plaque meningiomas; (2) associated cysts, present in 4% of intracranial meningiomas; and (3) a CSF-vascular cleft between tumor and normal cortex that may be absent in high-grade meningiomas invading the brain [9]. While no specific radiological criteria differentiate between grades I and II, grade III meningiomas are typically irregularly shaped and display diffuse growth, a higher relative cerebral blood volume, osteolysis, and invasion of the cortex [9, 11]. Cortical invasion is best characterized by the loss of a distinct border between tumor and cortex, particularly if the interface is also irregular [9, 11].

Meningiomas usually do not display significant vasogenic edema, except those of higher grades and certain subtypes [3, 9]. Although the aggressive meningiomas likely cause peritumoral edema by invading the brain, even grade I lesion scans may demonstrate edema without evidence of brain invasion. Peritumoral edema is observed in about 60% of meningiomas, regardless of tumor size [9]. Peritumoral edema has been correlated with angiogenesis and irregular tumor margins, factors that suggest a more aggressive phenotype [2]. Other imaging modalities, including apparent diffusion coefficient MRI sequences, have been incorporated to predict progression or recurrence in meningioma patients [2].

Another valuable imaging tool for diagnosing and describing meningiomas is the computed tomography (CT) scan, which is most useful for detecting calcification or skull bone changes. Meningioma calcification is present in nearly 20% of cases, similar to the prevalence of hyperostosis and osteolysis [9, 11]. Hyperostosis varies in presentation, regardless of tumor size, and does not predict tumor grade. However, hyperostosis is often associated with intraosseous tumor growth, especially among skull-based meningiomas [11]. While some suggest that hyperostosis is simply a reactive phenomenon, the strong, homogenous contrast enhancement within hyperostotic bone supports tumor infiltration as the biological rationale [9].

Various other imaging techniques reveal potentially important characteristics. Meningioma of grades II and III may be predicted using DTI measures, such as fractional anisotropy and mean diffusivity [9]. Magnetic resonance spectroscopy reveals changes in protein levels; for example, elevated lactate is associated with more aggressive behavior, regardless of histopathological characterization [9]. Lastly, gadolinium bolus magnetic resonance venography or catheter angiography can be used to image the invasion or obstruction of venous structures by meningiomas [9].

Although imaging studies can provide a great deal of information about the structure and behavior of meningiomas, the results are often not specific, as illustrated by the pervasiveness of the dural tail finding among other dural neoplasms [9]. This lack of specificity is a core factor for the continued reliance on histopathology as the gold standard for diagnosis.

Differential Diagnosis

Any diagnostic evaluation requires consideration of a differential diagnosis, usually driven by the imaging studies and clinical presentation. When tumor location and radiographic signature suggest meningioma, it remains crucial to consider other possibilities.

Perhaps the most probable alternative diagnosis is that of dural metastases. Those from primary tumors in the breast, lung, or prostate are nearly indistinguishable radiographically from meningiomas. Other diagnoses are either rare or different enough from meningiomas to not be typically considered. Granulomatous disease, such as sarcoidosis or tuberculosis, can evolve dural-based enhancing lesions. These etiologies generally produce multiple lesions, which is an uncommon presentation of meningioma. Immunoglobulin G4-related disease may present with pseudotumors causing dural thickening, mimicking meningiomas [9]. Dural hemangiomas are uncommon but can resemble meningiomas, though they are often T2 hyperintense radiographically [9]. Hemangiopericytomas are meningeal-based tumors that can appear quite similar, yet they do not calcify or cause hyperostosis [9].

Other diagnoses on the differential include conditions that resemble meningiomas of a specific location or grade. Focal idiopathic hypertrophic pachymeningitis, while rare, can cause enhancing lesions near the skull base, similar to skull base meningiomas. Dural lymphoma and granulocytic sarcoma may evolve enhancing dural masses, mimicking en plaque meningioma or meningiomatosis [9]. Lastly, osteogenic sarcoma and Ewing sarcoma can present similar to a high-grade, malignant meningioma [9].

The combination of clinical presentation and imaging studies can often aid in considering the differential diagnosis. The meningioma signature is an intradural, extra-axial mass with a long clinical history in a middle-aged, most likely female, patient. However, as above, many additional diagnoses should be considered [3]. Frequently, additional clinical management is determined by a definitive diagnosis.

Histopathology

The diagnosis of meningioma and the WHO grade are determined by histopathology, where cellular characteristics provide evidence of the behavior of the tumor. Histopathological analysis follows tissue sampling with surgical biopsy or resection.

Grade I meningiomas typically display a low mitotic rate, defined as less than 4 mitoses per 10 high-power fields (HPF) and an absence of brain invasion [11]. These tumors are often labeled "benign," and they are slow-growing, and nine morphologic subtypes exist: meningothelial, fibrous, transitional, psammomatous, angiomatous, microcystic, secretory, lymphoplasmacyte-rich, and metaplastic [15]. The histopathological distinction for grade II, or atypical, meningiomas is characterized by either increased mitotic activity relative to grade I, as defined by 4–19 mitoses per 10 HPF, evidence of brain invasion, or presence of at least three of the following features: hypercellularity, prominent nucleoli, small cells with high nuclear-to-cytoplasmic ratio, spontaneous necrosis without prior embolization, and uninterrupted, patternless growth or "sheeting" [9, 11, 15, 22]. Chordoid and clear cell meningiomas are also considered grade II due to their high rates of recurrence [15].

The most aggressive meningiomas are grade III, or anaplastic, tumors, defined as such by either elevated mitotic rates of over 20 mitoses per 10 HPF or clearly malignant cytological anaplasia, resembling that of carcinoma, melanoma, or high-grade sarcoma [9, 15]. Meningiomas are also considered grade III, if over half of the sample displays a papillary or rhabdoid variant, because such tumors are associated with poorer prognoses, multiple recurrences, and distant metastases [9, 11, 15]. As evident through definitions of grade, the mitotic index is a significant predictor for tumor aggression [15, 23, 24].

A significant association also exists between recurrence and histopathological classification, as shown by a 41.6% recurrence rate among grade II and 75% recurrence rate in grade III meningiomas [25]. Furthermore, the cellular marker Ki-67 proliferative index provides additional evidence of tumor aggression; an index above 3% is associated with meningioma progression and recurrence [15]. Overall, histopathological features and the final diagnosis is core component to determining the additional clinical management of many patients with meningiomas.

Surveillance and Treatment

The overall goal of surveillance and treatment of meningiomas is to effectively reduce morbidity and prolong survival. As meningioma grade predicts recurrence risk and overall prognosis, treatment and surveillance recommendations vary significantly based on the presumed or confirmed grade and clinical setting. Asymptomatic meningiomas thought to be grade I and with little or no radiographic mass effect may be observed, without resection or radiation therapy. Patients with meningiomas that produce mass effect and clinical symptoms, or have demonstrated rapid growth, should generally be offered surgery with or without radiation, followed by observation [11]. The National Comprehensive Cancer Network (NCCN) provides guidelines on the diagnostic algorithm, treatment options, and recommended surveillance [26]. Detailed surveillance and treatment recommendations, stratified by presumed diagnosis and known meningioma grade, are outlined below.

Presumed

Small, asymptomatic meningiomas are frequently diagnosed radiographically on scans obtained for other indications, and these tumors are often referred to as incidental. A radiographic diagnosis of meningioma requires the following features: (1) a dural-based mass, (2) homogenous enhancement, (3) a dural tail, and (4) a CSF cleft [26]. If the mass is noted an MRI without any prior imaging available, we generally obtain a repeat MRI brain with contrast in short order, within 1–3 months. Stable lesions should have repeat brain MRIs at 3, 6, and 12 months and then repeat imaging for 6–12 months for at least 5 years [26]. Repeat imaging intervals can be spread thereafter to up to every 3 years and even halted, as indicated, though we generally recommend annual surveillance indefinitely [26]. Follow-up imaging may be omitted entirely in cases of short life expectancy, so long as the radiological diagnosis was clear [11].

If the lesion is symptomatic, supportive care should be initiated. Patients with seizures should be treated with antiepileptic drug therapy, and corticosteroids should be considered for those with peritumoral edema [9]. In all patients with symptoms, treatment options should be considered, including surgery or empiric radiation treatment [2]. If surgical challenges exist, such as tumor location, patient age, or comorbidities, radiation may be considered as a first-line therapy [2, 12].

Grade I

The goal of surgery for all meningiomas is gross total resection. One classification system to describe the extent of meningioma resection was proposed in 1957 by Australian neurosurgeon Donald Simpson [27]. The Simpson classification stratifies the extent of resection into five grades. Simpson grade I is complete tumor removal, including the dural attachment and any abnormal bone. Simpson grade II is complete tumor removal and coagulation of the dural attachment. Simpson grade III is complete intradural tumor removal, without resection or coagulation of the dural attachment or extradural extensions. Simpson grade IV is partial tumor removal, and Simpson grade V is a simple decompression, with or without biopsy. Simpson grades I–III are classified as a gross total resection [12]. Preoperative planning may include MRI and neurovascular imaging, and tumor embolization prior to surgery may be considered in select cases [9].

Grade I meningiomas status post gross total resection should have a repeat MRI within 48 h of the operation or at 3 months post-surgery [2, 11]. Tumors should be imaged at least 3 months after surgery to allow time for treatment-related radiographic characteristics to resolve [9]. Proposed observation thereafter should include repeat brain MRIs at 3, 6, and 12 months and then repeat imaging for 6–12 months for at least 5 years. Tumors status post subtotal resection should be imaged postoperatively again either within 48 h or at 3 months after surgery. Adjuvant radiation should be considered, especially if the remaining lesion is symptomatic or located in a critical area [11, 26]. Otherwise, observation intervals as described above should be observed.

Grade II

Grade II meningiomas should undergo maximum possible resection, with postoperative imaging as above. For patients' status post gross total resection, adjuvant radiation should be considered [26]. Our practice has been to offer patients enrollment in a clinical trial or to recommend proceeding with radiation. Some controversy surrounds adjuvant radiation treatment for grade II meningiomas [9, 12]. We note that studies have shown improved survival outcomes and reduced recurrence rates with adjuvant radiation, regardless of the extent of resection [12, 28–31]. The timing of radiation is also important, with evidence favoring a short interval, as seen by better survival outcomes using postoperative SRS – within 6 months of surgery – as compared to SRS at recurrence or progression [12]. For grade II meningiomas status post subtotal resection, radiation is recommended [11, 26, 32, 33]. Subsequent surveillance should be as frequent as for grade I meningiomas, or more frequent, as clinically indicated. Serial re-resection is advised for tumor recurrence, with additional consideration for additional radiation treatment at each juncture [26].

Grade III

Following maximum possible resection, patients with grade III meningiomas should undergo adjuvant radiation [2, 12, 26]. Subsequent repeat imaging should be tailored to the patient, though an interval of every 3–6 months is the maximum suggested [11]. Retrospective data on patients with grade III meningiomas have demonstrated improved survival following adjuvant radiation [2]. While no systemic therapies have been proven, experimental agents continue to be explored [9, 11]. However, pharmacotherapies, including bevacizumab and somatostatin analogues, should only be considered when surgical and radiation treatment options have been exhausted [11, 26].

Survival

The prognosis for meningioma patients is largely driven by a variety of factors, including patient age, tumor location and grade, molecular and biological characteristics, and postoperative treatment. For example, patients over 60 or with parasellar or suprasellar tumors have worse outcomes, whereas those with more extensive resections and adjuvant radiation do better (9). Overall survival (OS) as a metric is strongly dependent upon the WHO grade classification. Progression-free survival (PFS) or recurrence-free survival (RFS) measure morbidity and predict mortality. RFS is shorter with smaller extent of resection, skull base location, male gender, lack of calcification, and reduced 1p and VEGF expression [2].

Grade I meningiomas have the best survival outcomes, as compared to those of higher grades. A meta-analysis of asymptomatic, untreated meningiomas smaller than 2.5 cm in diameter revealed no tumor growth for a period of 5 years after radiological diagnosis [9]. Grade I meningiomas have a reported mean OS of over 10 years and a 10-year PFS of 97.5% [9]. Tumors status post gross total resection have a 60–80% 10-year PFS, while tumors having undergone subtotal resection have a 10-year PFS of 50% [2]. Nearly 20% of grade I meningiomas recur, although the recurrence rates differ by extent of surgical resection and time frame [15]. After gross total resection, the grade I meningioma recurrence rate is 7–23% after 5 years, 20–39% after 10 years, and 24–60% after 15 years [9]. Tumors that have undergone subtotal resection have 5-year and 10-year recurrence rates of 40–50% and 55–100%, respectively [2, 11]. Grade I meningioma patients with recurrent tumors, regardless of extent of resection, and grade II meningioma patients having undergone a complete resection experience a 3-year PFS rate of 96% following radiation [2]. Patients who have recurred have 5-year PFS rates of 30% after surgery and 88% after surgery and adjuvant radiation and 8-year PFS rates of 11% after surgery and 78% after surgery and adjuvant radiation [9].

Patient outcome for grade II meningiomas is largely influenced by the extent of resection and subsequent treatment. The 5-year OS for grade II meningiomas is between 80 and 100%, but PFS varies by Simpson grade of surgical resection [34]. Patients receiving a grade I–III resection, or a gross total resection, have a PFS between 48 and 96 months, while those with grade IV resections have PFS between 47 and 59 months [9]. Patients with adjuvant radiation after subtotal resections have estimated 5-year PFS rates of 40–90%. The 10-year PFS rates for grade II meningiomas are 87% for those patients that underwent gross total resections and 17% for those with subtotal resections [2]. The 5-year recurrence rate is up to 30% for patients with gross total resections and 40% for patients with subtotal resections [11]. While some studies suggest that only 35% of grade II meningioma patients remain disease-free after 10 years, others report that 70% are disease-free at 10 years after combination treatment [9]. The Central Brain Tumor Registry of the United States (CBTRUS) categorizes survival by nonmalignant and malignant meningiomas, rather than by WHO grade. The 2018 CBTRUS revealed favorable 10-year survival estimates for nonmalignant meningiomas by age group (Fig. 5.2) [1].

Patients with grade III meningiomas unfortunately have worse outcomes. Median OS of patients with grade III meningiomas is 2–3 years and sometimes over 5 years, with a 5-year OS of 60% and 10-year relative survival of 53.5% [1].

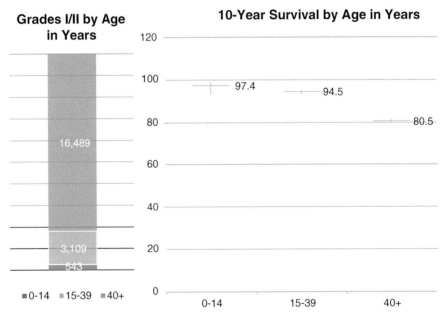

Fig. 5.2 WHO grades I/II meningioma survival by age in years. The Central Brain Tumor Registry of the United States (CBTRUS) dichotomizes survival for meningiomas of WHO grades I/II and grade III. For grade I/II meningiomas, 543 cases were aged 0–14, 3109 were aged 15–39, and 16,489 were aged 40 or older. The 10-year survival estimates were more favorable than those for grade III meningiomas. Ten-year survival estimates worsened with age and were 97.4%, 94.5%, and 80.5%, respectively. (Data from Ostrom et al. [1])

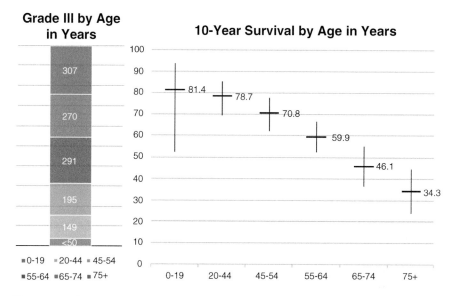

Fig. 5.3 WHO grade III meningioma survival by age in years. The Central Brain Tumor Registry of the United States (CBTRUS) dichotomizes survival for meningiomas of WHO grades I/II and grade III. For grade III meningiomas, fewer than 50 cases were in the ages 0–19, 149 were aged 20–44, 195 were aged 45–54, 291 were aged 55–64, 270 were aged 65–74, and 307 cases were aged 75 or older. Ten-year survival estimates worsened with age and were 81.4%, 78.7%, 70.8%, 59.9%, 46.1%, and 34.3%, respectively. (Data from Ostrom et al. [1])

Ten-year survival estimates decrease with age, reaching a 34% to 46% 10-year survival rate for patients over 65 (Fig. 5.3) [1]. The 5-year PFS rate for grade III meningiomas status post gross total resection is 28% [2, 9]. This outcome is improved when patients receive adjuvant radiation, with studies reporting 5-year PFS rates of 12–57%, 27–40%, and even up to 80% [9, 11]. Unfortunately, patients with grade III meningiomas that have only undergone subtotal resections experience a 5-year PFS rate of 0% [2]. Even grade III meningioma patients that have received gross total resections, including some with adjuvant treatments, have a 5-year recurrence rate of 78% [12]. The mean time to recurrence is an estimated 39 months for grade III meningiomas, as compared to a mean time to recurrence of 60.5 months for their counterparts of lower grades [35].

Future Avenues

Although the survival outcomes for grade I meningioma patients are favorable, the lack of congruence among treatment regimens for higher-grade meningiomas contributes to short PFS and high recurrence rates. Novel approaches to diagnostic imaging, tumor genetics, and pharmacotherapy have expanded our understanding of meningioma behavior, with promising results for improved management.

Hormonal expression in meningiomas has been studied as a means for radiographic differentiation. Using peptide ligands, like Gallium-68-DOTATATE, as positron emission tomography (PET) tracers, the expression of somatostatin receptor 2 in the tumor can be radiologically discriminated from healthy tissue [11]. Fast-growing tumors with transosseous expansion bind more strongly to Gallium, suggesting a potential avenue for radionuclide-based therapy [2, 36]. While this imaging tool has shown benefits in the diagnosis and grading of meningiomas, recent advances in understanding other prognostic factors have informed our predictions of tumor recurrence, the key marker for survival.

Genetic alterations exist in nearly 80% of meningiomas, and specific mutations are present among tumors of a particular location or subtype. Genomic instability is a significant factor in associated with tumor grade; for example, chromosome 1p and 14q loss affect half of grade II meningiomas and nearly all grade III meningiomas [2]. Other genetic clues include increased telomerase activation and microRNA dysregulation in higher-grade meningiomas [2]. Co-methylation of homeobox genes and aberrant hypermethylation have been implicated in tumorigenesis and associated with grade II and III meningiomas [2]. These methylation patterns, regardless of WHO grade, retain high sensitivity and specificity to predict tumor recurrence [2]. While skull base lesions show SMO or PIK3CA mutations, AKT1 is often found among meningothelial and transitional subtypes, and KLF4 and TRAF7 mutations are present in secretory meningiomas [11, 15].

The association between meningiomas and the NF2 gene on chromosome 22 is well-described in the literature [2]. NF2-mutated tumors often have a specific localization and comprise over half of sporadic cases [3, 15]. The majority of young patients with sporadic meningioma have causative genetic predispositions, 40% of which are NF2 mutations [37]. The most common cytogenetic abnormality, however, is the loss of chromosome 22, found in 60–80% of meningioma cases [3, 38].

Consideration of four classes of systemic therapies is currently recommended: alpha interferon, somatostatin receptor agonists, VEGF inhibitors, and everolimus [26]. Bevacizumab, an antiangiogenic VEGF inhibitor, has shown improved PFS rates in meningioma patients with recurrent or progressive disease [2, 39]. With Gallium-68-DOTATATE PET imaging as a predictive marker for optimal meningioma targets, somatostatin receptor-targeted radionuclide therapy has had some favorable impact in a subset of these tumors [40]. Octreotide and everolimus have been used in recurrent meningiomas of all grades, resulting in acceptable toxicity and a nearly 60% 6-month PFS [2]. The high prevalence of progesterone receptor expression in meningiomas has also prompted studies using endocrine manipulations [38, 41–43].

Optune, a device that administers tumor-treating electromagnetic fields, is being studied, with or without bevacizumab, in recurrent grade II and III meningiomas [2]. Trabectedin, a DNA-binding alkylating agent, has demonstrated benefit in recurrent, high-grade meningiomas [2, 11]. Preclinical studies have considered pegvisomant, valproic acid, bortezomib, and aminolevulinic acid as potential pharmacotherapies [2]. Overall, however, drugs with antiangiogenic properties have produced the most encouraging outcomes [11].

Modifications in radiation therapy have also been considered. A study of hypofractionated stereotactic radiotherapy, in comparison to other radiotherapy approaches, has reported comparable toxicity and local control rates [44]. The confirmation of these preliminary results through controlled, prospective trials is necessary to advance treatment options and improve the clinical management of meningiomas.

References

1. Ostrom QT, Gittleman H, Truitt G, Boscia A, Kruchko C, Barnholtz-Sloan JS. CBTRUS statistical report: primary brain and other central nervous system tumors diagnosed in the United States in 2011–2015. Neuro Oncol. 2018;20(suppl_4):iv1–86.
2. Shaikh N, Dixit K, Raizer J. Recent advances in managing/understanding meningioma. F1000Res. 2018;7:490.
3. Lacruz CR, Saenz de Santamaria J, Bardales RH. Central nervous system intraoperative cytopathology. Essentials in cytopathology series. New York: Springer Nature; 2018.
4. Wiemels J, Wrensch M, Claus EB. Epidemiology and etiology of meningioma. J Neuro-Oncol. 2010;99(3):307–14.
5. Sun T, Plutynski A, Ward S, Rubin JB. An integrative view on sex differences in brain tumors. Cell Mol Life Sci. 2015;72(17):3323–42.
6. Kshettry VR, Ostrom QT, Kruchko C, Al-Mefty O, Barnett GH, Barnholtz-Sloan JS. Descriptive epidemiology of World Health Organization grades II and III intracranial meningiomas in the United States. Neuro-Oncology. 2015;17(8):1166–73.
7. Blitshteyn S, Crook JE, Jaeckle KA. Is there an association between meningioma and hormone replacement therapy? J Clin Oncol. 2008;26(2):279–82.
8. Fan ZX, Shen J, Wu YY, Yu H, Zhu Y, Zhan RY. Hormone replacement therapy and risk of meningioma in women: a meta-analysis. Cancer Causes Control. 2013;24(8):1517–25.
9. Fogh SE, Johnson DR, Barker FG II, Brastianos PK, Clarke JL, Kaufmann TJ, et al. Case-based review: meningioma. NeuroOncol Practice. 2016;3(2):120–34.
10. Baldi I, Engelhardt J, Bonnet C, Bauchet L, Berteaud E, Gruber A, et al. Epidemiology of meningiomas. Neurochirurgie. 2018;64(1):5–14.
11. Goldbrunner R, Minniti G, Preusser M, Jenkinson MD, Sallabanda K, Houdart E, et al. EANO guidelines for the diagnosis and treatment of meningiomas. Lancet Oncol. 2016;17(9):e383–91.
12. Rogers L, Barani I, Chamberlain M, Kaley TJ, McDermott M, Raizer J, et al. Meningiomas: knowledge base, treatment outcomes, and uncertainties. A RANO review. J Neurosurg. 2015;122(1):4–23.
13. Bowers DC, Moskowitz CS, Chou JF, Mazewski CM, Neglia JP, Armstrong GT, et al. Morbidity and mortality associated with meningioma after cranial radiotherapy: a report from the childhood cancer survivor study. J Clin Oncol. 2017;35(14):1570–6.
14. Peyre M, Stemmer-Rachamimov A, Clermont-Taranchon E, Quentin S, El-Taraya N, Walczak C, et al. Meningioma progression in mice triggered by Nf2 and Cdkn2ab inactivation. Oncogene. 2013;32(36):4264–72.
15. Harter PN, Braun Y, Plate KH. Classification of meningiomas-advances and controversies. Chin Clin Oncol. 2017;6(Suppl 1):S2.
16. Preusser M, Brastianos PK, Mawrin C. Advances in meningioma genetics: novel therapeutic opportunities. Nat Rev Neurol. 2018;14(2):106–15.
17. Hortobagyi T, Bencze J, Varkoly G, Kouhsari MC, Klekner A. Meningioma recurrence. Open Med (Wars). 2016;11(1):168–73.
18. Maillo A, Orfao A, Sayagues JM, Diaz P, Gomez-Moreta JA, Caballero M, et al. New classification scheme for the prognostic stratification of meningioma on the basis of chromosome 14 abnormalities, patient age, and tumor histopathology. J Clin Oncol. 2003;21(17):3285–95.

19. Louis DN, Perry A, Reifenberger G, von Deimling A, Figarella-Branger D, Cavenee WK, et al. The 2016 World Health Organization classification of tumors of the central nervous system: a summary. Acta Neuropathol. 2016;131(6):803–20.
20. Yano S, Kuratsu J. Kumamoto brain tumor research G. indications for surgery in patients with asymptomatic meningiomas based on an extensive experience. J Neurosurg. 2006;105(4):538–43.
21. Islim AI, Mohan M, Moon R, Kolamunnage-Dona R, Rathi N, Mills SJ, et al. A risk calculator to predict the need for an intervention within a patient's estimated lifetime for incidentally-found asymptomatic meningiomas. Neuro Oncol. 2018;20(Suppl_3, 1):iii222. https://doi.org/10.1093/neuonc/noy139.026.
22. Perry A, Scheithauer BW, Stafford SL, Lohse CM, Wollan PC. "Malignancy" in meningiomas: a clinicopathologic study of 116 patients, with grading implications. Cancer. 1999;85(9):2046–56.
23. Stafford SL, Perry A, Suman VJ, Meyer FB, Scheithauer BW, Lohse CM, et al. Primarily resected meningiomas: outcome and prognostic factors in 581 Mayo Clinic patients, 1978 through 1988. Mayo Clin Proc. 1998;73(10):936–42.
24. Pasquier D, Bijmolt S, Veninga T, Rezvoy N, Villa S, Krengli M, et al. Atypical and malignant meningioma: outcome and prognostic factors in 119 irradiated patients. A multicenter, retrospective study of the Rare Cancer Network. Int J Radiat Oncol Biol Phys. 2008;71(5):1388–93.
25. Violaris K, Katsarides V, Karakyriou M, Sakellariou P. Surgical outcome of treating grades II and III meningiomas: a report of 32 cases. Neurosci J. 2013;2013:706481.
26. NCCN Clinical Practice Guidelines in Oncology. Central nervous system cancers, Version 3.2019, (2019).
27. Simpson D. The recurrence of intracranial meningiomas after surgical treatment. J Neurol Neurosurg Psychiatry. 1957;20(1):22–39.
28. Walcott BP, Nahed BV, Brastianos PK, Loeffler JS. Radiation treatment for WHO grade II and III meningiomas. Front Oncol. 2013;3:227.
29. Yang SY, Park CK, Park SH, Kim DG, Chung YS, Jung HW. Atypical and anaplastic meningiomas: prognostic implications of clinicopathological features. J Neurol Neurosurg Psychiatry. 2008;79(5):574–80.
30. Aghi MK, Carter BS, Cosgrove GR, Ojemann RG, Amin-Hanjani S, Martuza RL, et al. Long-term recurrence rates of atypical meningiomas after gross total resection with or without post-operative adjuvant radiation. Neurosurgery. 2009;64(1):56–60.
31. Coke CC, Corn BW, Werner-Wasik M, Xie Y, Curran WJ Jr. Atypical and malignant meningiomas: an outcome report of seventeen cases. J Neuro-Oncol. 1998;39(1):65–70.
32. Hwang KL, Hwang WL, Bussiere MR, Shih HA. The role of radiotherapy in the management of high-grade meningiomas. Chin Clin Oncol. 2017;6(Suppl 1):S5.
33. Achey RL, Gittleman H, Schroer J, Khanna V, Kruchko C, Barnholtz-Sloan JS. Nonmalignant and malignant meningioma incidence and survival in the elderly, 2005-2015, using the Central Brain Tumor Registry of the United States. Neuro-Oncology. 2019;21(3):380–91.
34. Palma L, Celli P, Franco C, Cervoni L, Cantore G. Long-term prognosis for atypical and malignant meningiomas: a study of 71 surgical cases. J Neurosurg. 1997;86(5):793–800.
35. Ildan F, Erman T, Gocer AI, Tuna M, Bagdatoglu H, Cetinalp E, et al. Predicting the probability of meningioma recurrence in the preoperative and early postoperative period: a multivariate analysis in the midterm follow-up. Skull Base. 2007;17(3):157–71.
36. Sommerauer M, Burkhardt JK, Frontzek K, Rushing E, Buck A, Krayenbuehl N, et al. 68Gallium-DOTATATE PET in meningioma: a reliable predictor of tumor growth rate? Neuro-Oncology. 2016;18(7):1021–7.
37. Pathmanaban ON, Sadler KV, Kamaly-Asl ID, King AT, Rutherford SA, Hammerbeck-Ward C, et al. Association of genetic predisposition with solitary schwannoma or meningioma in children and young adults. JAMA Neurol. 2017;74(9):1123–9.
38. Prados MD, Berger MS, Wilson CB. Primary central nervous system tumors: advances in knowledge and treatment. CA Cancer J Clin. 1998;48(6):331–60, 21.

39. Franke AJ, Skelton Iv WP, Woody LE, Bregy A, Shah AH, Vakharia K, et al. Role of bevaci-zumab for treatment-refractory meningiomas: a systematic analysis and literature review. Surg Neurol Int. 2018;9:133.

40. Seystahl K, Stoecklein V, Schuller U, Rushing E, Nicolas G, Schafer N, et al. Somatostatin receptor-targeted radionuclide therapy for progressive meningioma: benefit linked to 68Ga-DOTATATE/-TOC uptake. Neuro-Oncology. 2016;18(11):1538–47.

41. Ji Y, Rankin C, Grunberg S, Sherrod AE, Ahmadi J, Townsend JJ, et al. Double-blind phase III randomized trial of the antiprogestin agent mifepristone in the treatment of unresectable meningioma: SWOG S9005. J Clin Oncol. 2015;33(34):4093–8.

42. Chamberlain M. What lessons are imparted from SWOG S9005 for recurrent meningioma? J Clin Oncol. 2016;34(15):1825.

43. Kruser TJ. Systemic therapy in Unresectable meningioma before radiotherapy. J Clin Oncol. 2016;34(15):1826–7.

44. Nguyen EK, Nguyen TK, Boldt G, Louie AV, Bauman GS. Hypofractionated stereotactic radio-therapy for intracranial meningioma: a systemic review. Neurooncol Pract. 2019;6(5):346–53. https://doi.org/10.1093/nop/npy053.

Surgical Considerations for Newly Diagnosed Meningiomas

6

Christopher S. Hong and Jennifer Moliterno

Introduction

Meningiomas are the most common primary intracranial tumors, comprising nearly one-third of all brain tumors with a peak incidence at 45 years of age and predilection toward females [1]. Located extradurally and thought to arise from various layers of the meninges, the vast majority of meningiomas are typically slow-growing (i.e., WHO grade I). However, a smaller subset are higher grade (i.e., WHO grades II and III), and similar to glial tumors, can arise either de novo or progress from lower-grade meningiomas, and in both cases exhibiting faster growth rates with increased recurrence rates despite treatment [2]. To date, surgery remains the mainstay treatment for all types of meningiomas, and as such, optimal surgical management of the patient with a newly diagnosed meningioma is paramount toward achieving the best patient outcomes. This chapter reviews surgical considerations for patients with newly diagnosed meningiomas, including indications for surgical intervention, aspects of perioperative care, nuances to surgical approaches based on tumor location, and post-operative management based on tumor histopathology, as well as genomic analysis.

C. S. Hong
Department of Neurosurgery, Yale School of Medicine, New Haven, CT, USA
e-mail: christopher.hong@yale.edu

J. Moliterno (✉)
Yale New Haven Hospital and Smilow Cancer Hospital, New Haven, CT, USA

Yale Brain Tumor Center at Smilow Cancer Hospital, New Haven, CT, USA

Section of Neurosurgical Oncology, Yale School of Medicine, New Haven, CT, USA
e-mail: jennifer.moliternogunel@yale.edu

© Springer Nature Switzerland AG 2020
J. Moliterno, A. Omuro (eds.), *Meningiomas*,
https://doi.org/10.1007/978-3-030-59558-6_6

Indications for Surgery

Currently, the mainstay treatment for meningiomas and only potential for cure in a majority of them remains complete surgical resection, and therefore the neurosurgeon is often the first specialist offering advice for a newly diagnosed meningioma. Meningiomas are commonly incidental findings found on cranial imaging as the use of magnetic resonance imaging (MRI) becomes more commonplace in general medical practice. The fact that the vast majority of meningiomas tend to be slow-growing, or WHO grade I tumors, neurosurgeons are often faced with the decision as to whether and when to intervene on these tumors, particularly for patients who are asymptomatic. This decision-making relies heavily upon an understanding of the natural history, incorporating the recent molecular insights into meningioma biology that may influence rates of tumor growth, into patient care.

As a general rule, any patient who presents with a tumor with associated mass effect and/or related symptoms (i.e., seizures, weakness) warrants prompt neurosurgical evaluation and possible intervention. Exact timing of early surgery at the time of initial diagnosis can be tailored based on how debilitated the patient is with regard to the tumor, its size and mass effect, extent of edema, or concern for malignancy (Fig. 6.1). Tumors in certain locations, such as those arising near the optic canal and nerve or in the cerebellopontine angle (CPA), may necessitate relatively earlier surgical intervention, despite possibly relatively smaller sizes, given close proximity to and compression of nearby critical neurovascular structures. Though there are no hard and fast rules, certain radiographic characteristics, such as the presence of peritumoral edema, bony invasion, and/or areas of tumor necrosis (without prior embolization), can be seen in certain WHO grade I tumors, but can also confer concern for a more aggressive meningioma histology and thus favor early surgical intervention [3–7].

For other initial encounters with meningiomas that are relatively small, heavily calcified, and/or asymptomatic with little or no mass effect, surveillance with serial imaging might be a reasonable approach. At our institution, we typically monitor these patients with serial MRIs, beginning quite conservatively at 3 months and then stretching out over time. Details of surveillance depend on a host of factors, including patient age, tumor size, location, tumor radiographic features, and observed growth rate over time. Similar to those for upfront surgery, indications for operative intervention during surveillance include the development of symptoms and/ or a relatively quicker growth rate than anticipated with or without mass effect or edema based on serial imaging. Data for meningioma growth rates remain mixed with some studies reporting annual growth rates of up to 1 cm per year, while others have shown that meningiomas may not grow at all for several years following diagnosis [8–10]. This of course does not apply to all meningiomas as they can vary considerably with their behavior, underscoring the need for serial imaging and

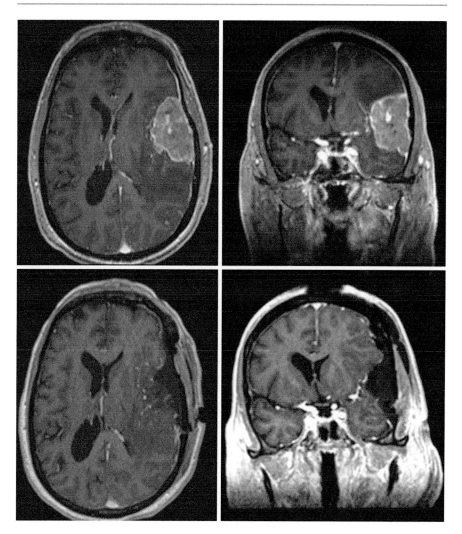

Fig. 6.1 A 59-year-old male presented with episodes of acute right-sided paresthesias and visual-spatial difficulties thought to represent seizures. Representative (**a**) axial and (**b**) coronal images of T1-weighted post-contrast MRI demonstrated a left sphenoid wing meningioma with surrounding vasogenic edema causing significant midline shift, suggestive of potential higher-grade pathology. Given his relatively acute and progressive symptom onset, coupled with the size, mass effect and edema, and potential concern for higher-grade pathology, the patient underwent surgery during the same hospital admission. Intraoperatively, the tumor was noted to be invasive of normal brain but was ultimately removed in its entirety and all dura and bony involvement excised. Representative (**c**) axial and (**d**) coronal images of post-operative T1-weighted post-contrast MRI demonstrated no residual enhancing disease. Final histopathology was consistent with WHO grade II, and whole-exome sequencing revealed the tumor to be *NF2* mutant

tailored care for each patient. Age and medical comorbidities also factor heavily into the decision to pursue elective surgery. Because relatively younger and healthier patients, as compared to older individuals, carry a potential increased risk of symptom development given their relative life span and thus increased number of years for tumor growth, careful consideration for surgical intervention should be given [11]. Furthermore, for older and/or debilitated patients who exhibit reason for concern during surveillance, or for tumors located purely within areas such as the cavernous sinus, radiosurgery may be a better approach and beyond the scope of this chapter.

Once the decision to pursue surgery has been made, whether initially or delayed and whether the patient is symptomatic or there is concern about the aggressiveness of the tumor, the typical goal is to remove as much tumor as safely as possible. Even in instances where complete resection is not possible, as is often the case with tumors arising from the dura along the skull base, increased extent of resection (EOR) has been correlated with decreased tumor recurrence rates. Thus, the goal of the neurosurgical management of most patients with most meningiomas remains maximal safe resection, or removing as much tumor as safely as possible, while minimizing morbidity and preserving neurological function.

Indeed, the Simpson grade of meningioma resection, first described in 1957, is a commonly used reference to predict likelihood of symptomatic recurrence at 10 years after surgery (Table 6.1) [12]. This scale incorporates not only the extent of tumor removal but also resection of the associated dura and bone. It ranges from a prediction of a 9% risk for symptomatic recurrence at 10 years (i.e., Simpson grade I as defined as complete removal of tumor, including underlying bone and associated dura) to 100% risk of symptomatic recurrence at 10 years across all grades (i.e., Simpson grade V as defined as simple decompression with biopsy). Indeed, large-scale clinical series have supported the clinical utility of Simpson grading in predicting tumor recurrence [13–15] which can also be useful in determining the need for adjuvant radiotherapy in incompletely resected tumors and/or atypical meningiomas [16, 17]. As such, a more aggressive approach with the goal of complete surgical resection of the tumor, dural attachment, and involved bone, when safely possible, may especially be warranted in younger patients to prevent future tumor recurrence. Surgery in older patients should be tailored based on age and comorbidities, considering these general recurrence rates.

Table 6.1 Simpson grading of meningioma resection

Grade	Definition	Recurrence rate over 10 years (%)
I	Total resection of tumor, dural attachments, and bone	9
II	Total resection of tumor, coagulation of dural attachments	19
III	Total resection of tumor without resection or coagulation of dural attachments or bone	29
IV	Partial resection of tumor	40
V	Simple decompression and/or biopsy	100

Concern and consideration for a clinically more aggressive meningioma due to certain radiographic features at initial presentation or higher than expected growth rate during serial imaging are important. High-grade meningiomas, consisting of atypical and anaplastic tumors, are distinct entities due to their aggressive clinical behavior. As defined as WHO II or III tumors, and comprising approximately 20% of all intracranial meningiomas, they carry an increased risk of recurrence despite maximal resection compared to their WHO grade I counterparts [18]. Recurrence rates for WHO II/III meningiomas have been reported between 9% and 50% after gross total resection (GTR), as compared to 36–83% after subtotal resection (STR) [19]. Additionally, STR in these higher-grade tumors seems to portend worsened overall survival as compared to GTR [20, 21]. Indeed, STR for atypical (WHO grade II) and malignant (WHO grade III) meningiomas reduced 5-year overall survival rates from 91.3% to 78.2% and 64.5% to 41.1%, respectively, in one large database study [22]. Thus, the surgical approach toward any meningioma, but especially higher-grade ones, remains maximal safe resection.

In practice, the definitive knowledge of dealing with a more aggressive meningioma at the time of initial surgery is currently being developed, but some features that correlate have already been identified. In addition to the aforementioned radiographic features, tumor location has been shown to correlate with underlying genomic alterations, which in turn affects the clinical behavior and thereby surgical decision-making. Utilizing genomic analyses from 300 meningioma samples, Clark et al. demonstrated that the clinical and anatomic features of meningiomas, including their site of origin, are determined by their molecular subtype as defined by the underlying driver somatic mutation [23]. NF2 mutant meningiomas showed increasing medial-to-lateral and anterior-to-posterior gradients along the skull base and convexities. Indeed, there were very few NF2 mutant meningiomas along the midline skull base, or anterior to the coronal suture, but rather occurred more laterally along the convexities. Instead, almost all meningiomas within the midline skull base, originating from the olfactory groove or planum sphenoidale, harbored a somatic mutation in one of the molecules involved in Hedgehog signaling, including Smoothened receptor (SMO) or SUFU. Other non-NF2 mutant tumors, including those with TRAF7 mutations concurrent with a recurrent mutation in KLF4 or PI3K pathway molecule mutations, localized to the anterior skull base. Further work by the same group identified POLR2A mutations in meningiomas, originating from the tuberculum sellae region [24].

Furthermore, the underlying driver mutations correlated with histology and biological potential for being atypical or malignant, For example, non-NF2 mutants were typically of meningothelial histology and uniquely WHO grade I [24]. Among these, all secretory meningiomas were TRAF7/KLF4 co-mutant, with significant clinical implications (see below). Tumors with NF2 mutations typically exhibit fibrous histopathology and have a greater likelihood to be atypical due to chromosomal instability or co-occurring mutations in the SMARCB1 gene [2]. These de novo NF2 mutant atypical meningiomas demonstrate a hypermethylated phenotype, leading to a more dedifferentiated cellular state [2]. Indeed, due to these biological factors, *NF2* mutant meningiomas, even though more commonly originating in more surgically accessible lateral convexity regions, are often associated with more aggressive clinical behavior.

Taken together, recent advances in understanding the genomic landscape of meningiomas, classifying them into mutually exclusive molecular subgroups, which can be predicted by their intracranial (or spinal) locations, have now allowed neurosurgeons to predict their overall clinical behavior. This pre-operative prognostication has important inferences in deciding treatment. Likewise, specific genetic findings may guide perioperative management in these patients as, for example, *KLF4/TRAF7* mutations in lateral skull base meningiomas are associated with malignant post-operative edema, while concurrent loss of *NF2* and a *SMARCB1* mutation may necessitate increased post-operative surveillance and/or need for adjuvant therapy.

In short, the anatomical origin of meningiomas can now provide insight into the likely underlying genomic subtype and even short- and long-term clinical behavior, with significant implications for surgical decision-making, and can be factored into the process.

Surgical Considerations for Multiple Meningiomas

Approximately 5–10% of patients harbor multiple meningiomas at the time of diagnosis, typically due to an associated underlying genetic predisposition (i.e., neurofibromatosis type 2, Cowden syndrome, Werner syndrome) [25, 26]. However, multiple meningiomas may also occur in non-syndromic patients, often limited to a single hemisphere, and may derive from subarachnoid spread of a tumor clone versus tumor formation from multiple separate foci [26–28]. The therapeutic approach toward treating patients with multiple meningiomas is similar to those with single lesions, comprised of surgery for tumors causing symptoms, exhibiting faster growth, and/or significant mass effect or peritumoral edema [8, 29]. In patients with multiple meningiomas, smaller, asymptomatic tumors can typically be observed. Although no relationship between increased number of meningiomas and faster growth rates has been suggested [30], more recent studies have shown the majority of these tumors to be *NF2* mutant, which is associated with a more aggressive clinical course. As such, the current data suggest a similar approach for patients with multiple meningiomas as those who harbor a single tumor, with incorporation of as many meningiomas into a single approach at the time of surgery when feasible, specifically focusing on the one(s) where surgery is indicated (Fig. 6.2).

A subset of patients with multiple meningiomas may present with this condition secondary to a history of prior cranial radiation therapy. Radiation-induced meningiomas are known to occur after both high- and low-dose radiation exposure to the brain, often presenting as multiple lesions at time of diagnosis and limited to occurrence within the original irradiated field [31, 32]. While the surgical approach

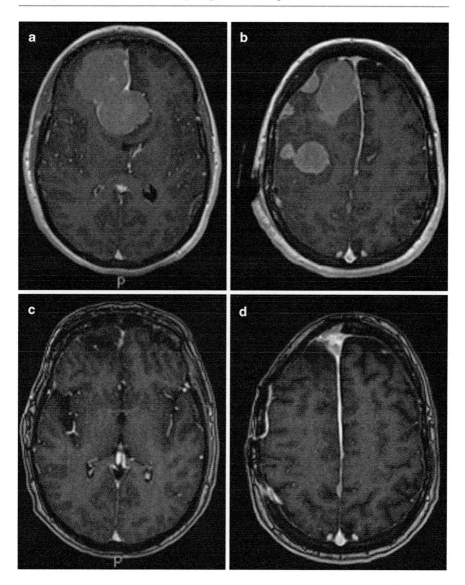

Fig. 6.2 A 49-year-old female presented with a generalized seizure secondary to multiple (at least ten) meningiomas arising from the right hemisphere, shown on representative (**a**) axial slices from a T1-weighted post-contrast MRI with the (**b**) largest along the right parafalcine region, measuring 5x8cm. She underwent a staged resection, with the first surgery aimed at removal of dominant tumor and at least four other smaller convexity lesions. A second operation removed the remaining tumors that exhibited subsequent growth. (**c**, **d**) Representative axial T1-weighted post-contrast MRI after resection showed no residual enhancing disease. Final pathology demonstrated WHO grade I with tumor-specific mutations in *NF2* as well as a germline mutation in *TP53*, rendering a diagnosis of Li-Fraumeni syndrome

for these patients remains focused on removal of dominant, symptomatic lesions, radiation-induced meningiomas often exhibit higher WHO grade on histopathology, increased bony invasion, and greater rates of recurrence despite maximal surgical resection, ranging from 18.7 to 25.6%, compared to sporadic counterparts [31–34]. As such, patients with suspected radiation-induced meningiomas based on relevant past medical history may warrant a more aggressive approach, including a lower threshold to operate, more aggressive bony and dural removal when surgically feasible, and closer surveillance after surgery.

Pre-operative Evaluation and Surgical Planning

Once it has been determined that a patient should undergo surgery for resection of a meningioma, various pre-operative factors must be taken into consideration to enhance the chances for successful surgical resection. To minimize risk of recurrence, the goal of surgery remains maximizing EOR safely with removal of as much tumor, involved dura and bone, when feasible. Understanding each tumor's relationship to adjacent neurovascular structures, including its vascular supply, and determining the safest surgical corridor for resection are crucial in pre-operative planning. Conventional MRI with contrast delineates basic characteristics of the tumor, including size, extent of peritumoral edema, dural involvement, and vascularity. Understanding the brain interface, sometimes characterized by a CSF cleft between tumor and surrounding brain parenchyma, is critically important. The absence of this finding might suggest brain invasion and potential higher-grade meningioma and thus increased risk of complications, residual tumor, and recurrence [35, 36]. Additionally, routine computed tomography (CT) can be helpful to better visualize whether the adjacent bone is infiltrated with tumor. The addition of contrast to CT may be helpful, as strong enhancement within the hyperostotic bone has been correlated with greater likelihood of tumor invasion and thus guides the need for more aggressive bony removal and reconstruction [37].

Additional imaging adjuncts should be considered to understand the relationship of critical vasculature structures to the meningioma. Early devascularization of the tumor itself is imperative, as is the preservation of unrelated, but nearby and often intimately associated, vasculature. In general, meningiomas are supplied by branches of the external carotid artery, meningeal branches from the internal carotid artery, or the vertebrobasilar system. Meningiomas arising from the convexities, sphenoid wing, or parasagittal region are supplied by branches off of the middle meningeal arteries, while tumors along the anterior skull base are typically fed by branches of the ethmoidal arteries from the external carotid artery as well as dural branches from the internal carotid artery. Within the posterior fossa, petroclival and tentorial meningiomas generally derive blood supply from the posterior meningeal artery and anterior inferior cerebellar artery off of the vertebral artery, as well as branches off of the external carotid artery including the ascending pharyngeal artery, the middle meningeal artery, the accessory meningeal artery, and the occipital artery. More specifically, laterally positioned tumors within the posterior fossa are typically fed by branches of the occipital and ascending pharyngeal arteries from the external carotid artery, while more medially located tumors are fed by meningeal branches off of the vertebral artery or from the posterior meningeal artery arising from the ascending pharyngeal artery. More centrally located meningiomas such as those arising from the clivus or tentorium are vascularized by various sources, such as the cavernous segment of the internal carotid artery, specifically the tentorial artery, and the middle meningeal artery with dedicated clival feeders. As such, dedicated arterial imaging via computed tomography angiography (CTA), or formal catheter angiography sometimes, may be particularly useful to understanding the relationship of the major feeders, as well as major branches of the intracranial vessels to the tumor, importantly distinguishing between vessel displacement and encasement [38]. Consequentially, the surgical approach may be tailored to optimize maintaining visualization and potential control of these major vessels.

Pre-operative embolization may be considered for highly vascularized meningiomas perhaps at high risk for significant intraoperative blood loss due to a potential inability to gain control of the blood supply early on in the surgery. Advances in modern endovascular techniques have led to wider spread use of pre-operative embolization and may facilitate higher rates of GTR, decreased blood loss, and shorter operating times in select tumors [39, 40]. While complication rates are typically low (i.e., reported under 5%), adverse events are not insignificant and may lead to ischemic injury to surrounding brain and stroke, exacerbate local mass effect leading to significant swelling and even herniation, and cause intratumoral hemorrhage, especially depending on which vessels are embolized (i.e., ICA feeders versus ECA feeders) [41–45]. Pre-operative risk factors that have been proposed to predict higher likelihood of post-operative complications include previous intratumoral hemorrhage, intratumoral cystic changes, larger tumors >6 cm, and atypical meningioma histology [46, 47]. For skull base meningiomas, embolization of ICA feeders may carry greater risk than ECA branches for intratumoral hemorrhage and incidence of stroke, while blindness may result from inadvertent occlusion of the ophthalmic artery during embolization of anterior skull base meningiomas [39]. Although outside the scope of this chapter, advances in both liquid and particle embolization materials have improved the accurate delivery of embolic agents to their intended targets while minimizing periprocedural complications.

To date, there is no general consensus on the optimal timing of surgery after embolization of meningiomas with a range of time periods reported, from 1 day to over 2 months after embolization, and there are reportedly similar rates of histopathological necrosis and post-operative blood transfusion requirements [42, 48]. Likewise, while no robust guidelines exist regarding indications for pre-operative embolization, generally giant meningiomas with large, multidirectional vascularization and/or deep-seated tumors where intraoperative visualization may be obscured may be ideal candidates for this procedure. Patients should be carefully monitored after embolization prior to surgery, given the risk of increased local mass effect from increased edema, ischemic injury to normal brain, or peritumoral hemorrhage. In our institution, though we have the benefit from a hybrid operating room with biplane angiography capabilities which can help minimize deleterious effects related to acute swelling, we rarely embolize meningiomas pre-operatively as the blood supply can typically be addressed and eradicated early on microsurgically.

In certain meningioma locations, such as near the falx or tentorial edge, dedicated venous imaging with magnetic resonance venography (MRV) or CTV is critical to determine the patency of the nearby venous sinuses, as well as the relationship of major cortical draining veins [49]. Understanding the degree of sinus involvement is essential, as is for those tumors involving the superior sagittal sinus (SSS), as a partially occluded sinus may be opened to obtain more complete tumor resection and preserve sinus patency. In contrast, a completely occluded sinus may be resected entirely along the extent of tumor involvement. Preservation of collateral venous brain drainage is imperative, and an MRV and/or formal catheter venogram may be helpful to better elucidate drainage.

Finally, cranial reconstruction must be considered in the pre-operative planning for meningioma surgery. The majority of meningiomas exhibit some degree of radiographic bony hyperostosis, which may correlate with tumor invasion of the bone at the histopathological level [50]. In cases where gross evidence of bony invasion by the tumor into overlying bone is absent, bony removal may simply be accomplished by burr-drilling along the underside of the bone flap prior to plating back on the native bone. Indeed, drilling down the inner table of the bone during meningioma surgery is the practice of the senior author. However, for tumors with significant bony hyperostosis in situ and particularly for intraosseous meningiomas, such as those occurring along the sphenoid wing with bowing into the orbit, complete removal of bone is necessary to prevent recurrence and improve symptoms (Fig. 6.3) [51, 52]. As such, in these cases, cranial reconstruction is necessary for both treatment and cosmetic purposes and is typically performed with titanium mesh [53, 54] or customized implants with plastic polymers (polyether ether ketone). It is the senior author's practice to include a plastic and reconstructive surgeon to assist in creating and implanting custom-made prostheses made in advance of especially large meningioma surgery, accomplished by defining a pre-operatively planned craniectomy to create the implant pre-operatively [52, 55]. For smaller and more straightforward cases, titanium mesh can be used.

Technical Nuances to Meningioma Surgery

All surgeries for meningioma begin with the use of antibiotics and hyperosmolar therapy, as well as mild hyperventilation at the beginning of the case. Loading patients with an anti-epileptic drug in the operating room is standard in our practice, especially for tumors that may involve the brain, although there is no level I evidence to support its use empirically [56, 57]. Patients' heads are always securely affixed to the table, and positioning is based on the location of the tumor, often considering vascular access and control in tumors encasing intracranial vessels and/or along the skull base.

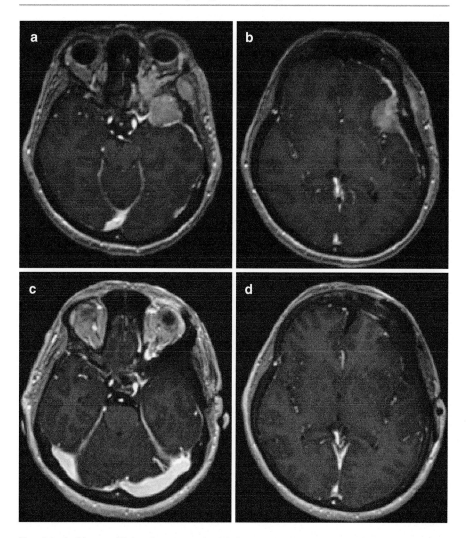

Fig. 6.3 A 64-year-old female presented with 2 months of progressive left-sided visual loss. T1-weighted post-contrast MRI showed a (**a**) 4.5 cm left sphenoid wing intraosseous tumor with bowing into the optic canal and orbit and (**b**) nearby involvement of critical brain arteries and veins. Tumor resection was achieved via a left frontotemporal craniotomy with removal of the lateral orbital wall, followed by orbital reconstruction with split calvarial bone grafts and an overlying cranioplasty accompanied by a temporalis muscle rotation advancement flap. Post-operative imaging demonstrates (**c**) gross total resection with optic nerve and orbital decompression and orbital reconstruction, as well as (**d**) cranial reconstruction with preservation of blood vessels. The patient's vision significantly improved following surgery. Pathology was consistent with an *NF2*-mutated atypical meningioma

CSF Diversion

We have found that the use of cerebrospinal fluid drainage (CSF), whether from the microsurgical dissection and opening of cisterns or with an external ventricular drain or lumbar drain, can be invaluable to the success of meningioma surgery, particularly those that are located deep and along the skull base. Release of CSF can greatly facilitate brain relaxation, negating the need for brain retraction and optimizing total tumor resection. Indeed, with the exception of intraventricular meningiomas or the use of a subtemporal approach, all of our meningioma surgeries are performed without retractors. Opening of the optic carotid cistern and proximal Sylvian fissure, for instance, during sphenoid wing meningioma surgeries can lead to sufficient brain relaxation, facilitating access and tumor removal with minimal, if any brain manipulation. Tumors that are located more laterally can often obscure the cistern and compress the fissure and can be hidden beneath potentially eloquent frontal and temporal lobes. In those cases, pre-operative placement of a lumbar drain is preferred. Similarly, removal of parafalcine tumors, or those located along the olfactory groove or planum or tentorial leaflet, for instance, often require the use of CSF diversion for access (Fig. 6.4). An external ventricular drain can be helpful with large petroclival meningiomas as associated tonsillar herniation can often preclude opening of the cisterna magna and cerebellar relaxation. It is important to note

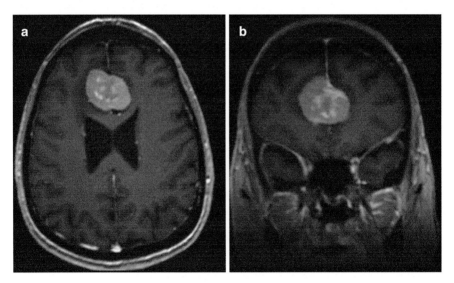

Fig. 6.4 A 65-year-old female presented with memory difficulties, and workup revealed a 3.6 cm parafalcine meningioma, shown on representative (**a**) axial and (**b**) coronal slices on a T1-weighted post-contrast MRI, causing mass effect on the bilateral frontal lobes. Pre-operative vascular imaging demonstrated splaying of the anterior cerebral arteries along the outside of the tumor capsule. During surgery, a lumbar drain was placed, allowing for CSF drainage and brain relaxation, which enabled surgical resection of the tumor and the falx without retraction of the brain. Representative (**c**) axial and (**d**) coronal slices on post-operative imaging showed gross total resection of the tumor

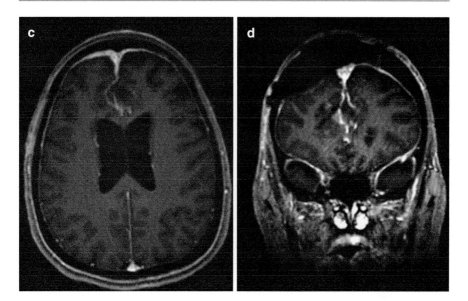

Fig. 6.4 (continued)

that the craniotomy must be performed with the bone flap removed prior to draining CSF. Careful review with anesthesia at the beginning of the case is important to ensure safety of its use.

Neurophysiology Monitoring

Intraoperative neurophysiology monitoring is a key adjunct to utilize in surgery for meningiomas involving critical neurovascular structures, such as important arteries, cranial nerves, and eloquent brain. Monitoring somatosensory evoked potentials (SSEPs) and motor evoked potentials (MEPs) is routinely used to localize the central sulcus during surgery of convexity meningiomas near the motor region, as well as for other brain tumors in this area [58]. Additionally, during resection of sphenoid wing meningiomas, for instance, monitoring of SSEPs and MEPs, as well as electroencephalography (EEG), can be important in understanding the preservation of the supply from major branches of the anterior and middle cerebral arteries, as well as critical vessels such as the anterior choroidal artery. It is important to understand the nuances of its use, as neuromonitoring can give a false sense of security as often times once the loss of potential is encountered, the damage has already been done. For meningiomas located within the CPA or along the petrous bone or clivus, neuromonitoring is essential to preserve function of nearby cranial nerves, particularly the facial and lower cranial nerves. Brainstem auditory evoked potentials are imperative for attempts at "hearing preservation surgery" and can also be useful adjunct to elucidate brainstem integrity [59]. Similarly, neuromonitoring can be beneficial when removing tumors in close proximity to the primary motor or sensory cortices, though more sophisticated techniques such as intraoperative mapping of the motor cortex by direct cortical electrical stimulation are not often needed given these tumors are not intraparenchymal [60].

Microsurgical Techniques

There are various intraoperative techniques that may be utilized at the time of surgery to optimize the greatest EOR. The use of neuronavigation is standard on all of our meningioma cases and allows for a more focused craniotomy, as well as avoidance of certain structures, such as the torcula or frontal sinus. For larger tumors, neuronavigation also helps to ensure that all of the diseased dura is included within the craniotomy, allowing for its later excision. Once the dura is opened, CSF is released, and the tumor is encountered, our practice is typically to begin by eradicating the tumor's blood supply. Often times, tumor debulking must first be performed, as larger tumors can obscure its dural base and feeders. Prior to obtaining control of the blood supply, meningiomas can be quite vascular, and control with bipolar cautery can be helpful, but often times futile until the blood supply is better controlled. Packing off larger tumors with thrombin-soaked cotton balls can be helpful to allow debulking until the vascular supply is eradicated. Once this is accomplished, devascularized tumors can often be easily removed en bloc or with the use of an ultrasonic aspirator device.

Tumor removal proceeds by careful dissection of the tumor capsule along the arachnoid plane, and the operative microscope can be helpful for visualization. Establishing and maintaining the brain-tumor interface is key, especially along the eloquent cortex and specifically with the ependymal lining in the case of intraventricular tumors. This can be understandably challenging with more invasive and higher-grade tumors. Relatively small tumors can typically be removed en bloc after circumferential dissection. Along the capsule, feeding arteries can be quite hypertrophied and in certain locations can be confusing with important normal vasculature, especially perforator arteries. Following the vessel and ensuring that it does not simply loop along the capsule is fundamentally important. We have found that the use of temporary aneurysm clips on these vessels while watching for potential neuromonitoring changes can help to differentiate feeders from "en passant" arteries, providing security prior to taking any of these arteries. Larger intracranial arteries that are embedded and encased within the meningioma can be skeletonized. The level of aggressiveness of the surgery should be decided based on the consistency and potential pathological grade of the tumor, as well as patient factors, including age and comorbidities. We find identifying these vessels in normal anatomy, either proximally or distally to their encasement, provides the safest understanding and protection of the involved vasculature. The vascular Doppler can be useful while working within the tumor, as can the intraoperative ultrasound (iUS). Intraoperative judgment to decide whether some residual tumor should be left in order to avoid injury, for example, to small perforators, is of fundamental importance (Fig. 6.5).

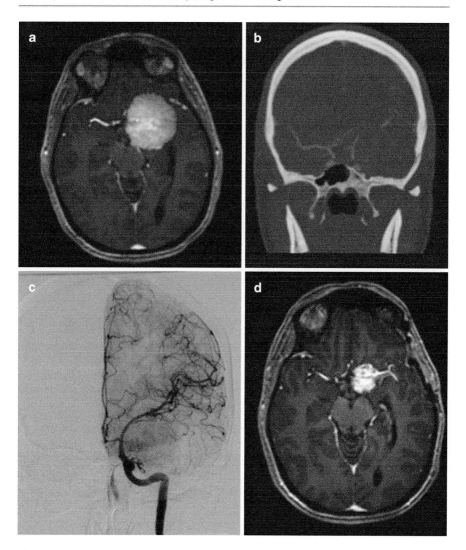

Fig. 6.5 A 50-year-old female presented with olfactory auras, which on further workup revealed a large 5 cm left-sided sphenoid wing meningioma, demonstrated on a representative (**a**) axial slice of a T1-weighted post-contrast MRI. (**b**) A pre-operative CTA showed tumor encasement of the internal carotid artery and M1 segment, confirmed on (**c**) digital subtraction angiography which also revealed prominent blood supply from the meningohypophyseal trunk off of the cavernous carotid segment. The tumor was maximally debulked with aid of a lumbar drain to minimize brain retraction and judicious use of an intraoperative Doppler ultrasound to identify important vasculature, namely, the middle cerebral artery and other major arteries within the tumor. (**d**) Postoperative T1-weighted post-contrast MRI revealed expected residual tumor and preservation of the encased normal vasculature, including perforators. Histology was consistent with an *NF2*-mutated atypical meningioma

As mentioned, certain meningiomas can involve or alter venous anatomy and function. Most notably, parafalcine tumors can frequently involve the SSS. Our typical practice is to remove the diseased segment, ensuring collateral venous drainage is preserved. When the tumor is observed to grow into, but not occlude, the superior sagittal sinus, there are multiple strategies that may be employed. Firstly, any adjacent venous channels that may have formed over time from the partially occluded sinus should be noted, and great care should be taken to preserve these collaterals. It is important not to ligate the sinus, which traditionally has been reported to be safe if performed in the anterior third of the sinus to avoid significant venous infarction [61]. The sinus may also be resected and then re-approximated primarily or with a patch, particularly if only one wall is involved. Residual tumor may be left with the caveat that regrowth is likely, especially depending on how much. Importantly, a staged approach, allowing for further growth of venous collaterals with planned future complete sinus ligation and tumor removal, can be considered. With this approach, residual tumor has to be monitored and radiosurgery considered. An understanding of nearby venous anatomy is also essential for meningiomas in other locations, such as tentorial or petroclival ones. These tumors are typically removed through a transpetrosal approach, which might require ligation of the petrosal sinus, retraction and protection of the vein of Labbe, as well as understanding the basal temporal veins.

Frank bony involvement, as seen in intraosseous tumors, must be completely removed to decrease tumor recurrence and to enable improvement of function. This can be most notable in sphenoid wing meningiomas. Here, bony decompression, particularly of the orbit, is necessary to help reconstruct and diminish proptosis and preserve the optic nerve, as well as lessen the likelihood of tumor recurrence. Our practice is typically to perform these cases along with head and neck/oculoplastic and plastic and reconstruction surgeons to ensure all goals of surgery are met. A pterional craniotomy is usually performed, and a high-speed drill bit is used to drill down the hyperostotic sphenoid wing and infiltrated bone. This is continued until periorbital fat is exposed. Unroofing the optic canal can be decided based on the degree of its involvement and/or dysfunction, but should be carefully considered in every case.

After the tumor has been successfully and safely removed to the greatest extent, attention then turns toward hemostasis and closure. Special attention should be taken when leaving any residual tumor as this mass can have the propensity to bleed post-operatively [62, 63]. Care should be taken to ensure blood has been irrigated out, especially within the ventricle and posterior fossa. Likewise, during closure, excision of the involved dura is performed. For those tumors, for instance, convexity meningiomas in which they are abutting and involving easily accessible dura, a relatively wide margin can be readily removed. For skull base tumors, however, in which complete removal of involved dura is not possible, coagulation with electrocautery is essential to achieve higher Simpson grade resection and thus reduce the chance of future tumor recurrence. A dural patch can be sutured into place when feasible to reduce the incidence of pseudomeningocele formation. Similarly, drilling of the inner table of the associated bone flap, as mentioned above, or use of a cranioplasty can be performed at this time.

Post-Operative Considerations

Once surgery is completed, various factors must be taken into consideration, including post-operative intensive care unit and inpatient management, need for adjuvant therapy, and long-term follow-up. While the use of perioperative anti-epileptic medications (AEDs) in brain tumors continues to remain largely surgeon-specific and a topic of ongoing debate [64, 65], certain meningioma characteristics have been reported to increase the risk of new-onset seizures in the post-operative setting, including non-skull base locations, especially in the parietal area, larger tumor size, and brain invasion [56, 66–68]. In addition, patients with recurrent meningiomas can develop tumor-related epilepsy [69], especially post-operatively, thereby necessitating immediate post-op and longer-term AED therapy. Indeed, it is our practice to routinely utilize perioperative AEDs, typically loaded in the operating room and continued for approximately 1 week after surgery for meningioma patients who present without seizures.

In addition to routine use of glucocorticosteroids to manage any post-operative edema after meningioma resection, we routinely use mildly hypertonic saline as an adjunct therapy during inpatient care up until time of discharge. Steroid use is effective in reducing brain tumor-related vasogenic edema but may be ineffective in other conditions, such as traumatic brain injury, which typically leads to cytotoxic edema [70]. As post-operative edema after brain tumor surgery may represent a combination of vasogenic and cytotoxic edema related to the surgical intervention, we have found that the addition of mildly hypertonic saline to a standard dexamethasone taper has reduced the likelihood of new post-operative deficits related to edema around the resection bed and has allowed for the reduction of steroids quicker and thus prevention of possible side effects. There is no current data to support this practice, but anecdotally this seems to offer some benefit with no significant side effects. Hyperosmolar therapy can be reserved for patients with substantial and significant peritumoral edema.

Management of meningioma patients after surgery may be simple with periodic surveillance to more complex and multidisciplinary with the need for adjunct therapy and even reoperations in the future. The approach is often personalized for each individual. For the meningioma patient after surgery, the objective of the multidisciplinary "Brain Tumor Board" which exists at leading institutions in the United States, including ours, is to determine the next steps for post-operative care. These recommendations are typically based on EOR, clinical characteristics (i.e., age, comorbidities) and function of the patient, histopathology and WHO grade, as well as a focus on the underlying tumor genomics, as is in our Precision Brain Tumor Board. For patients undergoing GTR or near total resection of WHO grade I meningiomas, we typically perform surveillance with follow-up imaging, beginning 3 months after surgery, expanding the timeframe in between scans. Patients with a higher-grade histology are typically referred for adjuvant radiotherapy, regardless of EOR [71]. However, the indications for adjuvant radiation in WHO II and III meningiomas continue to remain unclear and beyond the scope of this chapter. In addition, all tumors, including meningiomas, undergo whole-exome sequencing at our institution, which allows for possible some insight into follow-up and potential use of adjuvant therapy based on what was discussed earlier in this chapter.

Conclusions

Neurosurgical intervention remains the mainstay for treatment for most meningiomas. For a newly diagnosed meningioma, surgery is pursued initially if the tumor is large, and/or results in significant mass effect or symptoms, and/or there is concern for a higher-grade pathology. Similar factors contribute to surgical decision-making if observation and surveillance is initially pursued, with patient factors such as age and comorbidities taken into account. Radiographic features, such as location, correlate with the underlying genomic subgroup, affecting the clinical behavior, and can prove to be useful in whether and when to operate, as well as post-operative follow-up. Once surgery is decided, dedicated arterial and venous imaging as well as planning whether any bony reconstruction is needed is important to optimize the chances for maximal, safe tumor resection. Beyond the standard intraoperative surgical adjuncts used in tumor surgery, the use of a lumbar drain and neuromonitoring may be helpful in making the surgery as safe as possible. After surgery, patients may benefit from perioperative anti-epileptic therapy and hypertonic saline use in addition to routine glucocorticosteroids to manage post-operative edema and minimize new-onset seizures. In addition to routine histopathological study, comprehensive tumor genomic profiling yields greater insights into the expected clinical behavior of meningiomas after surgery, regardless of EOR. Lastly, input from a multidisciplinary tumor board is essential toward establishing the need for adjuvant therapy and post-operative surveillance, particularly after more complex and higher-grade meningioma resection.

References

1. Wara WM, Sheline GE, Newman H, Townsend JJ, Boldrey EB. Radiation therapy of meningiomas. Am J Roentgenol Radium Therapy, Nucl Med. 1975;123(3):453–8.
2. Harmanci AS, Youngblood MW, Clark VE, Coskun S, Henegariu O, Duran D, et al. Integrated genomic analyses of de novo pathways underlying atypical meningiomas. Nat Commun. 2017;8:14433.
3. Spille DC, Sporns PB, Hess K, Stummer W, Brokinkel B. Prediction of high-grade histology and recurrence in meningiomas using routine preoperative magnetic resonance imaging - a systematic review. World Neurosurg. 2019;128:174–81.
4. Spille DC, Hess K, Sauerland C, Sanai N, Stummer W, Paulus W, et al. Brain invasion in meningiomas: incidence and correlations with clinical variables and prognosis. World Neurosurg. 2016;93:346–54.
5. Lee KJ, Joo WI, Rha HK, Park HK, Chough JK, Hong YK, et al. Peritumoral brain edema in meningiomas: correlations between magnetic resonance imaging, angiography, and pathology. Surg Neurol. 2008;69(4):350–5; discussion 5.

6. Hale AT, Wang L, Strother MK, Chambless LB. Differentiating meningioma grade by imaging features on magnetic resonance imaging. J Clin Neurosci. 2018;48:71–5.
7. Adeli A, Hess K, Mawrin C, Streckert EMS, Stummer W, Paulus W, et al. Prediction of brain invasion in patients with meningiomas using preoperative magnetic resonance imaging. Oncotarget. 2018;9(89):35974–82.
8. Nakamura M, Roser F, Michel J, Jacobs C, Samii M. The natural history of incidental meningiomas. Neurosurgery. 2003;53(1):62–70; discussion -1.
9. Jadid KD, Feychting M, Hoijer J, Hylin S, Kihlstrom L, Mathiesen T. Long-term follow-up of incidentally discovered meningiomas. Acta Neurochir. 2015;157(2):225–30; discussion 30.
10. Fountain DM, Soon WC, Matys T, Guilfoyle MR, Kirollos R, Santarius T. Volumetric growth rates of meningioma and its correlation with histological diagnosis and clinical outcome: a systematic review. Acta Neurochir. 2017;159(3):435–45.
11. Oya S, Kim SH, Sade B, Lee JH. The natural history of intracranial meningiomas. J Neurosurg. 2011;114(5):1250–6.
12. Simpson D. The recurrence of intracranial meningiomas after surgical treatment. J Neurol Neurosurg Psychiatry. 1957;20(1):22–39.
13. Oya S, Kawai K, Nakatomi H, Saito N. Significance of Simpson grading system in modern meningioma surgery: integration of the grade with MIB-1 labeling index as a key to predict the recurrence of WHO Grade I meningiomas. J Neurosurg. 2012;117(1):121–8.
14. Nanda A, Bir SC, Maiti TK, Konar SK, Missios S, Guthikonda B. Relevance of Simpson grading system and recurrence-free survival after surgery for World Health Organization grade I meningioma. J Neurosurg. 2017;126(1):201–11.
15. Stafford SL, Perry A, Suman VJ, Meyer FB, Scheithauer BW, Lohse CM, et al. Primarily resected meningiomas: outcome and prognostic factors in 581 Mayo Clinic patients, 1978 through 1988. Mayo Clin Proc. 1998;73(10):936–42.
16. Pollock BE, Stafford SL, Link MJ. Gamma knife radiosurgery for skull base meningiomas. Neurosurg Clin N Am. 2000;11(4):659–66.
17. Park S, Cha YJ, Suh SH, Lee IJ, Lee KS, Hong CK, et al. Risk group-adapted adjuvant radiotherapy for WHO grade I and II skull base meningioma. J Cancer Res Clin Oncol. 2019;145(5):1351–60.
18. Louis DN, Perry A, Reifenberger G, von Deimling A, Figarella-Branger D, Cavenee WK, et al. The 2016 World Health Organization classification of tumors of the central nervous system: a summary. Acta Neuropathol. 2016;131(6):803–20.
19. Chohan MO, Ryan CT, Singh R, Lanning RM, Reiner AS, Rosenblum MK, et al. Predictors of treatment response and survival outcomes in meningioma recurrence with atypical or anaplastic histology. Neurosurgery. 2018;82(6):824–32.
20. Moliterno J, Cope WP, Vartanian ED, Reiner AS, Kellen R, Ogilvie SQ, et al. Survival in patients treated for anaplastic meningioma. J Neurosurg. 2015;123(1):23–30.
21. Kumar N, Kumar R, Khosla D, Salunke PS, Gupta SK, Radotra BD. Survival and failure patterns in atypical and anaplastic meningiomas: a single-center experience of surgery and postoperative radiotherapy. J Cancer Res Ther. 2015;11(4):735–9.
22. Aizer AA, Bi WL, Kandola MS, Lee EQ, Nayak L, Rinne ML, et al. Extent of resection and overall survival for patients with atypical and malignant meningioma. Cancer. 2015;121(24):4376–81.
23. Clark VE, Erson-Omay EZ, Serin A, Yin J, Cotney J, Ozduman K, et al. Genomic analysis of non-NF2 meningiomas reveals mutations in TRAF7, KLF4, AKT1, and SMO. Science. 2013;339(6123):1077–80.
24. Clark VE, Harmanci AS, Bai H, Youngblood MW, Lee TI, Baranoski JF, et al. Recurrent somatic mutations in POLR2A define a distinct subset of meningiomas. Nat Genet. 2016;48(10):1253–9.
25. Kerr K, Qualmann K, Esquenazi Y, Hagan J, Kim DH. Familial syndromes involving meningiomas provide mechanistic insight into sporadic disease. Neurosurgery. 2018;83(6):1107–18.

26. Araujo Pereira BJ, Nogueira de Almeida A, Pires de Aguiar PH, Paiva WS, Teixeira MJ, Nagahashi Marie SK. Multiple intracranial meningiomas: a case series and review of the literature. World Neurosurg. 2019;122:e1536–e41.

27. Stangl AP, Wellenreuther R, Lenartz D, Kraus JA, Menon AG, Schramm J, et al. Clonality of multiple meningiomas. J Neurosurg. 1997;86(5):853–8.

28. Ohla V, Scheiwe C. Meningiomatosis restricted to the left cerebral hemisphere with acute clinical deterioration: case presentation and discussion of treatment options. Surg Neurol Int. 2015;6:64.

29. Sheehy JP, Crockard HA. Multiple meningiomas: a long-term review. J Neurosurg. 1983;59(1):1–5.

30. Jaaskelainen J. Seemingly complete removal of histologically benign intracranial meningioma: late recurrence rate and factors predicting recurrence in 657 patients. A multivariate analysis. Surg Neurol. 1986;26(5):461–9.

31. Al-Mefty O, Topsakal C, Pravdenkova S, Sawyer JR, Harrison MJ. Radiation-induced meningiomas: clinical, pathological, cytokinetic, and cytogenetic characteristics. J Neurosurg. 2004;100(6):1002–13.

32. Elbabaa SK, Gokden M, Crawford JR, Kesari S, Saad AG. Radiation-associated meningiomas in children: clinical, pathological, and cytogenetic characteristics with a critical review of the literature. J Neurosurg Pediatr. 2012;10(4):281–90.

33. Strojan P, Popovic M, Jereb B. Secondary intracranial meningiomas after high-dose cranial irradiation: report of five cases and review of the literature. Int J Radiat Oncol Biol Phys. 2000;48(1):65–73.

34. Morgenstern PF, Shah K, Dunkel IJ, Reiner AS, Khakoo Y, Rosenblum MK, et al. Meningioma after radiotherapy for malignancy. J Clin Neurosci. 2016;30:93–7.

35. Ildan F, Tuna M, Gocer AP, Boyar B, Bagdatoglu H, Sen O, et al. Correlation of the relationships of brain-tumor interfaces, magnetic resonance imaging, and angiographic findings to predict cleavage of meningiomas. J Neurosurg. 1999;91(3):384–90.

36. Enokizono M, Morikawa M, Matsuo T, Hayashi T, Horie N, Honda S, et al. The rim pattern of meningioma on 3D FLAIR imaging: correlation with tumor-brain adhesion and histological grading. Magn Reson Med Sci. 2014;13(4):251–60.

37. Huang RY, Bi WL, Griffith B, Kaufmann TJ, la Fougere C, Schmidt NO, et al. Imaging and diagnostic advances for intracranial meningiomas. Neuro Oncol. 2019;21(Supplement_1):i44–61.

38. Zhao X, Yu RT, Li JS, Xu K, Li X. Clinical value of multi-slice 3-dimensional computed tomographic angiography in the preoperative assessment of meningioma. Exp Ther Med. 2013;6(2):475–8.

39. Rosen CL, Ammerman JM, Sekhar LN, Bank WO. Outcome analysis of preoperative embolization in cranial base surgery. Acta Neurochir. 2002;144(11):1157–64.

40. Oka H, Kurata A, Kawano N, Saegusa H, Kobayashi I, Ohmomo T, et al. Preoperative superselective embolization of skull-base meningiomas: indications and limitations. J Neuro-Oncol. 1998;40(1):67–71.

41. Sluzewski M, van Rooij WJ, Lohle PN, Beute GN, Peluso JP. Embolization of meningiomas: comparison of safety between calibrated microspheres and polyvinyl-alcohol particles as embolic agents. AJNR Am J Neuroradiol. 2013;34(4):727–9.

42. Borg A, Ekanayake J, Mair R, Smedley T, Brew S, Kitchen N, et al. Preoperative particle and glue embolization of meningiomas: indications, results, and lessons learned from 117 consecutive patients. Neurosurgery. 2013;73(2 Suppl Operative):ons244–51; discussion ons52.

43. Yoon N, Shah A, Couldwell WT, Kalani MYS, Park MS. Preoperative embolization of skull base meningiomas: current indications, techniques, and pearls for complication avoidance. Neurosurg Focus. 2018;44(4):E5.

44. Singla A, Deshaies EM, Melnyk V, Toshkezi G, Swarnkar A, Choi H, et al. Controversies in the role of preoperative embolization in meningioma management. Neurosurg Focus. 2013;35(6):E17.

45. Friconnet G, Espindola Ala VH, Lemnos L, Saleme S, Duchesne M, Salle H, et al. Pre-surgical embolization of intracranial meningioma with Onyx: a safety and efficacy study. J Neuroradiol. 2020;47(5):353–7.
46. Kallmes DF, Evans AJ, Kaptain GJ, Mathis JM, Jensen ME, Jane JA, et al. Hemorrhagic complications in embolization of a meningioma: case report and review of the literature. Neuroradiology. 1997;39(12):877–80.
47. Bendszus M, Monoranu CM, Schutz A, Nolte I, Vince GH, Solymosi L. Neurologic complications after particle embolization of intracranial meningiomas. AJNR Am J Neuroradiol. 2005;26(6):1413–9.
48. Ng HK, Poon WS, Goh K, Chan MS. Histopathology of post-embolized meningiomas. Am J Surg Pathol. 1996;20(10):1224–30.
49. Zimmerman RD, Fleming CA, Saint-Louis LA, Lee BC, Manning JJ, Deck MD. Magnetic resonance imaging of meningiomas. AJNR Am J Neuroradiol. 1985;6(2):149–57.
50. Goyal N, Kakkar A, Sarkar C, Agrawal D. Does bony hyperostosis in intracranial meningioma signify tumor invasion? A radio-pathologic study. Neurol India. 2012;60(1):50–4.
51. Chen TC. Primary intraosseous meningioma. Neurosurg Clin N Am. 2016;27(2):189–93.
52. Broeckx CE, Maal TJJ, Vreeken RD, Bos RRM, Ter Laan M. Single-step resection of an intraosseous meningioma and cranial reconstruction: technical note. World Neurosurg. 2017;108:225–9.
53. Kuttenberger JJ, Hardt N. Long-term results following reconstruction of craniofacial defects with titanium micro-mesh systems. J Craniomaxillofac Surg. 2001;29(2):75–81.
54. Janecka IP. New reconstructive technologies in skull base surgery: role of titanium mesh and porous polyethylene. Arch Otolaryngol Head Neck Surg. 2000;126(3):396–401.
55. Bianchi F, Signorelli F, Di Bonaventura R, Trevisi G, Pompucci A. One-stage frame-guided resection and reconstruction with PEEK custom-made prostheses for predominantly intraosseous meningiomas: technical notes and a case series. Neurosurg Rev. 2019;42(3):769–75.
56. Islim AI, McKeever S, Kusu-Orkar TE, Jenkinson MD. The role of prophylactic antiepileptic drugs for seizure prophylaxis in meningioma surgery: a systematic review. J Clin Neurosci. 2017;43:47–53.
57. Islim AI, Ali A, Bagchi A, Ahmad MU, Mills SJ, Chavredakis E, et al. Postoperative seizures in meningioma patients: improving patient selection for antiepileptic drug therapy. J Neuro-Oncol. 2018;140(1):123–34.
58. Cedzich C, Taniguchi M, Schafer S, Schramm J. Somatosensory evoked potential phase reversal and direct motor cortex stimulation during surgery in and around the central region. Neurosurgery. 1996;38(5):962–70.
59. Simon MV. Neurophysiologic intraoperative monitoring of the vestibulocochlear nerve. J Clin Neurophysiol. 2011;28(6):566–81.
60. Ebeling U, Schmid UD, Reulen HJ. Tumour-surgery within the central motor strip: surgical results with the aid of electrical motor cortex stimulation. Acta Neurochir. 1989;101(3–4):100–7.
61. Shrivastava RK, Segal S, Camins MB, Sen C, Post KD. Harvey Cushing's Meningiomas text and the historical origin of resectability criteria for the anterior one third of the superior sagittal sinus. J Neurosurg. 2003;99(4):787–91.
62. Gerlach R, Raabe A, Scharrer I, Meixensberger J, Seifert V. Post-operative hematoma after surgery for intracranial meningiomas: causes, avoidable risk factors and clinical outcome. Neurol Res. 2004;26(1):61–6.
63. Bosnjak R, Derham C, Popovic M, Ravnik J. Spontaneous intracranial meningioma bleeding: clinicopathological features and outcome. J Neurosurg. 2005;103(3):473–84.
64. Tomasello F. Meningiomas and postoperative epilepsy: it is time for a randomized controlled clinical trial. World Neurosurg. 2013;79(3–4):431–2.
65. Ngwenya LB, Chiocca EA. Do meningioma patients benefit from antiepileptic drug treatment? World Neurosurg. 2013;79(3–4):433–4.

66. Mantle RE, Lach B, Delgado MR, Baeesa S, Belanger G. Predicting the probability of meningioma recurrence based on the quantity of peritumoral brain edema on computerized tomography scanning. J Neurosurg. 1999;91(3):375–83.
67. Hess K, Spille DC, Adeli A, Sporns PB, Brokinkel C, Grauer O, et al. Brain invasion and the risk of seizures in patients with meningioma. J Neurosurg. 2018;130(3):789–96.
68. Chen WC, Magill ST, Englot DJ, Baal JD, Wagle S, Rick JW, et al. Factors associated with pre- and postoperative seizures in 1033 patients undergoing supratentorial meningioma resection. Neurosurgery. 2017;81(2):297–306.
69. Chow SY, Hsi MS, Tang LM, Fong VH. Epilepsy and intracranial meningiomas. Zhonghua Yi Xue Za Zhi (Taipei). 1995;55(2):151–5.
70. Roberts I, Yates D, Sandercock P, Farrell B, Wasserberg J, Lomas G, et al. Effect of intravenous corticosteroids on death within 14 days in 10008 adults with clinically significant head injury (MRC CRASH trial): randomised placebo-controlled trial. Lancet. 2004;364(9442):1321–8.
71. Reddy AK, Ryoo JS, Denyer S, McGuire LS, Mehta AI. Determining the role of adjuvant radiotherapy in the management of meningioma: a surveillance, epidemiology, and end results analysis. Neurosurg Focus. 2019;46(6):E3.

Endoscopic and Minimally Invasive Meningioma Surgery

7

S. Bulent Omay and Theodore H. Schwartz

Rationale and Background

In the last 15 years, several minimally invasive approaches have been developed that can be used in the removal of skull base meningiomas. Meningiomas of the anterior skull base have been the target for most endoscopic and minimally invasive approaches. We will focus on these lesions as we discuss how these approaches can be utilized in meningioma surgery. The minimally invasive techniques discussed will include EEA (endoscopic endonasal approach), SKM (supraorbital keyhole minicraniotomy) which involves an eyebrow incision and utilizes endoscopic visualization, and TOA (transorbital approach) which uses the four quadrants of the orbit as a natural access corridor.

Meningiomas of the anterior skull base most frequently cause symptoms by exerting mass effect on the frontal lobes, optic nerves, chiasm, and olfactory nerves. They may cause hydrocephalus and sometimes extensively involve the bony skull base. These tumors have been traditionally approached through transcranial route including pterional, bifrontal, transbasal, and orbitozygomatic approaches. These approaches can sometimes involve retraction of normal brain, require manipulation of neurovascular structures, and can involve air sinuses that can potentially create postoperative sequelae related to wound healing and unwanted cosmetic outcomes [1–4].

S. B. Omay
Department of Neurosurgery, Yale School of Medicine, New Haven, CT, USA
e-mail: sacit.omay@yale.edu

T. H. Schwartz (✉)
Department of Neurosurgery, Otolaryngology and Neuroscience, Weill Cornell Medicine, New York Presbyterian Hospital, New York, NY, USA
e-mail: schwarh@med.cornell.edu

© Springer Nature Switzerland AG 2020
J. Moliterno, A. Omuro (eds.), *Meningiomas*,
https://doi.org/10.1007/978-3-030-59558-6_7

Endoscopic and minimally invasive surgery follows the concepts of keyhole approach in neurosurgery. This concept can be summarized by reducing the size of the craniotomy, making smaller dural openings, limiting cortical exposure, and minimizing normal brain manipulation. These key principles result in shorter hospital stay and minimize the risk of complications. This requires a conceptual change of predefined surgical corridors to individually tailored approaches [5].

Endoscopic, especially endonasal, approaches provide a direct access to skull base meningiomas that obviates the need for brain retraction. Also, it can take the neurosurgeon directly to pathology, without placing the optic nerves or carotid arteries between the surgeon and the tumor. EEA can provide complete, bilateral optic canal decompression without manipulation of a compressed optic nerve. Additionally, approaching these tumors from below enables the surgeon to remove the bone at the base of the tumor, which is a common site for meningioma recurrence and can interrupt the dural vascular supply early in the operation, minimizing blood loss [6].

The surgical treatment goals for meningiomas are not different when minimally invasive techniques are utilized. These goals include removal of the tumor, infiltrated dura, and bone. The skull base has a complex neurovascular anatomy that usually is intimately involved in the pathology. This will limit achieving these goals, and individual strategies have to be tailored based on the pathological anatomy, age of the patient, and availability of alternative treatment modalities [7] (Fig. 7.1).

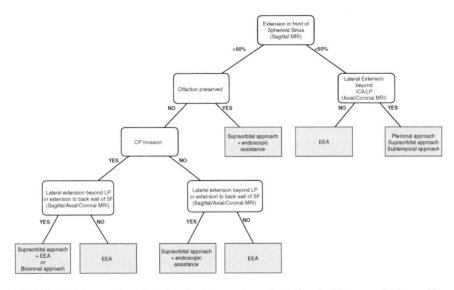

Fig. 7.1 Decision-making algorithm for the resection of anterior skull base meningiomas [7]. (Reprinted from Ottenhausen et al. [7], https://thejns.org/focus/view/journals/neurosurg-focus/44/4/article-pE1.xml, © 2018, with permission from Journal of Neurosurgery and AANS)

Endoscopic Endonasal Approach to Skull Base Meningiomas

EEA through the ethmoids and fovea ethmoidalis, cribriform plate, planum sphenoidale, tuberculum sella, sella, and clivus have developed as a useful alternative to conventional open cranial approaches [1]. The endoscope, by carrying the lens and light source closer to the focus of the operation, creates a panoramic, high-resolution image that surpasses the capability of the microscope. The anatomic and pathologic detail offered to the surgeon by the endoscope is even more enhanced by used of angled scopes [8].

Making a decision to utilize EEA in order to resect a meningioma of the anterior skull base requires a thorough understanding of the pathological anatomy of the lesion and the structures around the lesion, assessment of the size of the potential surgical corridor and its ability to provide bimanual dissection, and exposure adequate to remove the lesion. Reconstruction of the dura and skull base is an integral part of this thought process as well and should be planned ahead before the operation. The pathological anatomy of lesion and its surroundings, which include tumor location and its extent, degree of bony invasion and hyperostosis, vascularity of the tumor, brain edema and/or invasion and encasement of blood vessels, must be taken into consideration. Meningiomas usually present with a broad dural base, an enhancing dural tail, and hyperostosis and/or involvement of the neighboring bone. The involvement of the bone in meningiomas makes the endoscopic endonasal approach ideal for these lesions because it has the capability of removing all the involved bone in the initial phase of the approach. Tumor vasculature which is supplied by the dural base of the meningioma is again addressed by the endonasal approach earlier in the operation decreasing the amount of bleeding throughout the case. Tumors that do not extend laterally to the lamina papyracea or anteriorly to the frontal sinus are generally considered accessible for endonasal approaches [1].

In our experience, planum sphenoidale and tuberculum sella meningiomas are the best candidates for endonasal surgery [7]. Olfactory groove meningiomas can also be removed safely through an endonasal route; however, we prefer an eyebrow incision with a supraorbital craniotomy for larger tumors or those that abut the posterior wall of the frontal sinus [9] (Fig. 7.2). If a Simpson grade I resection (gross total resection with the associated tumor-infiltrated dura) is the goal of surgery, the endonasal approach must be paired with a close inspection of the relevant anatomy. Invasion of the medial optic canals should be appreciated before surgery, and, if necessary, the optic canals can be removed within the sphenoid sinus to ensure complete tumor removal. Nevertheless, in certain patients, aggressive debulking to alleviate symptoms followed by radiosurgery and fractionated radiation may be the preferred strategy [4].

Endoscopic endonasal approach also makes possible a less morbid decompression of the optic apparatus in frail or elderly patients who are losing vision in preparation for postresection radiation or observation. This approach also offers

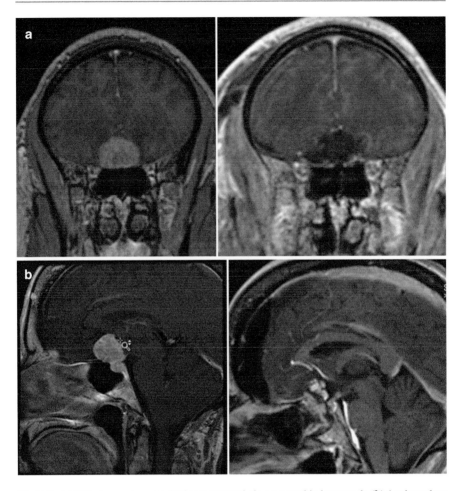

Fig. 7.2 (**a**) Olfactory groove meningioma resected via a supraorbital approach. (**b**) A tuberculum sella meningioma resected via EE with intradural fat graft, gasket seal and nasoseptal flap closure

the advantage below which is the ability to attack the dural vascular supply to the tumor early in the operation. Since not only the dura but also the bone at the base of the tumor is removed during the approach, the transtuberculum transplanum approach potentially offers a higher likelihood of curing these meningiomas. Endoscopic opening of the optic canals bilaterally can help in accessing all of the tumor remnants that are located inferior to the optic nerve [4, 10]. A detailed neuro-ophthalmologic examination with visual field testing is recommended for patients with visual symptoms or optic apparatus compression on imaging. If the lesion is in vicinity of the pituitary gland, full endocrinological workup is usually indicated.

MRI of the brain and specifically a pituitary protocol MRI with fine coronal cuts is required for tumors of the sella. The location of the septations within the sphenoid sinus and the location of carotid arteries should be determined by CT or CTA as needed for all anterior skull base cases.

The pneumatization level of the sphenoid sinus, septal perforations, and spurs should be identified to establish quality and side of the nasoseptal flap [6].

Indications, Contraindications, and Considerations

Any anterior skull base meningioma exerting mass effect, causing neurologic, endocrinologic, or ophthalmologic symptoms, or any lesion which requires a tissue diagnosis is an indication for EEA to either resect or biopsy these lesions as necessary. Large tumors may not be completely resected using an endonasal approach. Depending on the age, comorbidities of the patient and the surgical goals, internal decompression, or staged resection with additional approaches may be utilized [11].

Lateral extension of the tumor relative to the orbits and the carotid artery creates a relative contraindication. Pathology which extends laterally over the orbits or lateral to or behind the carotid arteries is difficult to remove using EEA. The width of the planum sphenoidale, between the laminae papyracea, defines the preferred corridor by the EEA [6]. Visualization, with use of angled scopes, can be achievable, but resection of a lesion around a corner may not be technically feasible [12]. Encasement of neurovascular structures and cavernous sinus invasion is not a contraindication to EEA [13], but the possibility of radiosurgery and fractionated radiation to control the growth of residual unresectable meningioma should always be considered before tackling dissection of a tumor off a vital structure [12].

Undeniably, EEA has the disadvantage of a narrow working corridor reducing the measurability of surgical instruments. Careful analysis of the anatomy of the lesion and the skull base, combined with knowledge of the restrictions, can overcome these limitations.

Operating through the nose carries the theoretical risk of intracranial infection and CSF leak, given the challenge sterilizing the nose and reconstructing the dura and skull base from below, respectively. Surgeon's expertise with endoscopic techniques and knowledge of the limitations of the endonasal corridor affects operative quality and time which may significantly impact patient outcomes [1, 14].

Large tumors or tumors that are located laterally may not be resectable in a gross total fashion. But this should not be a contraindication. Endoscopic approaches may still have value, in these circumstanses, when age and condition of the patient may require other strategies such as internal decompression and/or staged resections [12].

Surgical Technique

Instruments

Endoscopic instruments are designed differently than microsurgical instruments. Bayoneted instruments are not usually preferred. Specially designed bipolar coagulation is used for intradural hemostasis. 18′ and 30′ endoscopes with 0-, 30-, and 45-degree lenses provide extended visualization, and scopes can be held by stationary holders or held by a second surgeon for a dynamic visualization. Dynamic visualization can help the neurosurgeon overcome the two- dimensionality of the visual output of the endoscope since the movement of the endoscope helps depth orientation. By bringing the lens and light source directly to the target, the endoscope provides a major advantage when compared to the microscope [6, 14].

The Approach

The head is placed in rigid fixation and registered with frameless neuronavigation, with the neck slightly extended to facilitate visualization of the cribriform plate and fovea ethmoidalis. The abdomen or thigh is prepared for harvesting autologous fat and fascia lata for multilayered skull base reconstruction. A long nasoseptal flap is harvested. A bilateral transethmoidal, transsellar, transtuberculum transplanum, transcribriform approach is performed depending on the location of the meningioma. This exposes the skull base from the back of the frontal sinus to the sella between the fovea ethmoidalis bilaterally to expose the meningioma. The anterior and posterior ethmoidal arteries are identified, cauterized, and transected at the junction between the fovea ethmoidalis and lamina papyracea. The skull base is drilled down to the dura circumferentially around the base of the tumor which is removed en bloc, exposing the attachment of the tumor. The dura is cauterized and internal decompression is performed. Once radical decompression is completed, the margins of the tumor can be mobilized into the cavity created in the center of the tumor. We generally remove the top of the tumor first, then open the canals and remove the lateral components, and then open below the superior intercavernous sinus and remove the bottom of the tumor. The closure is multilayer and has evolved at our institutions. We prefer a gasket seal closure in which an onlay of dural substitute or fascia lata is held in place with a rigid buttress of Medpore wedged into the bone defect [15, 16]. This construct is then covered with a nasoseptal flap and tissue sealant [17].

The Supraorbital Keyhole Craniotomy for Meningiomas

SKM is one of the minimally invasive techniques that can be utilized in the treatment of meningiomas. It has become increasingly popular due to its cosmetically appealing eyebrow (or eyelid) incisions and the ability to access the skull base through an incision on the forehead. It offers a corridor that can be used to treat most of the anterior cranial fossa meningiomas as well as parasellar ones [7]. It is usually used as a microscopic approach, but an endoscope can always be used to visualize and access areas which are otherwise hard to access with the microscope [5] (Fig. 7.3).

Fig. 7.3 The small size of the craniotomy in a supraorbital minicraniotomy approach

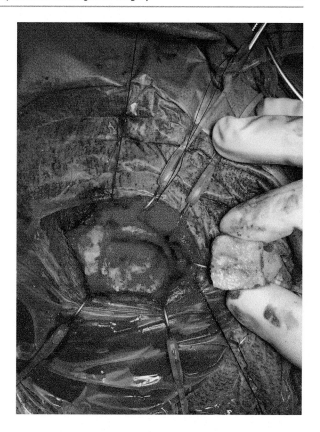

Indications, Contraindications, and Considerations

SKM offers the advantage of accessing neurovascular structures like the optic nerves and the chiasm and the ICAs from both a superior and an inferior perspective and is ideal for meningiomas that extend to superior or lateral to these structures. It can be performed with significantly reduced brain retraction when compared to traditional counterparts like the bicoronal or pterional approach [5, 7, 17].

SKM may not always provide the necessary maneuverability for midline meningiomas, especially if Simpson grade I resection is the surgical goal since it technically is hard to remove the tumor invading into the skull base at the midline especially at the level of the cribriform plate and crista galli. In addition, if a defect is created into the aerated nasal sinuses, it can be difficult to appreciate or repair [18]. Another limitation of SKM is limited visibility of the ipsilateral medial optic canal, although the contralateral medial optic canal is well-exposed [19].

Approach

The patient is placed in rigid head fixation and navigation is employed. Slight rotation and extension of the head is performed to facilitate the frontal lobe falling away from the skull base. An incision is made in the eyebrow in the direction of the follicles, and dissection is carried out through the orbicularis oculi muscle. A pericranial flap is raised. A single-piece craniotomy is performed, ideally including the orbital rim, from the keyhole to just medial to the supraorbital nerve. We prefer to remove the orbital rim to enlarge the working corridor and maximize upward visualization and facilitate exposure of the cribriform plate. Bony prominences on the roof of the orbit are flattened with high-speed drill. The dura is opened in a C-shape and reflected toward the orbit. CSF is drained either via a previously placed lumbar drain or through the subarachnoid opening until the brain is relaxed. The tumor is internally decompressed and sharply dissected off surrounding structures in a standard microsurgical fashion. Given the small opening, the most difficult aspect of the operation is the removal of the tumor deep in the cribriform plate and anterior along the crista galli in cases of olfactory groove meningiomas. To obtain adequate visualization of these areas, we may use endoscope assistance with a 45° endoscope. The base of the tumor has to be removed down to the bone. If a defect is anticipated, or if the tumor extends into the ethmoids, we prefer to combine the supraorbital keyhole approach with the endoscopic endonasal approach, so the defect can be patched from below, and a nasoseptal flap can be used [17].

The Transorbital Endoscopic Eyelid Approach for Meningiomas

The EEA together with SKA has achieved in proving a minimally invasive alternative to a variety of anterior skull base meningiomas except orbital and lateral sphenoid wing meningiomas that extended to anterior skull base, namely, spheno-orbital meningiomas, due to their lateral location [20] (Fig. 7.4). The lateral limit of the

Fig. 7.4 Hyperostosis of left lateral orbital wall and sphenoid bone from a spheno-orbital meningioma seen on 3D CT reconstruction

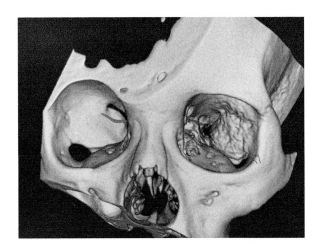

endoscopic endonasal approach has been the orbits, and the conventional open craniotomy techniques have been utilized to access these areas despite their cosmetic and functional disadvantages [21]. Gross total resection, with removal of the affected dura and drilling of the hyperostotic bone, might not be safely achieved in more than 50% of patients [22–24]. Progressive enlargement of those tumors is followed by compression of surrounding structures, such as the orbit, superior orbital fissure, optic canal, and cavernous sinus, which may lead to visual deterioration, disturbance of ocular movements, proptosis, and cosmetic alterations [22] (Fig. 7.5).

A variety of skull base approaches may be used for excision of those lesions, including the pterional, orbitozygomatic, and subfrontal approaches. Recently, a multiportal transorbital neuroendoscopic surgery (TONES) approach has been proposed as a new minimally invasive option to reach the lateral orbit and middle fossa [25, 26].

With the development of endoscopic techniques, the transorbital endoscopic approaches may replace a lateral craniotomy in selected cases. This selection should be based on symptom relief since gross total resection is often not achieved with ease with any of the approaches. Debulking of the hyperostosis and orbital decompression would be the primary goals of surgery, rather than complete tumor removal [20].

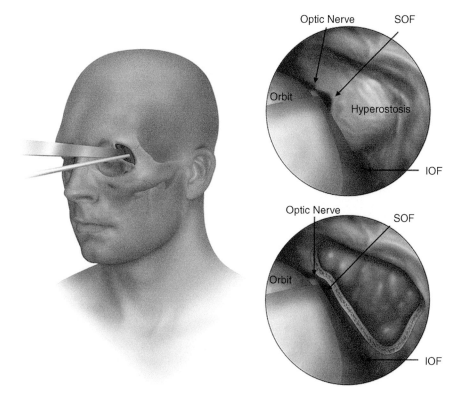

Fig. 7.5 Transorbital approach to spheno-orbital meningiomas [20]. ((C) Weill Cornell Medicine)

Indications, Contraindications, and Considerations

Spheno-orbital meningiomas that involve the lateral orbit are the typical indications in this tumor group. Like in other skull base approaches, concern for CSF exists as well as possibility of orbital damage, but so far there is not enough data for comparative analysis of these risks [20, 26, 27]. Like in other minimally invasive approaches, patient selection and balancing the surgical goals with the approach is of paramount importance.

Approach

After induction of general anesthesia, the patient is placed supine, and head is fixed after gentle elevation with a Mayfield head holder. A sterile protective corneal shield lubricated with ophthalmic ointment is placed in the eye. We employ oculoplastic to help with the initial aspects of the approach as well as the closure, but this is not required.

The orbicularis layer is opened after a superior eyelid approach along the length of the incision to expose the periosteum of the lateral orbital rim. The periorbita is elevated along the inner aspect of the lateral orbital rim using a freer elevator. The orbit may be protected by a silastic sheet. The hyperostotic bone of the orbit is exposed along the lateral orbit posteriorly to the level of the superior orbital fissure and superiorly under the anterior cranial fossa. CT image guidance is used to aid in identifying the orbital landmarks. Once adequate exposure is obtained, decompression of the hyperostotic bone and tumor removal are done using high-speed drills and Kerrison rongeurs. The medial landmarks were the superior and inferior orbital fissures. Any CSF leak can be closed with inlay and onlay of dural substitute. The relaxation of the orbit generally provides adequate pressure to prevent a CSF leak. The eyelid incision is closed using interrupted 6–0 nylon sutures [20].

Conclusion

Several minimally invasive approaches can be employed for removal of meningiomas, particularly those occurring along the anterior skull base. Patient selection is crucial in the successful application of these methods as well as surgeon's experience and proper instrumentation. When coupled with the right indication, an experienced minimally invasive neurosurgeon can achieve the expected oncologic results with minimal morbidity using one or a combination of these techniques.

References

1. Woodworth G, McCoul E, Anand V, Greenfiled J, Schwartz T. Endoscopic management of anterior cranial fossa meningiomas. Oper Tech Otolaryngol Head Neck Surg. 2011;22(4):254–62.
2. Patel SG, Singh B, Polluri A, Bridger PG, Cantu G, Cheesman AD, et al. Craniofacial surgery for malignant skull base tumors: report of an international collaborative study. Cancer. 2003;98(6):1179–87.

3. Origitano TC, Petruzzelli GJ, Leonetti JP, Vandevender D. Combined anterior and antero-lateral approaches to the cranial base: complication analysis, avoidance, and management. Neurosurgery. 2006;58(4 Suppl 2):ONS-327-36; discussion ONS-36-7.
4. Schwartz TH, Fraser JF, Brown S, Tabaee A, Kacker A, Anand VK. Endoscopic cranial base surgery: classification of operative approaches. Neurosurgery. 2008;62(5):991–1002; discussion -5.
5. Reisch R, Perneczky A, Filippi R. Surgical technique of the supraorbital key-hole craniotomy. Surg Neurol. 2003;59(3):223–7.
6. Khan O, Anand V, Raithatha R, Schwartz TH. Endoscopic surgery of the Sella and Suprasellar region. In: Sataloff RT, editor. Sataloff's comprehensive textbook of otolaryngology: head and neck surgery. New Delhi: Jaypee Brothers Medical Pub; 2016.
7. Ottenhausen M, Rumalla K, Alalade AF, Nair P, La Corte E, Younus I, et al. Decision-making algorithm for minimally invasive approaches to anterior skull base meningiomas. Neurosurg Focus. 2018;44(4):E7.
8. Schaberg MR, Anand VK, Schwartz TH, Cobb W. Microscopic versus endoscopic transnasal pituitary surgery. Curr Opin Otolaryngol Head Neck Surg. 2010;18(1):8–14.
9. Shetty SR, Ruiz-Treviño AS, Omay SB, Almeida JP, Liang B, Chen YN, et al. Limitations of the endonasal endoscopic approach in treating olfactory groove meningiomas. A systematic review. Acta Neurochir. 2017;159(10):1875–85.
10. Komotar RJ, Starke RM, Raper DM, Anand VK, Schwartz TH. Endoscopic endonasal versus open transcranial resection of anterior midline skull base meningiomas. World Neurosurg. 2012;77(5–6):713–24.
11. Silva D, Attia M, Kandasamy J, Alimi M, Anand VK, Schwartz TH. Endoscopic endonasal transsphenoidal "above and below" approach to the retroinfundibular area and interpeduncular cistern--cadaveric study and case illustrations. World Neurosurg. 2014;81(2):374–84.
12. Schwartz TH, Anand VK. The endoscopic endonasal transsphenoidal approach to the suprasellar cistern. Clin Neurosurg. 2007;54:226–35.
13. Khan OH, Anand VK, Schwartz TH. Endoscopic endonasal resection of skull base meningiomas: the significance of a "cortical cuff" and brain edema compared with careful case selection and surgical experience in predicting morbidity and extent of resection. Neurosurg Focus. 2014;37(4):E7.
14. Schwartz TH, Anand VJ. Endonasal transplanum approach to the anterior cranial fossa. In: Snyderman C, Gardner P, editors. Master techniques in otolaryngology-head and neck surgery. Philadelphia: LWW; 2014.
15. Leng LZ, Brown S, Anand VK, Schwartz TH. "Gasket-seal" watertight closure in minimal-access endoscopic cranial base surgery. Neurosurgery. 2008;62(5 Suppl 2):ONSE342-3; discussion ONSE3.
16. Garcia-Navarro V, Anand VK, Schwartz TH. Gasket seal closure for extended endonasal endoscopic skull base surgery: efficacy in a large case series. World Neurosurg. 2013;80(5):563–8.
17. Banu MA, Mehta A, Ottenhausen M, Fraser JF, Patel KS, Szentirmai O, et al. Endoscope-assisted endonasal versus supraorbital keyhole resection of olfactory groove meningiomas: comparison and combination of 2 minimally invasive approaches. J Neurosurg. 2016;124(3):605–20.
18. Borghei-Razavi H, Truong HQ, Fernandes-Cabral DT, Celtikci E, Chabot JD, Stefko ST, et al. Minimally invasive approaches for anterior skull base meningiomas: supraorbital eyebrow, endoscopic endonasal, or a combination of both? Anatomic study, limitations, and surgical application. World Neurosurg. 2018;112:e666–e74.
19. Singh H, Essayed WI, Jada A, Moussazadeh N, Dhandapani S, Rote S, et al. Contralateral supraorbital keyhole approach to medial optic nerve lesions: an anatomoclinical study. J Neurosurg. 2017;126(3):940–4.
20. Almeida JP, Omay SB, Shetty SR, Chen YN, Ruiz-Treviño AS, Liang B, et al. Transorbital endoscopic eyelid approach for resection of sphenoorbital meningiomas with predominant hyperostosis: report of 2 cases. J Neurosurg. 2018;128(6):1885–95.
21. Altay T, Patel BC, Couldwell WT. Lateral orbital wall approach to the cavernous sinus. J Neurosurg. 2012;116(4):755–63.
22. Oya S, Sade B, Lee JH. Sphenoorbital meningioma: surgical technique and outcome. J Neurosurg. 2011;114(5):1241–9.

23. Ringel F, Cedzich C, Schramm J. Microsurgical technique and results of a series of 63 spheno-orbital meningiomas. Neurosurgery. 2007;60(4 Suppl 2):214–21; discussion 21–2.
24. Moe KS, Bergeron CM, Ellenbogen RG. Transorbital neuroendoscopic surgery. Neurosurgery. 2010;67(3 Suppl Operative):ons16–28.
25. Ramakrishna R, Kim LJ, Bly RA, Moe K, Ferreira M Jr. Transorbital neuroendoscopic surgery for the treatment of skull base lesions. J Clin Neurosci. 2016;24:99–104.
26. Dallan I, Castelnuovo P, Locatelli D, Turri-Zanoni M, AlQahtani A, Battaglia P, et al. Multiportal combined transorbital transnasal endoscopic approach for the management of selected skull base lesions: preliminary experience. World Neurosurg. 2015;84(1):97–107.
27. Bly RA, Morton RP, Kim LJ, Moe KS. Tension pneumocephalus after endoscopic sinus surgery: a technical report of multiportal endoscopic skull base repair. Otolaryngol Head Neck Surg. 2014;151(6):1081–3.

Comprehensive Treatment Strategies for Spinal Meningiomas

8

Robert J. Rothrock, Ori Barzilai, Yoshiya (Josh) Yamada, and Mark H. Bilsky

Key Points

1. Spinal meningioma is classically a WHO grade I psammomatous meningioma presenting in an elderly female in the thoracic spine.
2. Observation is a valid management strategy in an asymptomatic patient with an incidentally discovered, non-compressive tumor.
3. The goal of surgery is gross total resection along with the dural attachment (Simpson grade I) or gross total resection with cauterization of the dural attachment (Simpson grade II).
4. Stereotactic radiosurgery provides durable local control as both adjuvant and salvage therapies.
5. Rates of recurrence are directly related to both WHO grade and the initial extent of resection (EOR).

Introduction

Spinal meningiomas are the second most common intradural extramedullary tumor and are commonly encountered in neurosurgical practice. In the era of widespread access to magnetic resonance imaging (MRI), these tumors can be encountered incidentally, leaving patients and referring providers anxious for treatment recommendations. This chapter will systematically address considerations for diagnosis and management of spinal meningioma.

R. J. Rothrock · O. Barzilai · M. H. Bilsky (✉)
Department of Neurosurgery, Memorial Sloan-Kettering Cancer Center, New York, NY, USA
e-mail: bilskym@mskcc.org

Y. (J.) Yamada
Department of Radiation Oncology, Memorial Sloan-Kettering Cancer Center, New York, NY, USA

© Springer Nature Switzerland AG 2020
J. Moliterno, A. Omuro (eds.), *Meningiomas*,
https://doi.org/10.1007/978-3-030-59558-6_8

Part I:Epidemiology, Pathology, and Diagnosis of Spinal Meningioma

Epidemiology

Although seen routinely in neurosurgical practice, spinal meningioma is a rare clinical entity. The incidence of intradural extramedullary spinal tumors is estimated to be 0.74 in 100,000 person-years [1]. Spinal meningiomas are thought to represent approximately 12% of overall meningiomas and account for 40–45% of all benign intradural extramedullary tumors [1, 2]. Similar to intracranial meningiomas, the female to male ratio is 3:1 [3] with a peak incidence in the sixth and seventh decades [2]. Although more common in women, male sex has been associated with a higher rate of recurrence of spinal meningioma following surgery [4].

Risk factors for spinal meningioma include prior radiation exposure as well as syndromic predisposition, such as neurofibromatosis type 2 (NF2) [5, 6]. Patients with these risk factors tend to present with spinal meningiomas at a younger age [4]. Spinal meningiomas have a predilection for the thoracic spine, but have been described in all areas of the spine, including cervical, lumbar, and sacral [7, 8].

Histology and Pathophysiology

Meningiomas are thought to arise from arachnoid cap cells, which form the outer layer of the arachnoid, and facilitate the drainage of cerebrospinal fluid (CSF) into dural sinuses and veins [9]. This hypothesis arose from the observation that normal arachnoidal cap cell clusters in older patients can form whorls and psammoma bodies identical to those found in meningiomas. However, the cell of origin for meningiomas has not been clearly defined. Others have proposed the possibility of fibroblastic origin, having to do with the mesodermal features observed in these tumors, and that they have sometimes arisen independently from dural attachment [10]. Meningiomas display both mesenchymal and epithelial-like features, which help establish diagnosis [9].

Several stereotypic genetic alterations have been identified within spinal meningioma, but few have altered clinical practice. The most common is loss of heterozygosity of the 22q12.2 chromosomal region of the neurofibromatosis type 2 (NF2) gene, which can be found in 40 to 70% of sporadic meningioma as well as most NF2-associated meningiomas [9, 11]. Other chromosomally related genes that have been implicated include the beta-adaptin BAM22 gene and the tissue inhibitor of metalloproteinase 3 (TIMP3) gene [12, 13]. Additional genes have been associated with progression from low- to higher-grade meningioma, such as the 4.1 family member *DAL1* and the tumor suppressor in Lung Cancer-1 (*TSLC1*) gene [14, 15].

The World Health Organization defines three grades of meningioma and a far greater number of histologically distinct morphologies [16]. Classically, the psammomatous subtype is the most common spinal meningioma, usually thoracic in location and predominantly observed in elderly female patients. Psammomatous meningiomas express bone-related proteins, such as osteopontin, which are thought to contribute to their relatively high degree of calcification [17]. Conversely, clear cell meningiomas are found in younger patients and also predominantly thoracic in location [18]. Although they are histologically low grade, they are clinically more aggressive with higher rates of recurrence.

For the surgeon, the most important histopathological distinction remains grade I versus grade II/III tumors, the latter of which exhibit cellular atypia, pial invasion, and more aggressive clinical behavior (i.e., recurrence and local invasion) [19]. Like their intracranial counterparts, spinal meningiomas are most commonly WHO grade I, but can also be atypical (WHO grade II/III). WHO grade III meningiomas, i.e., anaplastic meningioma, are differentiated by 20 or more mitoses per 10 high-power fields or the presence of frank anaplasia – defined as carcinoma-, melanoma-, or sarcoma-like histology [9].

Within grade I spinal tumors, the presence of a clear dural tail on preoperative imaging has been associated with high-grade transformation and invasive, recurrent behavior [20]. WHO grade on initial pathology correlates with recurrence rates, with WHO grade I spinal meningioma undergoing a Simpson grade I or II resection demonstrating 0% recurrence at 10 years in one series [21]. In addition, given the indolent course of WHO grade I tumors, even with recurrence, symptoms typically develop slowly [22].

Imaging

Magnetic resonance imaging (MRI) is the preferred diagnostic imaging modality for spinal meningioma [23]. Diagnostic consideration is raised with the presence of an intradural extramedullary lesion. Spinal meningiomas are 90% intradural extramedullary lesions, with only 10% manifesting either extradural or dumbbell (intradural/extradural) in location [24]. Partial or complete calcification is highly suggestive of meningioma, but is only seen in approximately 5% of cases [25, 26]. MRI characteristically reveals avid enhancement with administration of gadolinium contrast. In addition, meningiomas are more specifically hypo- or isointense on T2-weighted imaging compared to schwannomas, which are typically hyperintense [27].

Although the presence of a dural origin or tail to a lesion is specific to meningioma, this is observed less frequently than in intracranial meningioma [23]. Common to all meningiomas, the blood supply is usually localized to the dural origin of the lesion. Large meningiomas may demonstrate significant intratumoral vasculature. Although rare, meningiomas may be fully extradural or even intramedullary [28, 29]. In one case in our institutional series, a primary meningioma was resected in the extrapleural space over 6 cm from the closest dural margin.

Computed tomography (CT) can be a useful adjunct to delineate the degree of tumoral calcification or remodeling of local bony structures, both of which can be suggestive of a diagnosis of meningioma [30]. CT can also be used to assess bone quality in patients who will require spinal instrumentation as an element of surgery.

Spinal angiography can be utilized in cases of hypervascular tumors as suggested by MRI, both to visualize the main vascular supply and to perform preoperative embolization [31]. For lower thoracic tumors, spinal angiography may be important for determining the origin of the artery of Adamkiewicz, which is the dominant radiculomedullary feeding artery. This vessel commonly originates on the left side at T9 or T10, in 75% and 50% of cases, respectively; however, the location is variable [32]. Sacrifice of the artery of Adamkiewicz can be neurologically devastating to a patient, but alterations can be made to a surgical approach if the origin is determined preoperatively.

Terminology for Spinal Meningioma

The Simpson grade of resection describes the amount of residual tumor left after surgery [33]. Simpson grade I describes complete resection of the meningioma as well as its dural attachment. Grade II describes gross total resection of the meningioma with coagulation of the dural attachment. Grade III refers to gross total resection of tumor without coagulation of the dural attachment or any extradural component. Grade IV refers to subtotal tumor resection, and grade V is a biopsy or simple decompression surgery. The clinical importance of the Simpson grade for the purpose of intracranial neurosurgery is the direct correlation with rates of tumor recurrence if residual tumor is left behind [34]. Unlike the case of intracranial convexity meningiomas, it is often not feasible to obtain a Simpson grade I resection of a spinal meningioma given the high morbidity resulting from spinal CSF leak, which is more complicated with dural resection. Thus, Simpson grade II resection is often the primary surgical goal [21].

The McCormick grade describes the level of functional impairment from intradural tumor-associated myelopathy [35]. Originally developed in reference to spinal intramedullary ependymoma, this scale is now utilized for many intradural tumor studies. McCormick grade I refers to a neurologically "normal" patient with unimpaired and independent gait allowing for mild spasticity or reflexes on exam. Grade II describes functionally independent gait in the presence of focal neurologic deficit or mild difficulty with balance (also severe pain). Grade III requires a cane or assistive device for ambulation with more severe neurologic deficit and/or bilateral upper extremity impairment. Grade IV describes a severely disabled patient who requires a wheelchair for mobility and with a severe/dense neurologic deficit.

Natural History of Spinal Meningioma

Defining the natural history of spinal meningioma has become more feasible with increasing use of MRI imaging and incidental discovery of clinically silent intradural extramedullary tumors [36]. While it can be difficult to determine the histopathology of a tumor simply from imaging, the presence of a clear dural tail on MRI reliably denotes a spinal meningioma [27, 37]. Interestingly, some studies have shown a higher growth rate for meningioma versus schwannoma over 5-year serial imaging follow-up [38]. Even with tumoral growth, however, there is no assurance that a relatively slow-growing spinal meningioma will become symptomatic. For those lesions that do become symptomatic in the presence of serial imaging and history, surgery is offered more promptly, especially with clinical deterioration.

Differential Diagnosis

The main differential diagnosis for an intradural extramedullary lesion on seen on MRI includes schwannoma, meningioma, neurofibroma, solitary fibrous tumor/hemangiopericytoma, malignant peripheral nerve sheath tumor, leptomeningeal metastasis (solid or hematopoietic), as well as paraganglioma and myxopapillary ependymoma depending on location [39]. In the absence of a history of cancer or a multisystemic syndrome, the main considerations are schwannoma, meningioma, and neurofibroma, with the first two being the more common. As described earlier, the presence of a dural tail or calcification is considered more specific for meningioma. Since both schwannoma and meningioma tend to avidly enhance with gadolinium, T2-weighted imaging is considered to be a differentiating factor, with hypointensity favoring meningioma. Using this method, however, only yields 80% sensitivity and 75% specificity [27]. In cases where both schwannoma and meningioma are considerations, operative planning should account for both scenarios. Intraoperative findings often help differentiate the two entities, but histopathology is the gold standard for final diagnosis.

In patients presenting with suspected spinal meningioma at a young age, a diagnosis of NF2 should be considered, especially if multiple lesions are seen on MRI and without the stigmata of NF1 (which may instead favor multiple schwannoma/neurofibroma). Multiple intradural extramedullary lesions should also raise consideration for schwannomatosis, which is more common in persons of Japanese and Ashkenazi Jewish descent [40]. Discovery of multiple lesions should also prompt imaging of the entire neuraxis.

Part II: Management of Spinal Meningioma

Management of a suspected spinal meningioma is often dependent on the manner of discovery. Incidental lesions are usually managed expectantly with serial imaging, whereas lesions presenting with a neurologic deficit or severe biologic pain are typically operated at presentation.

Observation

With the increased use of CT and MRI, many intradural extramedullary lesions are incidentally discovered. Unlike intracranial meningiomas, spinal tumors do not usually penetrate the pia and do not result in spinal cord edema by direct invasion. Intramedullary spinal cord edema results from the compressive effects of the tumor and may not be manifest radiographically until the tumor is resected [41]. Whereas relatively small intracranial meningiomas can cause significant vasogenic edema (and become symptomatic), spinal meningiomas become symptomatic once they exhibit mass effect directly on the neural elements. For incidentally discovered suspected meningiomas, clinical and radiographic observation with serial visits and MRI is often the best management strategy. Even if growing on serial imaging, consideration must be given to the patient's age, comorbidities, and the relative size of the tumor if he or she is asymptomatic.

Surgical Indications

Surgical resection is indicated in patients with a progressive neurologic deficit, unremitting biologic pain or radiculopathy directly attributable to the tumor, or progressive growth on serial imaging with radiographic spinal cord compression. Biologic pain describes inflammatory pain directly caused by the tumor, as opposed to mechanical pain which is caused by spinal instability. Biologic pain from a spinal tumor usually occurs at night when the body's endogenous steroid production is at its lowest. Similarly, biologic pain improves with the administration of exogenous steroids [42].

Surgery is not performed for diagnosis alone, given that the main differential considerations are also benign. One notable exception is in the case of a conus medullaris or filum terminale tumor in which myxopapillary ependymoma is a consideration. In this case there is a risk of tumor leptomeningeal seeding with delayed intervention [43]. Progressive neurologic deficit is usually in the form of clinical myelopathy for cervical or thoracic tumors and multi-nerve distribution radiculopathy in the case of lumbar tumors. Because meningiomas are slow-growing tumors, they are extremely unlikely to present with an acute compression syndrome and require emergent surgery.

Surgical Goals

The goal of surgery is gross total resection if feasible (Simpson grade I), but at least Simpson grade II resection, given the durable low rates of recurrence with these results. In cases of ventral tumor where gross total resection is not safely achievable, small amounts of tumor should be left rather than cause a new or worsened neurologic deficit. Residual tumor can be observed and treated with stereotactic radiation if interval growth is seen.

Surgical Approach and Considerations

The surgical approach is determined by the location of the tumor. A posterior laminectomy or posterolateral approach can be employed for virtually all spinal meningiomas. Ventrally located cervical tumors are a category where some authors have advocated for resection using an anterior approach via a vertebrectomy [44]. Even though direct visualization of the tumor may be easier via an anterior approach, primary dural closure and reconstruction of dural defects is extremely difficult. Despite potential benefits, this approach is rarely indicated. Recently, some authors have advocated for the use of minimal access surgery, including tubular retractor systems, especially in patients presenting at an advanced age [45]. The potential advantages include decreased muscle dissection and a better, watertight fascial closure. At present, this approach has not been widely adopted for meningiomas, but remains an area of active investigation in select centers.

Resection Techniques

Localization of the tumor is critically important. If available, intraoperative CT is a reliable localization technique. In the absence of this modality, the lumbar and cervical spine levels can typically be imaged with cross-table lateral plain radiographs or fluoroscopy. Thoracic tumors can be reliably localized using an anterior-posterior (AP) fluoroscopic image with a marker that lines up with the rib and pedicle at the level of interest. The correct level is identified counting from either the T1 or T12 ribs.

Following exposure and radiographic confirmation of the level, laminectomy is performed with a high-speed drill using a 3 mm matchstick or diamond burr and 2 mm Kerrison Rongeur. Rarely, a posterolateral resection (i.e., laminectomy with unilateral facetectomy and pedicle resection) is required for exposure. Intraoperative ultrasound is used to ensure that the laminectomy has encompassed the superior and inferior extent of the tumor. All bone edges are waxed, and a hemostatic agent is placed in the lateral gutters.

At this point, the operating microscope or alternatively the exoscope is employed for dural opening and tumor resection. The durotomy is created with a 15 blade over a Woodson dental tool used to protect the intradural neural elements and tacked back with dural sutures. The dural opening is typically straightforward with the exception of calcified meningiomas. The calcified component can be dissected from the dura using micro-instruments, such as Rhoton 2 and 6 dissectors. Bisecting the dural calcification with a 1 mm side cutting or diamond drill bit allows for the safe removal of the tumor while preserving the dura and preventing spinal cord injury [46]. The soft tissue component of the meningioma is often deep to the calcified mass, providing a safe margin of resection.

Following dural opening, the arachnoid is opened sharply, and the tumor is explored to define the interface with the spinal cord. WHO grade I spinal meningiomas rarely violate the pia providing a plane of dissection. Defining the spinal cord margin is considerably more difficult in grade II/III meningioma, which may be invasive into the spinal cord. For ventrally located cervical and thoracic meningiomas with limited exposure, the dentate ligament may be sectioned to allow for slight rotation of the spinal cord during resection. This can be accomplished with 7-0 Prolene stitches placed through the dentate ligament and secured to the contralateral dura with a small vascular clip.

Safe resection is facilitated by intratumoral debulking using an ultrasonic aspirator and sharp resection. The tumor is dissected from the ventral spinal cord using Rhoton 2 and 6 instruments. Following decompression of the spinal cord, the meningioma is resected off the dural attachment using sharp dissection. This margin may be hypervascular, and bipolar cautery is used for hemostasis. Typically, the inner layer of the dura is resected with an 11 blade, and the dura is bipolar-cauterized to achieve a Simpson grade II resection. In some centers, the dura is resected to achieve a Simpson grade I resection.

Dural closure is accomplished with a 4-0 Surgilon or Prolene running suture. For cases in which dural resection is undertaken, reconstruction may best be accomplished with Dura-Guard (Baxter International, Minnesota) using a running 4-0 Surgilon stitch. Dura-Guard is a bovine pericardial patch graft that sews water tight and, in our experience, has little infection risk even when abutting contaminated spaces. Following dural closure, thrombin glue and gel foam are placed over the dura. A subfascial Jackson-Pratt drain is left in place to bulb suction for 24 h. The wound is closed in multiple layers to obliterate the dead space. The paraspinal muscles are closed with 2-0 Vicryls followed by a running 0 PDS in the fascia. The subcutaneous tissue is closed with 0 Vicryls and a 3-0 Monocryl running subcuticular stitch and a 3-0 Nylon running stitch for the skin (Fig. 8.1).

Immediate Postoperative Management

Several postoperative management issues require special attention. For 24 h, the head of bed (HOB) is raised no higher than 30 degrees to provide time for reconstitution of CSF. After 24 h, the HOB is slowly elevated, and patients are evaluated for headaches associated with intracranial hypotension. If headaches occur, the HOB is returned flat, and a more graduated head elevation is pursued. For persistent headaches in the absence of a known CSF leak, patients are placed on Fioricet and encouraged to ambulate. The subfascial Jackson-Pratt drain is kept on bulb suction for 24 h while the head of bed is low and then taken off suction and left in place for an additional 72 h.

Typically, patients are started on Decadron 3 days prior to surgery to reduce inflammation associated with the tumor and to provide neural protection. Postoperatively, patients are placed on 6 mg Decadron 4 times a day. A rapid taper is performed every other day until 2 mg Decadron daily is achieved. At this time, 2 mg daily is continued for 5 days to prevent the sequelae of chemical meningitis.

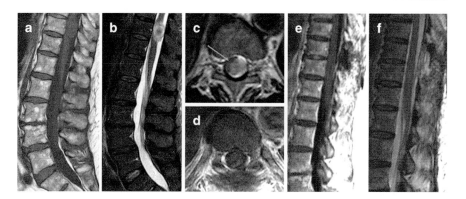

Fig. 8.1 A 65-year-old female presenting with worsening ataxic gait and leg buckling. (**a**) T1-weighted MRI demonstrates a large isointense intradural extramedullary mass at T11. (**b**) STIR MRI demonstrates heterogeneous signal intradural extramedullary mass at T11. (**c**) Axial T2 demonstrates 90% canal compromise with high-grade cord compression. Green arrow highlights crescentic-appearing compressed spinal cord. Preoperative differential diagnosis included meningioma and schwannoma (tumor appeared to extend toward left T11–T12 foramen). Patient underwent bilateral T10 to T11 midline laminectomy and intradural tumor resection with Simpson grade I resection. Final pathology was WHO grade I meningioma. (**d**) Postoperative axial T1 postcontrast MRI demonstrates gross total resection. (**e, f**) Postoperative sagittal T1 post-contrast and T2-weighted MRI demonstrate gross total resection of tumor and re-expansion of the spinal cord. The patient's gait improved postoperatively, and she returned to work 3 months following surgery

Instrumentation

The use of spinal instrumentation is rarely required, but is increasingly being used for specific indications. Instrumentation is not commonly required for lumbar and mid-thoracic tumor resection. There is evidence for the use of instrumentation for multilevel cervical laminectomies, laminectomies performed at the cervicothoracic or thoracolumbar junctions, or laminectomies performed across the thoracic apex to decrease risk of delayed spinal deformity [47, 48]. In cases of laterally located tumors, resection of the facet joint or a portion of the pedicle may be required to adequately visualize the tumor resection, and in these cases spinal instrumentation is recommended [49]. In the case of multilevel cervical exposure without violation of the facet joints, laminoplasty is an option [50]. Laminoplasty is likely effective in preventing development of delayed spinal deformity, but importantly is likely not effective in treating an already present spinal deformity in the context of intradural tumor resection [51].

Surgical Adjuvants

Intraoperative neurophysiologic monitoring (IOM) is often used as an adjuvant in the resection of intradural extramedullary tumors, including somatosensory evoked potentials (SSEP), electromyography (EMG), and motor evoked potentials (MEPs).

Epidural D-wave monitoring is not routinely employed in our center for these tumor types. MEPs are useful in avoiding iatrogenic injury if rotation of the spinal cord via the dentate ligaments is necessary for tumor resection. Intraoperative corrections to blood pressure and hypothermia can be made to address changes in MEP's that may not be specifically related to manipulation of the spinal cord, but may improve neurologic outcomes. Changes in IOM, most importantly loss of MEPs, might influence a surgeon to leave behind residual tumor in favor of avoiding potential iatrogenic injury during resection [52, 53].

Role of Radiation/Radiosurgery

Stereotactic body radiation therapy (SBRT) also known as stereotactic radiosurgery (SRS) has been described as initial therapy, adjuvant therapy, and salvage therapy for spinal meningioma [54]. In the case of meningioma, upfront radiosurgery is usually not the preferred treatment, given that small, non-compressive lesions are typically observed and larger symptomatic lesions should be resected. SRS can be considered as upfront treatment in patients who have major medical contraindications to open surgery. In addition, ideally, a 2–3 mm margin between tumor and spinal cord is required for an effective tumoricidal dose of radiation to the tumor [55]. Thus, SBRT is well suited to patients who have already undergone surgical resection and who are more likely to have a safe margin. Definitive SBRT dose is considered 21 Gy delivered in 3 fractions [56]. Local 5-year control rates with SBRT for intradural tumors, including meningiomas, are reported from 70% to 100% [56].

Adjuvant SBRT or radiation therapy is considered when a significant amount of tumor is knowingly left at the time of surgery (i.e., Simpson grade III or higher). Adjuvant radiation is also considered in cases of WHO grade II or III meningioma, given the more aggressive clinical behavior and rates of recurrence [57]. As mentioned previously, SBRT is also used for salvage treatment in the case of recurrent tumor on serial imaging (Fig. 8.2).

Image-modulated radiation therapy (IMRT) and conventional fractionated radiation therapy have also been used in the treatment of spinal meningioma, but SBRT is the current preferred modality [58].

Chemotherapy

Chemotherapy is not commonly employed for treatment of spinal meningioma. In cases of invasive, atypical meningioma (WHO III), multiple agents have been employed including hydroxyurea, interferon α-2B, long-acting Sandostatin, and even multidrug sarcoma protocols [59]. Chemotherapy is used for salvage therapy in cases of highly aggressive tumors.

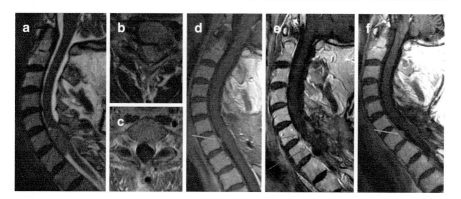

Fig. 8.2 A 58-year-old male presenting with neck pain, worst at night, without clinical myelopathy (biologic pain). (**a**) T2-weighted MRI demonstrating a large isointense intradural extramedullary mass at C6–C7. (**b**) Axial T2 demonstrates 90% canal compromise with high-grade cord compression. Patient underwent bilateral C6 to T1 midline laminectomy and intradural tumor resection with Simpson grade II resection (ventral dural base coagulated). Final pathology was WHO grade I meningioma. (**c, d**) Postoperative T1 post-contrast MRI demonstrates small known residual ventral dural attachment tumor. (**e**) Follow-up T1 post-contrast MRI at 1 year demonstrates recurrent/progressive tumor. Patient was treated with conventional fractionated radiation (54 Gy in 30 fractions). (**f**) Follow-up T1 post-contrast MRI 3 years after radiation shows durable local control with decrease in previously seen tumor volume. The patient remained neurologically intact at 5-year follow up

Part III: Outcomes for Spinal Meningioma

Surgical Outcomes

Surgical outcomes in patients undergoing resection of spinal meningioma are favorable, especially with Simpson grade I or II resection. Nakamura et al. reported a consecutive series of 43 patients who underwent Simpson grade I resection of spinal meningioma with 12.1-year follow-up, at which time 0 patients had tumor recurrence [20]. Of 19 patients who had grade II resection, 6 patients (30%) had recurrence at 12-year follow-up. All patients with grade II resection had a ventral tumor location at initial surgery. Overall tumor recurrence at 12 years combining both Simpson grade I and II resection patients was 9.7% In a review of the literature combining 581 cases, Gottfried et al. reported postoperative clinical improvement of McCormick grade in 53% to 95% of patients following surgery for spinal meningioma [2]. Perioperative mortality was low (0–3%) as were rates of CSF leakage (0–4%).

Recurrence

As discussed earlier, rates of recurrence are low with Simpson grade I resection, but are more significant with Simpson grade II resection and higher (i.e., residual tumor at time of surgery). A relatively high percentage (45%) of recurrent spinal meningioma are not fully resectable, due either to tumor invasion or to scar tissue at the site of previous resection, favoring treatment with radiation therapy [7]. In patients without direct compressive symptoms from recurrence, we advocate for SBRT as the salvage treatment of choice in the setting of recurrent spinal meningioma. SBRT has durable high rates of local control in the setting of spinal meningioma [54].

Conclusion

Spinal meningiomas frequently present in elderly patients, in whom surgical intervention can have broader implications. Observation should be utilized when appropriate. Surgical treatment should be definitive, with a goal of gross total resection. In cases where full resection cannot be safely achieved, stereotactic radiosurgery can offer high rates of local control.

References

1. Schellinger KA, Propp JM, Villano JL, McCarthy BJ. Descriptive epidemiology of primary spinal cord tumors. J Neuro-Oncol. 2008;87(2):173–9.
2. Gottfried ON, Gluf W, Quinones-Hinojosa A, Kan P, Schmidt MH. Spinal meningiomas: surgical management and outcome. Neurosurg Focus. 2003;14(6):e2.
3. Preston-Martin S. Descriptive epidemiology of primary tumors of the spinal cord and spinal meninges in Los Angeles County, 1972–1985. Neuroepidemiology. 1990;9:106–11.
4. Maiti TK, Bir SC, Patra DP, Kalakoti P, Guthikonda B, Nanda A. Spinal meningiomas: clinicoradiological factors predicting recurrence and functional outcome. Neurosurg Focus. 2016;41(2):E6. https://doi.org/10.3171/2016.5.FOCUS16163.
5. Kok JL, Teepen JC, van Leeuwen FE, Tissing WJE, Neggers SJ, van der Pal HJ; DCOG-LATER Study Group, et al. Risk of benign meningioma after childhood cancer in the DCOG-LATER cohort: contributions of radiation dose, exposed cranial volume, and age. Neuro Oncol. 2018. https://doi.org/10.1093/neuonc/noy124.
6. Campian J, Gutmann DH. CNS tumors in Neurofibromatosis. J Clin Oncol. 2017;35(21):2378–85. https://doi.org/10.1200/JCO.2016.71.7199.
7. Solero CL, Fornari M, Giombini S, Lasio G, Oliveri G, Cimino C, Pluchino F. Spinal meningiomas: review of 174 operated cases. Neurosurgery. 1989;25(2):153–60.
8. Roux FX, Nataf F, Pinaudeau M, Borne G, Devaux B, Meder JF. Intraspinal meningiomas: review of 54 cases with discussion of poor prognosis factors and modern therapeutic management. Surg Neurol. 1996;46(5):458–63; discussion 463–4.
9. Mawrin C, Perry A. Pathological classification and molecular genetics of meningiomas. J Neuro-Oncol. 2010;99:379–91.
10. Ng THK, Chan KH, Mann KS, Fung CF. Spinal meningioma arising from a lumbar nerve root. J Neurosurg. 1989;70:646–8.

11. Ruttledge MH, Sarrazin J, Rangaratnam S, Phelan CM, Twist E, Merel P, et al. Evidence for the complete inactivation of the NF2 gene in the majority of sporadic meningiomas. Nat Genet. 1994;6(2):180–4.
12. Barski D, Wolter M, Reifenberger G, Riemenschneider MJ. Hypermethylation and transcriptional downregulation of the TIMP3 gene is associated with allelic loss on 22q12.3 and malignancy in meningiomas. Brain Pathol. 2010;20:623–31.
13. Peyrard M, Fransson I, Xie Y-G, Han F-Y, Ruttledge MH, Swahn S, et al. Characterization of a new member of the human /−adaptin gene family from chromosome 22q12, a candidate meningioma gene. Human Mol Genet. 1994;3:1393–9.
14. Nunes F, Shen Y, Niida Y, Beauchamp R, Stemmer-Rachamimov AO, Ramesh V, et al. Inactivation patterns of NF2 and DAL-1/4.1B (EPB41L3) in sporadic meningioma. Cancer Genet Cytogenet. 2005;162(2):135–9.
15. Surace EI, Lusis E, Murakami Y, Scheithauer BW, Perry A, Gutmann DH. Loss of tumor suppressor in lung cancer-1 (TSLC1) expression in meningioma correlates with increased malignancy grade and reduced patient survival. J Neuropathol Exp Neurol. 2004;63(10):1015–27.
16. Louis DN, Perry A, Reifenberger G, von Deimling A, Figarella-Branger D, Cavenee WK, et al. The 2016 World Health Organization classification of tumors of the central nervous system: a summary. Acta Neuropathol. 2016;131(6):803–20. https://doi.org/10.1007/s00401-016-1545-1.
17. Hirota S, Nakajima Y, Yoshimine T, Kohri K, Nomura S, Taneda M, et al. Expression of bone-related protein messenger RNA in human meningiomas: possible involvement of osteopontin in development of psammoma bodies. J Neuropathol Exp Neurol. 1995;54(5):698–703.
18. Colen CB, Rayes M, McClendon J Jr, Rabah R, Ham SD. Pediatric spinal clear cell meningioma. Case report. J Neurosurg Pediatr. 2009;3:57–60.
19. Harter PN, Braun Y, Plate KH. Classification of meningiomas—advances and controversies. Chin Clin Oncol. 2017;6(Suppl 1):S2. https://doi.org/10.21037/cco.2017.05.02.
20. Nakamura M, Tsuji O, Fujiyoshi K, Hosogane N, Watanabe K, Tsuji T, et al. Long-term surgical outcomes of spinal meningiomas. Spine (Phila Pa 1976). 2012;37(10):E617–23. https://doi.org/10.1097/BRS.0b013e31824167f1.
21. Setzer M, Vatter H, Marquardt G, Seifert V, Vrionis FD. Management of spinal meningiomas: surgical results and a review of the literature. Neurosurg Focus. 2007;23(4):E14.
22. Tsuda K, Akutsu H, Yamamoto T, Nakai K, Ishikawa E, Matsumura A. Is Simpson grade I removal necessary in all cases of spinal meningioma? Assessment of postoperative recurrence during long-term follow-up. Neurol Med Chir (Tokyo). 2014;54(11):907–13.
23. Abul-Kasim K, Thurnher MM, McKeever P, Sundgren PC. Intradural spinal tumors: current classification and MRI features. Neuroradiology. 2008;50:301–14.
24. Sevick RJ. Diagnostic neuroradiology. 1994. First Edition. By Anne G. Osborn. Published by Mosby-Year Book, Inc. 936 pages. Can J Neurol Sci. 1995;22:78.
25. Doita M, Harada T, Nishida K, Marui T, Kurosaka M, Yoshiya S. Recurrent calcified spinal meningioma detected by plain radiograph. Spine (Phila Pa 1976). 2001;26(11):E249–52.
26. Zhu Q, Qian M, Xiao J, Wu Z, Wang Y, Zhang J. Myelopathy due to calcified meningiomas of the thoracic spine: minimum 3-year follow-up after surgical treatment. J Neurosurg Spine. 2013;18(5):436–42. https://doi.org/10.3171/2013.2.SPINE12609.
27. Takashima H, Takebayashi T, Yoshimoto M, Onodera M, Terashima Y, Iesato N, Tanimoto K, et al. Differentiating spinal intradural-extramedullary schwannoma from meningioma using MRI T weighted images. Br J Radiol. 2018;91(1092):20180262. https://doi.org/10.1259/bjr.20180262.
28. Bettaswamy G, Ambesh P, Das KK, Sahu R, Srivastava A, Mehrotra A, et al. Extradural spinal meningioma: revisiting a rare entity. J Craniovertebr Junction Spine. 2016;7(1):65–8. https://doi.org/10.4103/0974-8237.176630.
29. Sahni D, Harrop JS, Kalfas IH, Vaccaro AR, Weingarten D. Exophytic intramedullary meningioma of the cervical spinal cord. J Clin Neurosci. 2008;15:1176–9.

30. Lee JW, Lee IS, Choi KU, Lee YH, Yi JH, Song JW, et al. CT and MRI findings of calcified spinal meningiomas: correlation with pathological findings. Skelet Radiol. 2010;39(4):345–52. https://doi.org/10.1007/s00256-009-0771-1.

31. Shi HB, Suh DC, Lee HK, Lim SM, Kim DH, Choi CG, et al. Preoperative transarterial embolization of spinal tumor: embolization techniques and results. AJNR Am J Neuroradiol. 1999;20(10):2009–15.

32. Charles YP, Barbe B, Beaujeux R, Boujan F, Steib J-P. Relevance of the anatomical location of the Adamkiewicz artery in spine surgery. Surg Radiol Anat. 2011;33:3–9.

33. Simpson D. The recurrence of intracranial meningiomas after surgical treatment. J Neurol Neurosurg Psychiatry. 1957;20:22–39.

34. Nanda A, Bir SC, Maiti TK, Konar SK, Missios S, Guthikonda B. Relevance of Simpson grading system and recurrence-free survival after surgery for World Health Organization Grade I meningioma. J Neurosurg. 2017;126(1):201–11. https://doi.org/10.3171/2016.1.JNS151842.

35. McCormick PC, Torres R, Post KD, Stein BM. Intramedullary ependymoma of the spinal cord. J Neurosurg. 1990;72:523–32.

36. Nakamura M, Roser F, Michel J, Jacobs C, Samii M. The natural history of incidental meningiomas. Neurosurgery. 2003;53:62–71.

37. Liu WC, Choi G, Lee SH, Han H, Lee JY, Jeon YH, et al. Radiological findings of spinal schwannomas and meningiomas: focus on discrimination of two disease entities. Eur Radiol. 2009;19(11):2707–15. https://doi.org/10.1007/s00330-009-1466-7.

38. Ozawa H, Onoda Y, Aizawa T, Nakamura T, Koakutsu T, Itoi E. Natural history of intradural-extramedullary spinal cord tumors. Acta Neurol Belg. 2012;112(3):265–70. https://doi.org/10.1007/s13760-012-0048-7.

39. Koeller KK, Shih RY. Intradural extramedullary spinal neoplasms: radiologic-pathologic correlation. Radiographics. 2019;39:468–90.

40. Landi A, Dugoni DE, Marotta N, Mancarella C, Delfini R. Spinal schwannomatosis in the absence of neurofibromatosis: a very rare condition. Int J Surg Case Rep. 2011;2:36–9.

41. Salpietro FM, Alafaci C, Lucerna S, Lacopino DG, Tomasello F. Do spinal meningiomas penetrate the pial layer? Correlation between magnetic resonance imaging and microsurgical findings and intracranial tumor interfaces. Neurosurgery. 1997;41:254–8.

42. Chwistek M. Recent advances in understanding and managing cancer pain. F1000Res. 2017;6:945.

43. Kraetzig T, McLaughlin L, Bilsky MH, Laufer I. Metastases of spinal myxopapillary ependymoma: unique characteristics and clinical management. J Neurosurg Spine. 2018;28(2):201–8. https://doi.org/10.3171/2017.5.SPINE161164.

44. Payer M. The anterior approach to anterior cervical meningiomas: review illustrated by a case. Acta Neurochir. 2005;147:555–60; discussion 560.

45. Iacoangeli M, Gladi M, Di Rienzo A, Dobran M, Alvaro L, Nocchi N, et al. Minimally invasive surgery for benign intradural extramedullary spinal meningiomas: experience of a single institution in a cohort of elderly patients and review of the literature. Clin Interv Aging. 2012;7:557–64. https://doi.org/10.2147/CIA.S38923.

46. Ruggeri AG, Fazzolari B, Colistra D, Cappelletti M, Marotta N, Delfini R. Calcified spinal meningiomas. World Neurosurg. 2017;102:406–12. https://doi.org/10.1016/j.wneu.2017.03.045.

47. Ahmed R, Menezes AH, Awe OO, Mahaney KB, Torner JC, Weinstein SL. Long-term incidence and risk factors for development of spinal deformity following resection of pediatric intramedullary spinal cord tumors. J Neurosurg Pediatr. 2014;13(6):613–21. https://doi.org/10.3171/2014.1.PEDS13317.

48. Albert TJ, Vacarro A. Postlaminectomy kyphosis. Spine (Phila Pa 1976). 1998;23(24):2738–45.

49. Yasuoka S, Peterson HA, Laws ER, MacCarty CS. Pathogenesis and prophylaxis of postlaminectomy deformity of the spine after multiple level laminectomy. Neurosurgery. 1981;9:145–52. https://doi.org/10.1227/00006123-198108000-00006.

50. Dekker SE, Ostergard TA, Glenn CA, Cox E, Bambakidis NC. Posterior cervical laminoplasty for resection Intradural extramedullary spinal meningioma: 2-dimensional operative video. Oper Neurosurg (Hagerstown). 2019;16(3):392. https://doi.org/10.1093/ons/opy204.
51. Shi W, Wang S, Zhang H, Wang G, Guo Y, Sun Z, et al. Risk factor analysis of progressive spinal deformity after resection of intramedullary spinal cord tumors in patients who underwent laminoplasty: a report of 105 consecutive cases. J Neurosurg Spine. 2019;8:1–9. https://doi.org/10.3171/2018.10.SPINE18110.
52. Ghadirpour R, Nasi D, Iaccarino C, Giraldi D, Sabadini R, Motti L, et al. Intraoperative neurophysiological monitoring for intradural extramedullary tumors: why not? Clin Neurol Neurosurg. 2015;130:140–9. https://doi.org/10.1016/j.clineuro.2015.01.007.
53. Ghadirpour R, Nasi D, Iaccarino C, Romano A, Motti L, Sabadini R, et al. Intraoperative neurophysiological monitoring for intradural extramedullary spinal tumors: predictive value and relevance of D-wave amplitude on surgical outcome during a 10-year experience. J Neurosurg Spine. 2018;30(2):259–67. https://doi.org/10.3171/2018.7.SPINE18278.
54. Kufeld M, Wowra B, Muacevic A, Zausinger S, Tonn JC. Radiosurgery of spinal meningiomas and schwannomas. Technol Cancer Res Treat. 2012;11(1):27–34.
55. Tseng CL, Eppinga W, Charest-Morin R, Soliman H, Myrehaug S, Maralani PJ, et al. Spine stereotactic body radiotherapy: indications, outcomes, and points of caution. Global Spine J. 2017;7(2):179–97. https://doi.org/10.1177/2192568217694016.
56. Kalash R, Glaser SM, Flickinger JC, Burton S, Heron DE, Gerszten PC, et al. Stereotactic body radiation therapy for benign spine tumors: is dose de-escalation appropriate? J Neurosurg Spine. 2018;29(2):220–5. https://doi.org/10.3171/2017.12.SPINE17920.
57. Noh SH, Kim KH, Shin DA, Park JY, Yi S, Kuh SU, et al. Treatment outcomes of 17 patients with atypical spinal meningioma, including 4 with metastases: a retrospective observational study. Spine J. 2019;19(2):276–84. https://doi.org/10.1016/j.spinee.2018.06.006.
58. Gerszten PC, Chen S, Quader M, Xu Y, Novotny J Jr, Flickinger JC. Radiosurgery for benign tumors of the spine using the Synergy S with cone-beam computed tomography image guidance. J Neurosurg. 2012;117(Suppl):197–202. https://doi.org/10.3171/2012.8.GKS12981.
59. Moazzam AA, Wagle N, Zada G. Recent developments in chemotherapy for meningiomas: a review. Neurosurg Focus. 2013;35(6):E18. https://doi.org/10.3171/2013.10.FOCUS13341.

Radiation Therapy for Low Grade Meningiomas

9

Gabrielle W. Peters and Joseph N. Contessa

General Radiation Paradigm

Meningiomas can present with widely varying clinical scenarios, from benign and asymptomatic tumors to those with aggressive histologies and/or significant neuro-cognitive side effects. The choice of treatment modality for management depends on both clinical and histopathologic features. Radiation therapy (RT) is frequently indicated as the primary modality for definitive therapy (either with or without biopsy) as well as in the setting of postoperative treatment for residual or recurrent disease.

The mainstay of treatment for operable candidates is maximal safe resection, as detailed in the previous chapters. Dr. Simpson initially described the correlation of resection extent and disease recurrence in the 1950s [1–4], and this factor has been used for consideration of adjuvant therapy. Modern series have demonstrated no significant different in progression-free survival (PFS) for Simpson scores of 1–3; therefore recent clinical trials (such as RTOG 0539 and NRG BN003) use the term gross total resection (GTR) when referring to Simpson scores of 1–3, corresponding to removal of at least all gross tumor and in some cases resection of involved/adjacent dura or bone. Subtotal resection (STR) refers to Simpson scores of 4–5 [5–8], signifying that gross tumor remains intact and unresected. Moving forward in this

G. W. Peters (✉)
Yale Department of Therapeutic Radiology, New Haven, CT, USA
e-mail: gabrielle.welch@yale.edu

J. N. Contessa
Department of Therapeutic Radiology, Yale School of Medicine, Yale New Haven Hospital, New Haven, CT, USA
e-mail: joseph.contessa@yale.edu

© Springer Nature Switzerland AG 2020
J. Moliterno, A. Omuro (eds.), *Meningiomas*,
https://doi.org/10.1007/978-3-030-59558-6_9

Table 9.1 World Health Organization grading criteria of meningioma [12]

I	II	III
Not fulfilling criteria for grades II and III	≥4 mitoses per 10 hpf *or* ≥3 of the following Sheeting architecture Hypercellularity Prominent nucleoli Small cells with high N:C ratio Foci of spontaneous necrosis*or* Choroid or clear cell meningioma Brain invasion	>20 mitoses per hpf *or* Frank anaplasia, defined as loss of meningothelial differentiation in focal or diffuse pattern) resembling Sarcoma Carcinoma Melanoma*or* Papillary meningioma Rhabdoid meningioma

Adapted from Chan et al. [13]
hpf high-power field, *N:C* nuclear to cytoplasmic

chapter, these definitions will be applied to the terms GTR (Simpson scores of 1–3) and STR (Simpson scores of 4–5).

Histopathologic features are the second factor which guides meningioma management, and currently this is assessed with the World Health Organization (WHO 2016 grading system (Table 9.1). WHO grade I has traditionally been defined as "benign meningioma" (BM). However when a BM (histologically confirmed or presumed based on imaging characteristics) recurs, it may be treated as a higher-risk histology [9–11]. This approach is supported by inclusion of these patients on the RTOG 0539 trial, a phase II clinical study examining outcomes for adjuvant radiation that included patients with recurrent WHO grade I with any resection extent. Preliminary results, although limited by patient numbers, indicate these patients have a similar prognosis as those with newly diagnosed grade II disease and GTR [8].

Unfortunately, little randomized data exists for the comparison of therapeutic modalities and to provide level I evidence for guiding the radiation treatment paradigm for benign meningioma [14, 15]. Therefore large institutional experiences and limited phase I/II trials are predominantly used to inform practice [8, 16, 17]. In a select population of patients, definitive radiation offers comparable control rates to GTR (87–99%) [17]. Modern MRI allows for earlier diagnosis (primary and recurrent disease) and better radiographic characterization, improving our patient selection for definitive RT, and their outcomes are likely better than historical evidence suggests [18, 19]. This cohort includes patients with small lesions in confined spaces at risk of exerting mass effect or neurologic symptoms despite a slow growth rate. Definitive radiotherapy is also considered for patients who are not good surgical candidates, those with surgically inaccessible tumors, or those with either a risk of morbidity with surgery or a low probability of achieving meaningful resection. For patients with symptomatic or large meningiomas at risk of exerting mass effect on normal brain, a partial or subtotal resection should be considered. Tumor debulking is important in relieving mass effect, shrinking the radiation target volume, and creating space between gross disease and critical organs at risk (OARs) and may open the possibility for treatment with stereotactic radiosurgery (SRS). Neurological deficits prior to radiation stabilize or improve slightly for the majority of patients [20, 21], but complete resolution is less likely. Following radiotherapy, meningiomas typically remain stable, though a small percentage decrease in size [22, 23].

Efficacy of Primary Radiotherapy for Benign Meningioma

There is a large body of retrospective research demonstrating excellent local control with definitive RT for WHO grade I lesions located in surgically inaccessible sites and/or poor surgical candidates/medically inoperable. Outcomes for these patient approach that of primary surgical patients with greater than 90% local control, whether that is in the form of fractionated external beam radiation therapy (f-EBRT)

Table 9.2   Outcomes for definitive stereotactic radiosurgery in WHO grade I meningioma

Authors and year	Institution	No. of patients	Technique	Median marginal dose (Gy)	Recurrence-free survival (%)		Complication (%)
					5 years	10 years	
Pollock et al. 2012 & 2013 [39, 40]	Mayo Clinic	251	GK	15.8/16		99.4/93	12.4
Kuhn et al. 2013 [50]	Multi-institution	279	GK	12	81.8		N/a
Spiegelmann et al. 2010 [32]	Israel	42	LINAC	14	97.5	93%	16.7
Bledsoe et al. 2010ᵃ [42]	Mayo Clinic	116	GK	15.1	99	92	23
Skeie et al. 2010 [11]	Norway	100	GK	12.4	94.2	91.6	6
Colombo et al. 2009 [43]	Italy	199	CK	18.5	97		3
Ganz et al. 2009 [44]	Egypt	97	GK	12	100		3
Kondziolka et al. 2008 [45]	Pittsburgh	972	GK	14	97	87	8
Iwai et al. 2008 [46]	Japan	125	GK	12	93	83	7.2
Kollova et al. 2007 [47]	Czech Republic	331	GK	12.5	98		10

(continued)

Table 9.2 (continued)

Authors and year	Institution	No. of patients	Technique	Median marginal dose (Gy)	Recurrence-free survival (%) 5 years	Recurrence-free survival (%) 10 years	Complication (%)
Hasegawa et al. 2007 [51]	Japan	115	GK	13	94	92	12
Kreil et al. 2005 [52]	Austria	200	GK	12	98.5	95	2.5
DiBiase et al. 2004 [48]	New Jersey	127	GK	14	86.4		8.3
Roche et al. 2003 [49]	France	32	GK	13	100		14
Pollock et al. 2003 [53]	Mayo Clinic	62	GK	17.7	95		10
Lee et al. 2002 [54]	Pittsburgh	159	GK	13	93	93	5
Shin et al. 2001 [55]	Japan	42	GK	18	91.3	91.3	4.3
Stafford et al. 2001 [10]	Mayo Clinic	190	GK	16	93		13
Hakim et al. 1998 [56]	Boston	127	LINAC	15	89.3		4.7
Chang et al. 1997 [57]	Stanford	55	LINAC	15	94		8

GK Gamma Knife
[a]Population of patients with >10 cm³ tumor. 3- and 7-year outcomes given, rounded up to 5/10 year

Table 9.3 Outcomes for definitive fractionated radiation in WHO grade I meningioma

Authors and year	Institution	Site	No. of patients	Technique	Median dose (Gy)	Recurrence-free survival (%) 5 years	Recurrence-free survival (%) 10 years	Compli-cation (%)
Tanzler et al. 2011 [25]	Gainesville	NA	88	Photon	52.7	96	93	6.8
Korah et al. 2010 [24]	Emory	NA	41[a]	Photon	50.4		97	4
Onodera et al. 2011 [31]	Japan	Skull base	27	Photon	48–54	100		0
Minniti et al. 2011 [29]	Italy	Skull base	52	Photon	50	93		5.5
Arvold et al. 2009 [38]	Boston	ONSM	25	Photon	50.4	95		12
Litre et al. 2009 [20]	France	CSM	100	Photon	45	94		3

Table 9.3 (continued)

Authors and year	Institution	Site	No. of patients	Technique	Median dose (Gy)	Recurrence-free survival (%) 5 years	10 years	Complication (%)
Milker-Zabel et al. 2007 [58]	Germany	Skull base	94	Photon	57.6	93.6		4
Brell et al. 2006 [59]	Spain	CSM	30	Photon	52	94		6
Noel et al. 2005 [60]	France	NA	51	Photon/Proton	60.6	98		4
Torres et al. 2003 [61]	Los Angeles	NA	161[a]	Photon	48.4	90		5.2
Pitz et al. 2002 [35]	Germany	ONSM	15	Photon	54	100		0
Uy et al. 2002 [33]	Houston	NA	40	Photon	50.4	93		7
Turbin et al. 2002 [62]	Newark	ONSM	64	Photon	40–55		92	33
Debus et al. 2001 [63]	Germany	Skull base	180	Photon	56.8	98.4		1.6
Dufour et al. 2001 [64]	France	CSM	31	Photon	NA	92.8		7
Wenkel et al. 2000 [65]	Boston	NA	46[b]	Photon/Proton	59		88	9.3

[a]Included patients treated with SRS
[b]Included patients with recurrent meningioma

or stereotactic radiosurgery (SRS) [3, 11, 17, 20, 21, 24–49] (Tables 9.2 and 9.3). Radiation therapy is generally well tolerated with low risks for complications, and the most notable studies and toxicities associated with RT will be detailed further in the corresponding subsections.

Large patient series supporting the use of SRS have been reported since the late 1990s [10, 11, 32, 39, 43, 44, 46, 47, 49, 51–57, 66, 67], and this treatment modality has been primarily studied in lesions that have sufficient distance from critical OARs, such as the optic nerve and chiasm. SRS yields an expected local control (LC) at 5 years of 95–100% and 85–95% at 10 years. However, size limits the deliverable dose for single-fraction treatment due to the surrounding normal brain and OARs. Thus larger tumors are treated with lower RT doses, contributing to an inverse relationship between local control and tumor size. A threshold of 3–4 cm is used to consider treatment with either f-EBRT or SRS, and retrospective comparisons between the two techniques have demonstrated equivalent local control [68–71].

Fractionated radiation is utilized for larger tumors (>3–4 cm) or when a critical structure abuts the target volume. Based on numerous retrospective series, local control of WHO grade I meningioma following 50.4–55Gy in 1.8–2Gy fractions is greater than 90% at 10 years [16, 20, 22, 24, 25, 29, 31, 33–35, 38, 58–65]. Optic nerve sheath meningiomas (ONSM) have generally been studied separately from other intracranial meningiomas, and studies have demonstrated that control of 95–100% at 10 years may be expected. The majority of these patients will have stable or improved vision [21, 34–38]; however 5–10% may have worsening visual acuity/ocular motility. In comparison, two thirds of untreated ONSM patients have been reported to have deterioration of vision [37].

Candidates for Definitive Radiation Therapy

Greater than 90% of patients diagnosed with meningioma have WHO grade I (benign histology), whether histologically proven or radiographically presumed [13, 19]. Definitive RT to gross disease may be indicated for patients with ONSM and lesions in other surgically inaccessible locations, following debulking or subtotal resection, and/or in cases of medical inoperability. Both standard fractioned radiation therapy (SRT) and stereotactic radiosurgery (SRS) are reasonable in these cases; size/location of the lesion will determine the optimal approach. Certain genetic syndromes and collagen vascular diseases are relative contraindications for definitive radiation therapy (see "Radiation in the Setting of Genetic Diseases"). Patients with presumed or documented atypical histology will be covered separately.

For meningioma in eloquent areas of the brain or patients who cannot tolerate biopsy, a multidisciplinary review of clinical and imaging characteristics should be performed, and alternative diagnoses should be explored/excluded where possible. In some circumstances and with experienced radiologists, imaging features and location may be used to predict grade I disease [72]. For example, a well-circumscribed lesion with broad-based dural attachment and avid and homogeneous contrast enhancement on T1 post-contrast MRI is associated with grade I histology [17, 73, 74], while peritumoral edema and necrosis suggest atypical or alternative histology. Lesions at the skull base, cavernous sinus, and ONS are typically presumed benign, associated with excellent control using definitive radiotherapy [11, 20, 32, 34–36, 38, 43, 55, 59, 62, 64]. Parasagittal lesions and those along the falx should be approached cautiously as they are associated with higher grade [72, 75].

In the setting of multiple meningiomas, one should exclude hereditary syndromes and radiation-induced meningioma (RIM) as these scenarios should be approached with caution (see "Radiation in the Setting of Genetic Diseases").

A recurrent meningioma that grows slowly over the course of several years may be treated with primary radiotherapy. However, if the time to recurrence is short and/or growth rate is fast, this is likely to represent higher-grade disease and may have worse control rates with radiation alone and RT doses used for benign disease

[10–12]. These high-grade recurrences are outside the scope of this discussion and will be covered in another chapter.

Modalities of Radiation

Photon

Photon radiotherapy is the most commonly utilized form of radiation and can originate from naturally decaying radioactive sources, which is used in the Gamma Knife system with cobalt-60 (Co-60) decay, or by bombarding a high-density material (tungsten) with accelerated electrons to produce X-rays, which is the origin of linear accelerator (LINAC) X-rays. Both of these radiation sources produce megavoltage (MV) X-rays, 1.25 MV (Co-60) and 6–15 MV (LINACs), which cause ionizing reactions within the penetrated tissue. They can be used for conventionally fractionated radiation or stereotactic radiosurgery.

With photon irradiation, there will always be a component of exit dose to surrounding tissue; however with advancing technology such as intensity-modulated radiation therapy (IMRT) and volumetric modulated arc therapy (VMAT), more conformal treatments are possible which minimizes scatter radiation dose. With more conformal treatments, one must insure reproducible and immobilized patient position to limit intra- and infra-fractional movement. The degree of immobilization for treatment depends on the fractionation scheme used, and the combination of these factors determines target volume expansions. For those patients with intracranial meningioma, a thermoplastic mask (Aquaplast) is made at the time of CT simulation and will allow for reproducible setup. For those with spinal meningiomas, a moldable and vacuum-sealed cushion is used to immobilize the patient. These considerations are discussed further below.

Proton

Proton irradiation is a type of particle therapy that takes advantage of the inherent mass of a proton and its ability to terminally deposit without exit dose to surrounding tissues. It can be used in conventional fractionation regimens, similar to photons. Protons are most often generated with a cyclotron, and the energy ranges from 150 to 250 MeV. The beam passes through tissue with the majority of dose deposited at the end of its range, in a region called the Bragg peak [76]. The Bragg peak is a narrow region, but can be spread out by superimposing several beams of different energies to create a uniform dose distribution, allowing for clinical use in treating solid tumors [76–78].

The biologic effect of protons has been extensively studied and continues to be the subject of some debate. Most treatment facilities have adopted the relative biological effectiveness (RBE) of 1.1 for protons relative to therapeutic photons, meaning that protons have 10% higher effect in tissues [77]. For this reason, studies performed using proton irradiation decrease the delivered dose by a factor of 1.1, in order to respect normal tissue tolerance.

Patients with large skull base meningiomas, very young patients, or those requiring re-irradiation may realize a benefit from the ability to spare adjacent normal structures and minimize surrounding brain irradiation. The use of proton therapy for dose escalation in meningioma may have benefits for reducing side effects or escalating dose in select patients, but in patients who can be treated with either protons or photons, local control appears similar [15]. Regardless, the cost and size of this technology is high, making it a relatively scarce resource. Currently, proton therapy is available in 26 centers in the United States [79].

Stereotactic Radiosurgery (SRS)

Stereotactic radiosurgery, typically a form of photon irradiation, is a popular modality which permits treatment delivery in a single fraction, relies on advanced localization technology, and employs robust immobilization to allow for smaller tumor volume margins and higher dose per fraction. There are various ways of delivering SRS (Gamma Knife, CyberKnife, or an SRS-capable LINAC), each employing different immobilization and image guidance. SRS can also be delivered with stereotactic "hypo-fractionation" regimens in 3–5 treatment sessions [80]; however, great caution should be taken with this approach as optimal doses for fractionated radiosurgery have not been determined.

Traditionally, the optimal candidates for definitive SRS are those with meningiomas ≤3 cm in size (or volume ≤ 10 cm^3) with capacity to deliver ≥12Gy to the margin [44, 45, 48, 53, 55, 67], with some analyses demonstrating the dose necessary to obtain optimal tumor control is 14Gy at the tumor margin [53, 55]. While some modern series suggest that ≥12Gy portends similar outcomes, we typically aim to deliver ≥15Gy to the margin if normal tissue constraints are easily met. Additionally, recent advances in treatment planning, immobilization, and image guidance may allow safer treatments of larger targets (<4 cm) in a carefully selected patient population with limited adjacent normal brain or OARs and a low risk of WHO grade II disease [42, 44, 45, 47, 50].

The advantages to SRS include a steep dose fall off at the edge of the target and little minimal dose to surrounding normal tissues, same-day treatment planning and delivery, and acute side effects limited to slight headache related to the headframe used for Gamma Knife. However, when selecting patients within the presumed grade I meningioma cohort, physicians should take care to analyze the imaging prior to offering SRS, as OARs may be dose limiting and ultimately impact tumor control. There is evidence that doses greater than 16Gy and larger volume tumors have a higher risk of peritumoral edema [39, 47, 57, 81, 82]. Therefore, a dose of 12–16Gy is typically used, and patients with lesions >4 cm are typically not suitable candidates for this treatment.

Gamma Knife SRS

The modality referenced most in the literature is the Gamma Knife (GK) system, which employs 192 sources of cobalt-60 with rigid collimation options of 4, 8, and 16 mm apertures oriented in eight discrete segments [83]. The cobalt-60 sources emit characteristic megavoltage X-rays. The system traditionally utilizes a rigid stereotactic frame, though new versions of this system allow for a stiff Aquaplast mask combined with enhanced onboard image guidance via cone-beam computed tomography (CBCT) for patient alignment. These capabilities allow accurate treatment position (within 0.15–0.5 mm) and precise radiation delivery, translating into limited radiation to surrounding tissues. On the day of SRS, patients typically undergo a treatment planning MRI in the treatment position with stereotactic frame/thermoplastic mask and IV contrast which clearly delineates margins of the intracranial lesion. Same-day planning and treatment, along with rigid frame, minimizes the need for a planning target margin [84]. For inferiorly located skull base lesions, GK may not be an option due to limited head positions and fixed source locations. As mentioned previously this cannot be used with large lesions or those abutting the optic chiasm/brainstem. GK treatment plans are inherently heterogeneous with a relatively higher maximal

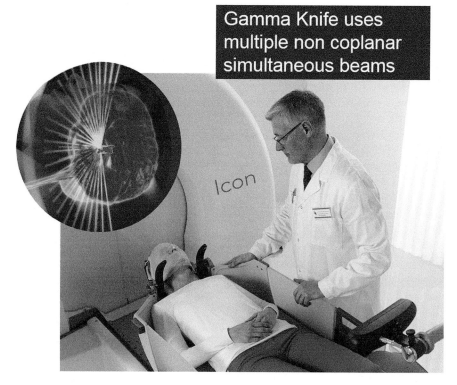

Fig. 9.1 Patient setup for Gamma Knife Treatment with frameless mask. (Image courtesy of Elekta)

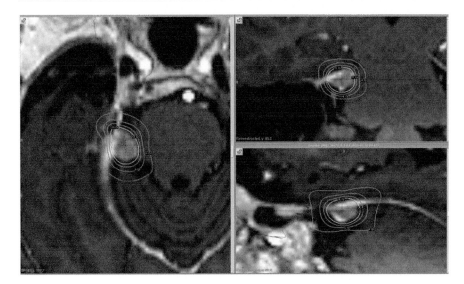

Fig. 9.2 Axial MRI image of a treatment plan delivering Gamma Knife SRS to a cavernous sinus meningioma

dose ("hot spot") in the center of the treatment field compared to the periphery (Figs. 9.1 and 9.2).

LINAC-Based Radiosurgery

Radiosurgery can been also be performed using a LINAC, an approach that has been used in select cases since the 1980s [32, 56, 57, 85]. With the advent of Aquaplast masks and advanced technology such as IMRT and VMAT, utilizing over 100 individual 0.5 cm multi-leaf collimators (MLCs) which can move simultaneously with a rotating LINAC gantry, physicians can now treat meningiomas of virtually any shape [86]. Onboard kilovoltage X-rays can be taken to ensure proper alignment of the patient, and the recently developed ExacTrac [87] technology allows for monitoring of the patient throughout the treatment. The main disadvantage of this modality is relatively more low-dose radiation in the surrounding tissue when compared to Gamma Knife or CyberKnife, and the treatment is typically not delivered on the same day as treatment planning. At centers treating with frameless SRS, a planning target margin may be necessary. The LINAC SRS plans are also more homogeneous is dose distribution, with a relatively lower "hot spot."

CyberKnife SRS

The CyberKnife (CK) system was developed in the 1990s as a frameless SRS option and employs a monoenergetic LINAC mounted on a robotic arm to allow for delivery of noncoplanar radiation beams. This system uses an Aquaplast mask similar to that for LINAC radiosurgery. During treatment, the system takes a series of orthogonal kilovoltage X-rays and compares the patient position on the CK table to the digitally reconstructed radiograph from the time of radiation planning. If at any time the patient is detected to be out of alignment, the CK LINAC will track patient motion, and the treatment couch will accommodate for any intrafractional motion. The disadvantage of this system is that the CK treatment head does not possess MLCs and requires fixed cones in varying sizes, and due to constant imaging/repositioning of the system, treatment times can be significantly longer when compared to the GK or LINAC.

Fractionated External Beam Radiation Therapy

Typical fractionated RT refers to the delivery of 1.8–2.0Gy of radiation daily, over the course of multiple weeks, achieving high total doses to preferentially kill tumor cells. This is most commonly delivered with a LINAC (photon irradiation) but can also delivered via cyclotron (proton therapy). Due to the higher prevalence of photon irradiation across the globe, it will be the default RT modality, unless otherwise specified.

Definitive EBRT for benign meningiomas is predominantly used for non-operable candidates with large tumors, or those abutting critical structures, as fractionation results in less normal tissue damage, widening the therapeutic window. The most commonly used dose fractionation for definitive RT for benign meningioma ranges from 50.4 to 54Gy in 1.8Gy fractions [20, 24, 25, 34, 35, 38, 59–65]. An exception is optic nerve sheath meningiomas in close proximity to the retina, where lowering dose and careful planning can preserve vision. Overall, the prescription should be modified based on surrounding OARs and is specified below in the radiation treatment planning section. Fractionated radiotherapy is given in precise manner using Aquaplast mask conformed to the patient's contour and used to minimize interfractional motion (Figs. 9.3 and 9.4).

Dose escalation above 55.8Gy has not proven efficacious for definitive treatment of benign meningioma, as evidenced by a phase III trial that randomized patients with subtotally resected or recurrent WHO grade I meningioma to 55.8Gy or 63Gy and showed that at 15 years, there was no difference in LC (85% vs 95% respectively; $p = 0.322$), although an overall survival trend favoring dose escalation (62% vs 75%; $p = 0.271$) was observed.

Radiation Effects

Modern MRI-/CT-based target and organ at risk (OAR) delineation is more accurate than historical standards; resulting improved disease control has improved and lower rates of toxicity [88]. The most common acute side effects of radiation for intracranial meningioma include fatigue, patchy hair loss (for superficial tumors), and less commonly nausea or headache. These symptoms resolve over weeks to

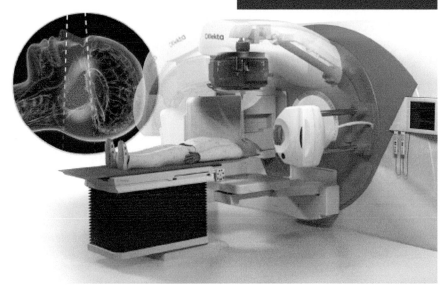

Fig. 9.3 Patient setup for treatment with LINAC-based radiotherapy. (Image courtesy of Elekta)

Fig. 9.4 Axial CT image of a treatment plan delivering fractionated radiotherapy to a cavernous sinus meningioma

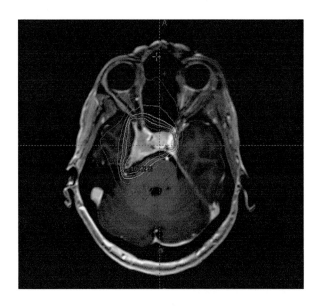

months after completion of therapy, although hair loss may be permanent. The incidence of post-radiation complications ranges from 2 to 20% for SRS and 0 to 15% f-EBRT [25, 26, 29], driven predominantly by the volume of irradiated tissue. Other factors associated with toxicity include location of the lesion, dose and fractionation delivered, RT modality, and degree of pre-treatment peritumoral edema [25, 39, 89]. Short-term complications include cerebral and/or peritumoral edema/necrosis, seizure, and neuropathies which may manifest during, months, or even years after radiotherapy. Peritumoral edema prior to radiation predicts for a higher risk of developing seizure, and radiation is associated with 4–17% risk of developing symptomatic edema (which may result in a variety of symptoms including seizure). This risk is slightly higher with SRS [17, 90]. Radiation necrosis is fairly uncommon with meningioma but has been reported [25].The risk of cranial nerve deficits following radiotherapy is up to 6% following SRS [29] which is associated with location of treated lesion, but is most commonly optic or trigeminal neuropathy. Depending on the location of meningioma treated, other effects such as changes in hearing and hypopituitarism may also occur. For patients with pre-treatment symptoms such as diplopia/cranial nerve deficits, headache, or exophthalmos, there may be resolution of deficits in 28–60% of patients, depending on duration and extent of organ involvement [20, 35, 52, 58–60, 63].

In the years following radiation, there is a small increased risk of cataracts, vascular complications/risk of stroke, and second malignancy. The risk of cataracts is dose dependent, and the latency period is 4–8 years. Cataracts associated with radiation therapy are removed in the same manner as an age-related cataract with little adverse effects on the patient [91]. There is limited evidence of a direct relationship between radiation and cerebrovascular accidents (CVA). The risk is believed to be primarily related to carotid artery stenosis, and this occurs at a rate of 1% with median time to onset of approximately 6 years [10, 15, 40]. Without a genetic tumor predisposition the incidence of a secondary malignancy ranges depending on age at radiation exposure and radiation dose. This risk ranges from 0.5 to 3% at 30 years for an adult, while children may have up to 30% risk at 30 years [92, 93]. The ability for SRS and proton therapy to minimize radiation to surrounding tissue is believed to decrease this risk [94]. This topic is further discussed in the following section.

Radiation-Induced Meningioma

The most *common* secondary brain tumor after cranial irradiation is meningioma, termed radiation-induced meningioma (RIM). The literature pertaining to adult/elderly patients is sparse, and RIMs are predominantly seen in pediatric patients, or those <30 years of age when receiving radiotherapy [93]. Many of these lesions are WHO grade II at diagnosis, and 10% of patients will develop multiple lesions [95, 96]. The criteria for radiation-induced brain tumors include occurring within the previously irradiated field, occurring with sufficient latency period since radiation, a different histologic type from original neoplasm, as well as lack of any genetic predisposition to the development of tumors [97].

These RIMs typically have a latency period of 20 years (range of 10–40 years); however atypical/anaplastic meningioma, or those arising within the high-dose (>30Gy) region, will occur in a shorter interval. There is also shorter interval for those with genetic syndromes such as NF2 [96]. Additionally, those who received higher doses of radiation had an increased probability of developing multiple and higher-grade lesions [96]. RIMs are believed to behave aggressively and recur more frequently, at a rate up to 26%, particularly distantly illustrating field effect [41, 98]. They are typically not included on clinical trials for those reasons.

Radiation in the Setting of Genetic Diseases

The genetic diseases most commonly associated with an increased risk of developing CNS tumors include neurofibromatosis (NF) (types 1 and 2), schwannomatosis, ataxia telangiectasia, Cowden syndrome, familial adenomatous polyposis, hereditary nonpolyposis colorectal cancer (HNPCC), Gorlin syndrome, von Hippel-Lindau disease, Turcot syndrome, Li-Fraumeni disease, tuberous sclerosis, and retinoblastoma [99]. Radiation is relatively contraindicated in ataxia telangiectasia, Li-Fraumeni syndrome, and Gorlin syndrome [100–102]; if it is unavoidable, then consideration for dose reduction and/or the high risk of severe late effects and second malignancy should be discussed.

The genetic syndrome most commonly associated with meningioma is NF2, which is caused by a mutation of a cell membrane-related protein (schwannomin) which also acts as a tumor suppressor [103, 104]. In patients with NF2, between 45 and 80% will develop meningioma [99, 103] and are more likely to arise at younger ages, in comparison to sporadic meningioma [105]. These patients are predisposed to synchronous or simultaneous multiple meningiomas, posing a challenge for delivery of radiation therapy and normal tissue sparing [103]. It is important to note that even solitary meningiomas in NF2 have proven to have poorer overall prognosis and survival, with more frequent atypical or anaplastic lesions [105, 106] and thus higher-grade disease should be ruled out when possible.

There is a paucity of data regarding the management of NF2 patients with radiation therapy, though it has been done with reasonable efficacy as evidenced by Wentworth et al. [107]. This is controversial due to the worry of increased risk of secondary malignancy [99] when radiation is utilized and warrants a frank discussion with the patient regarding the best treatment regimen. In these cases, surgery or active surveillance should be prioritized if possible, and for inoperable patients proton therapy or SRS may be reasonable approaches, depending on size and location of lesion.

Conclusion

For a selected patient population with confirmed or radiographically presumed WHO grade I meningioma, radiation therapy has demonstrated high rates of target control nearing that of surgical series. Physicians should compile all clinical and radiographic information, growth kinetics, and genetic predisposition in order to select the patients who will benefit most from definitive radiotherapy. With modern target delineation (using CT and MRI fusions) and daily image-guidance, radiation therapy for benign meningioma is effective, well-tolerated, and has limited long-term side effects.

References

1. Simpson D. The recurrence of intracranial meningiomas after surgical treatment. J Neurol Neurosurg Psychiatry. 1957;20(1):22–39.
2. Condra KS, Buatti JM, Mendenhall WM, Friedman WA, Marcus RB Jr, Rhoton AL. Benign meningiomas: primary treatment selection affects survival. Int J Radiat Oncol Biol Phys. 1997;39(2):427–36.
3. Stafford SL, Perry A, Suman VJ, Meyer FB, Scheithauer BW, Lohse CM, et al. Primarily resected meningiomas: outcome and prognostic factors in 581 Mayo Clinic patients, 1978 through 1988. Mayo Clin Proc. 1998;73(10):936–42.
4. Aizer AA, Bi WL, Kandola MS, Lee EQ, Nayak L, Rinne ML, et al. Extent of resection and overall survival for patients with atypical and malignant meningioma. Cancer. 2015;121(24):4376–81.
5. Sughrue ME, Sanai N, Shangari G, Parsa AT, Berger MS, McDermott MW. Outcome and survival following primary and repeat surgery for World Health Organization Grade III meningiomas. J Neurosurg. 2010;113(2):202–9.
6. Sughrue ME, Kane AJ, Shangari G, Rutkowski MJ, McDermott MW, Berger MS, et al. The relevance of Simpson Grade I and II resection in modern neurosurgical treatment of World Health Organization Grade I meningiomas. J Neurosurg. 2010;113(5):1029–35.
7. Oya S, Kawai K, Nakatomi H, Saito N. Significance of Simpson grading system in modern meningioma surgery: integration of the grade with MIB-1 labeling index as a key to predict the recurrence of WHO Grade I meningiomas. J Neurosurg. 2012;117(1):121–8.
8. Rogers L, Zhang P, Vogelbaum MA, Perry A, Ashby LS, Modi JM, et al. Intermediate-risk meningioma: initial outcomes from NRG Oncology RTOG 0539. J Neurosurg. 2018;129(1):35–47.
9. Bagshaw HP, Jensen RL, Palmer CA, Shrieve DC. Stereotactic radiation therapy and the management of atypical meningiomas: outcomes in the upfront and recurrent setting. Int J Radiat Oncol Biol Phys. 2015;93(3):S140.
10. Stafford SL, Pollock BE, Foote RL, Link MJ, Gorman DA, Schomberg PJ, et al. Meningioma radiosurgery: tumor control, outcomes, and complications among 190 consecutive patients. Neurosurgery. 2001;49(5):1029–38.
11. Skeie BS, Enger PO, Skeie GO, Thorsen F, Pedersen PH. Gamma knife surgery of meningiomas involving the cavernous sinus: long-term follow-up of 100 patients. Neurosurgery. 2010;66(4):661–8; discussion 8–9.
12. Louis DN, Perry A, Reifenberger G, von Deimling A, Figarella-Branger D, Cavenee WK, et al. The 2016 World Health Organization classification of tumors of the central nervous system: a summary. Acta Neuropathol. 2016;131(6):803–20.
13. Gunderson L, Tepper J. Clinical radiation oncology. 4th ed. Philadelphia: Elsevier; 2016.

14. Jenkinson MD, Javadpour M, Haylock BJ, Young B, Gillard H, Vinten J, et al. The ROAM/ EORTC-1308 trial: radiation versus observation following surgical resection of Atypical Meningioma: study protocol for a randomised controlled trial. Trials. 2015;16(1):519.
15. Sanford NN, Yeap BY, Larvie M, Daartz J, Munzenrider JE, Liebsch NJ, et al. Prospective, randomized study of radiation dose escalation with combined proton-photon therapy for benign Meningiomas. Int J Radiat Oncol Biol Phys. 2017;99(4):787–96.
16. Weber DC, Ares C, Villa S, Peerdeman SM, Renard L, Baumert BG, et al. Adjuvant post-operative high-dose radiotherapy for atypical and malignant meningioma: a phase-II parallel non-randomized and observation study (EORTC 22042-26042). Radiother Oncol. 2018;128(2):260–5.
17. Rogers L, Barani I, Chamberlain M, Kaley TJ, McDermott M, Raizer J, et al. Meningiomas: knowledge base, treatment outcomes, and uncertainties. A RANO review. J Neurosurg. 2015;122(1):4–23.
18. Shaikh N, Dixit K, Raizer J. Recent advances in managing/understanding meningioma. F1000Res. 2018;7:F1000 Faculty Rev-490.
19. Ostrom QT, Gittleman H, Liao P, Vecchione-Koval T, Wolinsky Y, Kruchko C, et al. CBTRUS Statistical Report: primary brain and other central nervous system tumors diagnosed in the United States in 2010–2014. Neuro Oncol. 2017;19(suppl_5):v1–88.
20. Litré CF, Colin P, Noudel R, Peruzzi P, Bazin A, Sherpereel B, et al. Fractionated stereotactic radiotherapy treatment of cavernous sinus meningiomas: a study of 100 cases. Int J Radiat Oncol Biol Phys. 2009;74(4):1012–7.
21. Paulsen F, Doerr S, Wilhelm H, Becker G, Bamberg M, Classen J. Fractionated stereotactic radiotherapy in patients with optic nerve sheath meningioma. Int J Radiat Oncol Biol Phys. 2012;82(2):773–8.
22. Minniti G, Amichetti M, Enrici RM. Radiotherapy and radiosurgery for benign skull base meningiomas. Radiat Oncol (London, England). 2009;4:42.
23. Pollock BE, Stafford SL, Link MJ, Brown PD, Garces YI, Foote RL. Single-fraction radiosurgery of benign intracranial meningiomas. Neurosurgery. 2012;71(3):604–13.
24. Korah MP, Nowlan AW, Johnstone PAS, Crocker IR. Radiation therapy alone for imaging-defined meningiomas. Int J Radiat Oncol Biol Phys. 2010;76(1):181–6.
25. Tanzler E, Morris CG, Kirwan JM, Amdur RJ, Mendenhall WM. Outcomes of WHO grade I meningiomas receiving definitive or postoperative radiotherapy. Int J Radiat Oncol Biol Phys. 2011;79(2):508–13.
26. Hamm K, Henzel M, Gross MW, Surber G, Kleinert G, Engenhart-Cabillic R. Radiosurgery/ stereotactic radiotherapy in the therapeutical concept for skull base meningiomas. Zentralblatt fur Neurochirurgie. 2008;69(1):14–21.
27. Metellus P, Batra S, Karkar S, Kapoor S, Weiss S, Kleinberg L, et al. Fractionated conformal radiotherapy in the management of cavernous sinus meningiomas: long-term functional outcome and tumor control at a single institution. Int J Radiat Oncol Biol Phys. 2010;78(3):836–43.
28. Bria C, Wegner RE, Clump DA, Vargo JA, Mintz AH, Heron DE, et al. Fractionated stereotactic radiosurgery for the treatment of meningiomas. J Cancer Res Ther. 2011;7(1):52–7.
29. Minniti G, Clarke E, Cavallo L, Osti MF, Esposito V, Cantore G, et al. Fractionated stereotactic conformal radiotherapy for large benign skull base meningiomas. Radiat Oncol (London, England). 2011;6:36.
30. Mahadevan A, Floyd S, Wong E, Chen C, Kasper E. Clinical outcome after hypofractionated stereotactic radiotherapy (HSRT) for benign skull base tumors. Comput Aided Surg. 2011;16(3):112–20.
31. Onodera S, Aoyama H, Katoh N, Taguchi H, Yasuda K, Yoshida D, et al. Long-term outcomes of fractionated stereotactic radiotherapy for intracranial skull base benign meningiomas in single institution. Jpn J Clin Oncol. 2011;41(4):462–8.
32. Spiegelmann R, Cohen ZR, Nissim O, Alezra D, Pfeffer R. Cavernous sinus meningiomas: a large LINAC radiosurgery series. J Neuro-Oncol. 2010;98(2):195–202.
33. Uy NW, Woo SY, Teh BS, Mai W-Y, Carpenter LS, Chiu JK, et al. Intensity-modulated radiation therapy (IMRT) for meningioma. Int J Radiat Oncol Biol Phys. 2002;53(5):1265–70.

34. Liu JK, Forman S, Hershewe GL, Moorthy CR, Benzil DL. Optic nerve sheath meningiomas: visual improvement after stereotactic radiotherapy. Neurosurgery. 2002;50(5):950–5; discussion 5–7.
35. Pitz S, Becker G, Schiefer U, Wilhelm H, Jeremic B, Bamberg M, et al. Stereotactic fractionated irradiation of optic nerve sheath meningioma: a new treatment alternative. Br J Ophthalmol. 2002;86(11):1265–8.
36. Eddleman CS, Liu JK. Optic nerve sheath meningioma: current diagnosis and treatment. Neurosurg Focus. 2007;23(5):E4.
37. Landert M, Baumert BG, Bosch MM, Lutolf UM, Landau K. The visual impact of fractionated stereotactic conformal radiotherapy on seven eyes with optic nerve sheath meningiomas. J Neuroophthalmol. 2005;25(2):86–91.
38. Arvold ND, Lessell S, Bussiere M, Beaudette K, Rizzo JF, Loeffler JS, et al. Visual outcome and tumor control after conformal radiotherapy for patients with optic nerve sheath meningioma. Int J Radiat Oncol Biol Phys. 2009;75(4):1166–72.
39. Pollock BE, Stafford SL, Link MJ, Garces YI, Foote RL. Single-fraction radiosurgery for presumed intracranial meningiomas: efficacy and complications from a 22-year experience. Int J Radiat Oncol Biol Phys. 2012;83(5):1414–8.
40. Pollock BE, Stafford SL, Link MJ. Stereotactic radiosurgery of intracranial meningiomas. Neurosurg Clin North Am. 2013;24(4):499–507.
41. Kuhn EN, Chan MD, Tatter SB, Ellis TL. Gamma knife stereotactic radiosurgery for radiation-induced meningiomas. Stereotact Funct Neurosurg. 2012;90(6):365–9.
42. Bledsoe JM, Link MJ, Stafford SL, Park PJ, Pollock BE. Radiosurgery for large-volume (> 10 cm3) benign meningiomas. J Neurosurg. 2010;112(5):951–6.
43. Colombo F, Casentini L, Cavedon C, Scalchi P, Cora S, Francescon P. Cyberknife radiosurgery for benign meningiomas: short-term results in 199 patients. Neurosurgery. 2009;64(2 Suppl):A7–13.
44. Ganz JC, Reda WA, Abdelkarim K. Gamma knife surgery of large meningiomas: early response to treatment. Acta Neurochir. 2009;151(1):1–8.
45. Kondziolka D, Mathieu D, Lunsford LD, Martin JJ, Madhok R, Niranjan A, et al. Radiosurgery as definitive management of intracranial meningiomas. Neurosurgery. 2008;62(1):53–8; discussion 8–60.
46. Iwai Y, Yamanaka K, Ikeda H. Gamma Knife radiosurgery for skull base meningioma: long-term results of low-dose treatment. J Neurosurg. 2008;109(5):804–10.
47. Kollova A, Liscak R, Novotny J Jr, Vladyka V, Simonova G, Janouskova L. Gamma knife surgery for benign meningioma. J Neurosurg. 2007;107(2):325–36.
48. DiBiase SJ, Kwok Y, Yovino S, Arena C, Naqvi S, Temple R, et al. Factors predicting local tumor control after gamma knife stereotactic radiosurgery for benign intracranial meningiomas. Int J Radiat Oncol Biol Phys. 2004;60(5):1515–9.
49. Roche PH, Pellet W, Fuentes S, Thomassin JM, Regis J. Gamma knife radiosurgical management of petroclival meningiomas results and indications. Acta Neurochir. 2003;145(10):883–8; discussion 8.
50. Kuhn EN, Taksler GB, Dayton O, Loganathan AG, Vern-Gross TZ, Bourland JD, et al. Patterns of recurrence after stereotactic radiosurgery for treatment of meningiomas. Neurosurg Focus. 2013;35(6):E14.
51. Hasegawa T, Kida Y, Yoshimoto M, Koike J, Iizuka H, Ishii D. Long-term outcomes of gamma knife surgery for cavernous sinus meningioma. J Neurosurg. 2007;107(4):745–51.
52. Kreil W, Luggin J, Fuchs I, Weigl V, Eustacchio S, Papaefthymiou G. Long term experience of gamma knife radiosurgery for benign skull base meningiomas. J Neurol Neurosurg Psychiatry. 2005;76(10):1425–30.
53. Pollock BE. Stereotactic radiosurgery for intracranial meningiomas: indications and results. Neurosurg Focus. 2003;14(5):e4.
54. Lee JY, Niranjan A, McInerney J, Kondziolka D, Flickinger JC, Lunsford LD. Stereotactic radiosurgery providing long-term tumor control of cavernous sinus meningiomas. J Neurosurg. 2002;97(1):65–72.

55. Shin M, Kurita H, Sasaki T, Kawamoto S, Tago M, Kawahara N, et al. Analysis of treatment outcome after stereotactic radiosurgery for cavernous sinus meningiomas. J Neurosurg. 2001;95(3):435–9.
56. Hakim R, Alexander E 3rd, Loeffler JS, Shrieve DC, Wen P, Fallon MP, et al. Results of linear accelerator-based radiosurgery for intracranial meningiomas. Neurosurgery. 1998;42(3):446–53; discussion 53–4.
57. Chang SD, Adler JR Jr. Treatment of cranial base meningiomas with linear accelerator radiosurgery. Neurosurgery. 1997;41(5):1019–25; discussion 25–7.
58. Milker-Zabel S, Zabel-du Bois A, Huber P, Schlegel W, Debus J. Intensity-modulated radiotherapy for complex-shaped meningioma of the skull base: long-term experience of a single institution. Int J Radiat Oncol Biol Phys. 2007;68(3):858–63.
59. Brell M, Villà S, Teixidor P, Lucas A, Ferrán E, Marín S, et al. Fractionated stereotactic radiotherapy in the treatment of exclusive cavernous sinus meningioma: functional outcome, local control, and tolerance. Surg Neurol. 2006;65(1):28–33.
60. Noel G, Bollet MA, Calugaru V, Feuvret L, Haie-Meder C, Dhermain F, et al. Functional outcome of patients with benign meningioma treated by 3D conformal irradiation with a combination of photons and protons. Int J Radiat Oncol Biol Phys. 2005;62(5):1412–22.
61. Torres RC, Frighetto L, De Salles AA, Goss B, Medin P, Solberg T, et al. Radiosurgery and stereotactic radiotherapy for intracranial meningiomas. Neurosurg Focus. 2003;14(5):e5.
62. Turbin RE, Thompson CR, Kennerdell JS, Cockerham KP, Kupersmith MJ. A long-term visual outcome comparison in patients with optic nerve sheath meningioma managed with observation, surgery, radiotherapy, or surgery and radiotherapy. Ophthalmology. 2002;109(5):890–9; discussion 9–900.
63. Debus J, Wuendrich M, Pirzkall A, Hoess A, Schlegel W, Zuna I, et al. High efficacy of fractionated stereotactic radiotherapy of large base-of-skull meningiomas: long-term results. J Clin Oncol. 2001;19(15):3547–53.
64. Dufour H, Régis J, Chinot O, Muracciole X, Métellus P, Grisoli F. Long-term tumor control and functional outcome in patients with cavernous sinus meningiomas treated by radiotherapy with or without previous surgery: is there an alternative to aggressive tumor removal? Neurosurgery. 2001;48(2):285–96.
65. Wenkel E, Thornton AF, Finkelstein D, Adams J, Lyons S, De La Monte S, et al. Benign meningioma: partially resected, biopsied, and recurrent intracranial tumors treated with combined proton and photon radiotherapy. Int J Radiat Oncol Biol Phys. 2000;48(5):1363–70.
66. Shafron DH, Friedman WA, Buatti JM, Bova FJ, Mendenhall WM. Linac radiosurgery for benign meningiomas. Int J Radiat Oncol Biol Phys. 1999;43(2):321–7.
67. Kondziolka D, Flickinger JC, Perez B. Judicious resection and/or radiosurgery for parasagittal meningiomas: outcomes from a multicenter review. Gamma Knife Meningioma Study Group. Neurosurgery. 1998;43(3):405–13; discussion 13–4.
68. Andrews DW, Suarez O, Goldman HW, Downes MB, Bednarz G, Corn BW, et al. Stereotactic radiosurgery and fractionated stereotactic radiotherapy for the treatment of acoustic schwannomas: comparative observations of 125 patients treated at one institution. Int J Radiat Oncol Biol Phys. 2001;50(5):1265–78.
69. Combs SE, Welzel T, Schulz-Ertner D, Huber PE, Debus J. Differences in clinical results after LINAC-based single-dose radiosurgery versus fractionated stereotactic radiotherapy for patients with vestibular schwannomas. Int J Radiat Oncol Biol Phys. 2010;76(1):193–200.
70. Meijer OW, Vandertop WP, Baayen JC, Slotman BJ. Single-fraction vs. fractionated linac-based stereotactic radiosurgery for vestibular schwannoma: a single-institution study. Int J Radiat Oncol Biol Phys. 2003;56(5):1390–6.
71. Anderson BM, Khuntia D, Bentzen SM, Geye HM, Hayes LL, Kuo JS, et al. Single institution experience treating 104 vestibular schwannomas with fractionated stereotactic radiation therapy or stereotactic radiosurgery. J Neuro-Oncol. 2014;116(1):187–93.
72. Sahm F, Schrimpf D, Stichel D, Jones DTW, Hielscher T, Schefzyk S, et al. DNA methylation-based classification and grading system for meningioma: a multicentre, retrospective analysis. Lancet Oncol. 2017;18(5):682–94.

73. William CO, Lister JR, Patrick WE. The natural history and growth rate of asymptomatic meningiomas: a review of 60 patients. J Neurosurg. 1995;83(2):222–4.
74. Watts J, Box G, Galvin A, Brotchie P, Trost N, Sutherland T. Magnetic resonance imaging of meningiomas: a pictorial review. Insights Imaging. 2014;5(1):113–22.
75. Magill ST, Young JS, Chae R, Aghi MK, Theodosopoulos PV, McDermott MW. Relationship between tumor location, size, and WHO grade in meningioma. Neurosurg Focus. 2018;44(4):E4.
76. Khan F. Clinical radiation generators. In: Physics of radiation therapy. 4th ed. Philadelphia: Lippincott Williams & Wilkins; 2010.
77. Khan F. Proton beam therapy. In: Physics of radiation therapy. 4th ed. Philadelphia: Lippincott Williams & Wilkins; 2010. p. 515–31.
78. Miller DW. A review of proton beam radiation therapy. Med Phys. 1995;22(11 Pt 2): 1943–54.
79. The National Association for Proton Therapy cited 2019. Available from: https://www.proton-therapy.org/map/.
80. Park HR, Lee JM, Park K-W, Kim JH, Jeong SS, Kim JW, et al. Fractionated gamma knife radiosurgery as initial treatment for large skull base meningioma. Exp Neurobiol. 2018;27(3):245–55.
81. Flickinger JC, Kondziolka D, Maitz AH, Lunsford LD. Gamma knife radiosurgery of imaging-diagnosed intracranial meningioma. Int J Radiat Oncol Biol Phys. 2003;56(3):801–6.
82. Milano MT, Usuki KY, Walter KA, Clark D, Schell MC. Stereotactic radiosurgery and hypo-fractionated stereotactic radiotherapy: Normal tissue dose constraints of the central nervous system. Cancer Treat Rev. 2011;37(7):567–78.
83. Bhatnagar JP, Novotny J, Niranjan A, Kondziolka D, Flickinger J, Lunsford D, et al. First year experience with newly developed Leksell Gamma Knife Perfexion. J Med Phys. 2009;34(3):141–8.
84. Subedi KS, Takahashi T, Yamano T, Saitoh J-I, Nishimura K, Suzuki Y, et al. Usefulness of double dose contrast-enhanced magnetic resonance imaging for clear delineation of gross tumor volume in stereotactic radiotherapy treatment planning of metastatic brain tumors: a dose comparison study. J Radiat Res. 2013;54(1):135–9.
85. Villavicencio AT, Black PM, Shrieve DC, Fallon MP, Alexander E, Loeffler JS. Linac radiosurgery for skull base meningiomas. Acta Neurochir. 2001;143(11):1141–52.
86. Rassiah-Szegedi P, Szegedi M, Sarkar V, Streitmatter S, Huang YJ, Zhao H, et al. Dosimetric impact of the 160 MLC on head and neck IMRT treatments. J Appl Clin Med Phys. 2014;15(6):4770.
87. Oh SA, Yea JW, Kang MK, Park JW, Kim SK. Analysis of the setup uncertainty and margin of the daily exactrac 6D image guide system for patients with brain tumors. PloS One. 2016;11(3):e0151709.
88. Goldsmith BJ, Wara WM, Wilson CB, Larson DA. Postoperative irradiation for subtotally resected meningiomas. A retrospective analysis of 140 patients treated from 1967 to 1990. J Neurosurg. 1994;80(2):195–201.
89. Pollock BE, Stafford SL, Link MJ, Garces Y, Foote RL. Single-fraction radiosurgery of benign cavernous sinus meningiomas. J Neurosurg. 2013;119(3):675–82.
90. Fatima N, Meola A, Pollom EL, Soltys SG, Chang SD. Stereotactic radiosurgery versus stereo-tactic radiotherapy in the management of intracranial meningiomas: a systematic review and meta-analysis. Neurosurg Focus. 2019;46(6):E2.
91. Ainsbury EA, Barnard S, Bright S, Dalke C, Jarrin M, Kunze S, et al. Ionizing radiation induced cataracts: recent biological and mechanistic developments and perspectives for future research. Mutat Res. 2016;770:238–61.
92. Evans DGR, Birch JM, Ramsden RT, Sharif S, Baser ME. Malignant transformation and new primary tumours after therapeutic radiation for benign disease: substantial risks in certain tumour prone syndromes. J Med Genet. 2006;43(4):289–94.
93. Mountford P, Temperton D. Recommendations of the international commission on radiological protection (ICRP) 1990. Eur J Nucl Med Mol Imaging. 1992;19(2):77–9.

94. Dracham CB, Shankar A, Madan R. Radiation induced secondary malignancies: a review article. Radiat Oncol J. 2018;36(2):85–94.
95. Galloway TJ, Indelicato DJ, Amdur RJ, Swanson EL, Morris CG, Marcus RB. Favorable outcomes of pediatric patients treated with radiotherapy to the central nervous system who develop radiation-induced meningiomas. Int J Radiat Oncol Biol Phys. 2011;79(1):117–20.
96. Yamanaka R, Hayano A, Kanayama T. Radiation-induced meningiomas: an exhaustive review of the literature. World Neurosurg. 2017;97:635–44.e8.
97. Cahan WG, Woodard HQ, Higinbotham NL, Stewart FW, Coley BL. Sarcoma arising in irradiated bone. Cancer. 1998;82(1):8–34.
98. Sadetzki S, Flint-Richter P, Ben-Tal T, Nass D. Radiation-induced meningioma: a descriptive study of 253 cases. J Neurosurg. 2002;97(5):1078.
99. Vijapura C, Aldin ES, Capizzano AA, Policeni B, Sato Y, Moritani T. Genetic syndromes associated with central nervous system tumors. Radiographics. 2017;37(1):258–80.
100. Golitz LE, Norris DA, Luekens CA Jr, Charles DM. Nevoid basal cell carcinoma syndrome: multiple basal cell carcinomas of the palms after radiation therapy. JAMA Dermatol. 1980;116(10):1159–63.
101. Ho AY, Fan G, Atencio DP, Green S, Formenti SC, Haffty BG, et al. Possession of ATM sequence variants as predictor for late normal tissue responses in breast cancer patients treated with radiotherapy. Int J Radiat Oncol Biol Phys. 2007;69(3):677–84.
102. Kony SJ, de Vathaire F, Chompret A, Shamsaldim A, Grimaud E, Raquin M-A, et al. Radiation and genetic factors in the risk of second malignant neoplasms after a first cancer in childhood. Lancet. 1997;350(9071):91–5.
103. Goutagny S, Kalamarides M. Meningiomas and neurofibromatosis. J Neuro-Oncol. 2010;99(3):341–7.
104. Créange A, Kalifa C, Rodriguez D, Doz F, Grill J, Guillamo JS, et al. Prognostic factors of CNS tumours in Neurofibromatosis 1 (NF1): a retrospective study of 104 patients. Brain. 2002;126(1):152–60.
105. Perry A, Giannini C, Raghavan R, Scheithauer BW, Banerjee R, Margraf L, et al. Aggressive phenotypic and genotypic features in pediatric and NF2-associated meningiomas: a clinicopathologic study of 53 cases. J Neuropathol Exp Neurol. 2001;60(10):994–1003.
106. Baser ME, Friedman JM, Aeschliman D, Joe H, Wallace AJ, Ramsden RT, et al. Predictors of the risk of mortality in neurofibromatosis 2. Am J Human Genet. 2002;71(4):715–23.
107. Wentworth S, Pinn M, Bourland JD, deGuzman AF, Ekstrand K, Ellis TL, et al. Clinical experience with radiation therapy in the management of neurofibromatosis-associated central nervous system tumors. Int J Radiat Oncol Biol Phys. 2009;73(1):208–13.

Part III

Treatment Options for more aggressive meningiomas

Low Grade Tumor Recurrence and Management of More Aggressive Meningiomas

Daniel M. Fountain and Thomas Santarius

Introduction

For the vast majority of patients with a meningioma, either it is an incidental finding and the patient does not require surgery or if the patient does require surgery, it is curative. This natural history is what most physicians associate with meningioma. However, there is a subset of aggressive meningiomas with significant morbidity and mortality. There are six features that, alone or more likely in combination, characterize aggressive meningiomas: anatomical location, size at initial presentation, speed of growth, infiltrative pattern of growth, migration along the meninges, and, rarely, formation of distant metastases. Aggressive meningiomas broadly incorporate meningiomas of a higher histological grade (atypical WHO grade II hereafter known as grade II, anaplastic WHO grade III, hereafter known as grade III) which can either progress from lower grades or arise de novo, or recurrent low grade (WHO grade I, hereafter known as grade I) meningioma that cannot be controlled by surgery to nonsurgical treatment. While 10-year recurrence rates for grade I meningiomas are 20–40% if resected totally, this increases to 55–100% following subtotal resection. Progression for grade II meningiomas within as little as 5 years can be as high as 40% in patients with subtotal resection [1]. Brain invasion is also a defining histological feature of grade II and III meningioma [2]. Although rare, this combination of recurrence requiring repeat surgeries, radiotherapy, and invasion of

D. M. Fountain (✉)
Manchester Centre for Clinical Neurosciences, Salford Royal NHS Foundation Trust, Salford, Manchester Greater Manchester, UK
e-mail: daniel.fountain@nhs.net

T. Santarius
Department of Clinical Neurosciences, Cambridge University Hospitals NHS Foundation Trust, Cambridge, Cambridgeshire, UK
e-mail: ts381@cam.ac.uk

© Springer Nature Switzerland AG 2020
J. Moliterno, A. Omuro (eds.), *Meningiomas*,
https://doi.org/10.1007/978-3-030-59558-6_10

surrounding anatomical structures results in gradual accumulation of morbidity and, ultimately, poor prognosis for patients with an aggressive meningioma.

This chapter will explore the natural history and current established management plans of patients with aggressive meningiomas including factors predicting this phenotype. The chapter will finish with a brief glance at future directions summarizing latest research identifying molecular and imaging signatures of aggressive meningiomas and future treatment options.

Characteristics of the "Aggressive Meningioma"

Demographics

The Simpson grade of resection was a classification system published in 1957 which has been central to clinical management of these patients including decisions regarding postoperative treatment and follow-up (Table 10.1) [3]. Recurrent grade I meningiomas are most commonly identified in follow-up MRI surveillance imaging in cases where gross total resection was performed (Simpson grades 1–3). This is to distinguish it from growth of a residual meningioma which was not removed (Simpson grades 4–5). Identified risk factors for recurrence in meningioma include brain invasion and increased mitotic index of the primary resected tumor [4]. The most significant predictor of recurrence of surgically treated grade I meningioma remains extent of resection of the initial tumor. Recent series have continued to confirm its relevance in predicting recurrence rates [5, 6]. A combination of Simpson grading and MIB-1 labeling index, a marker of cellular proliferation, can be used to differentiate grade I meningioma with a high risk of recurrence [7]. Meningiomas in the spine and parasagittal and convexity areas are associated with a lower risk of recurrence than meningiomas in the parasellar, sphenoid ridge, olfactory groove regions, though this is probably related to the frequency and the degree to which total resection can be achieved safely [8]. A lower initial age of presentation is also associated with a higher risk of recurrence [9].

Epidemiological data for aggressive meningioma are varied. A study from the Central Brain Tumor Registry of the United States (CBTRUS) covering the period

Table 10.1 Simpson grade of resection [3]

Simpson grade	Definition	Extent of resection
I	Gross total resection of tumor, dural attachment, abnormal bone	GTR
II	Gross total resection of tumor, coagulation of dural attachment	GTR
III	Gross total resection of tumor without resection or coagulation of dural attachments, or extradural extension (e.g., invaded sinus or hyperostotic bone)	GTR
IV	Partial resection of tumor	STR
V	Decompression, with or without biopsy	STR

Adapted from Simpson [3]

2004–2010 identified an annual age-adjusted incidence of grade II meningiomas which is around 0.28 per 100,000, while for grade III meningiomas, it is 0.09 per 100,000, together accounting for around 5% of newly diagnosed meningiomas [10]. Similarly, in a hospital-based study in Finland, 4.7% of all treated meningiomas were grade II and 1.0% grade III [11]. The majority of more recent studies (based on 2007 and 2016 versions of the WHO Classification of Tumours of the CNS) are derived from national registries [12–14]. For example, the CBTRUS study covering the period 2011–2015 of all primary brain tumors, reported of all meningiomas that 17.6% were grade II and 1.7% grade III [15]. Data from the National Cancer Registration and Analysis Service in the United Kingdom presented a similarly higher proportion of aggressive meningioma; of 15,417 patients undergoing surgery for meningioma, 18.4% were grade II and 2.1% grade III [16]. Although females have a significantly higher incidence of grade I and II meningiomas, this is not the case for grade III meningiomas [10]. Patients with meningioma associated with previous exposure to ionizing radiation are more likely to be grade II or grade III and multifocal, with a significantly higher rate of recurrence [17].

Imaging

Typical appearances for recurrent grade I and II meningioma include extra-axial T1-isointense T2-hyperintense homogeneously enhancing lesions at the site of or in proximity to the site of previous resection [18]. CT imaging can be helpful in assessing the extent of bone involvement. Grade III meningiomas are more likely to appear irregular and can have distant metastases [19]. Perfusion imaging has identified grade III tumors which are also more likely to have a higher relative cerebral blood volume than grade I or II meningiomas [20].

The initial size and speed of growth of a meningioma is intimately related to the potential for neurological deficit and can influence the speed at which treatment decisions are required. A systematic review of growth rates of meningioma did not identify robust evidence suggesting that growth rates can be used to predict histological grade. In retrospective studies, factors found to be predictive of a higher growth rate include histological grade, lower age at diagnosis, the presence of edema, and lack of calcification on MRI [21, 22]. The optimal threshold growth found to distinguish grade I from grade II meningioma was 3 cm^3/year which had a sensitivity of 88% and specificity of 74% [22]. A larger initial tumor volume was related to higher growth rates and is a predictor of a higher histological grade of meningioma [22]. Conceptually, the larger the tumor, the larger the interface between tumor and normal anatomy, hence the greater the chance of subtotal resection and the greater the risk of morbidity related to either surgery or radiotherapy. Such an effect is compounded if there a less apparent plane between the tumor and surrounding structures as are found in surgery for recurrent grade I and grade II and grade III meningioma. Finally, the presence of metastasis is more likely in patients with grade II and III meningiomas – in one series of 28 patients with metastases, 27 were grade II or III (96%) [19].

Current Management of Aggressive Meningiomas

Principles

As with any management decision for patients with a meningioma, a multidisciplinary team decision including neurosurgeons and neuro-oncologists is vital. Where the total of neurological and non-neurological (local and general medical) complications is deemed acceptable, surgery remains the treatment of choice for patients with aggressive meningiomas.

Surgery

Histological grade is confirmed following surgical resection performed in the vast majority of cases, with grade I histology confirmed in the absence of evidence of brain invasion and a low number of mitoses. Grade II meningiomas are defined by the presence of a higher mitotic count or specific histological features suggestive of a more aggressive phenotype, whereas grade III meningiomas have an even higher mitotic count or have specific histological appearances of a papillary or rhabdoid meningioma (Table 10.2) [2].

Technically, surgery for recurrent meningioma is more challenging, and the risk of neurological and non-neurological complications is much higher than at the first operation [23, 24]. This is due to distorted anatomy, scar tissue, invasion of brain and neurovascular structures, invasion of bone and air sinuses, diminished functional reserve of neural structured, as well as overall reduced healing capacity of the tissues compounded by previous radiotherapy and long-term use of steroids.

Table 10.2 2016 World Health Organization classification of meningiomas [2]

Grade	Features
I	Low mitotic rate <4 per 10 high-power fields (HPF) No brain invasion
II	Mitotic rate 4–19 per HPF OR brain invasion OR 3 out of 5 of: Spontaneous necrosis Sheeting (loss of whorling or fascicular architecture) Prominent nucleoli High cellularity Small cells (tumor clusters with high nuclear-cytoplasmic ratio).
III	Mitotic rate > 20 per HPF OR specifically: Papillary meningioma Rhabdoid meningioma

Adapted from Louis et al. [2]

One series of patients with anaplastic meningioma reported that patients underwent from one to nine surgeries with complications rising from 35% at the first surgery to 100% by the fourth surgery [25]. Consequently, patients require a longer time to recover, and if this is coupled with high speed of growth of the tumor, as seen in anaplastic meningiomas, this results in diminishing return with each subsequent operation [25].

Although there is evidence that grade III meningiomas demonstrate a higher relative cerebral blood volume, there is no current robust evidence supporting use of preoperative embolization of the tumor [1]. Overall, it is important to estimate, as accurately as possible, the returns from each operation by considering probabilities of complications and likely duration of recovery, to define specific aims of surgery and, certainly, pose the question whether to operate at all.

Adjuvant Treatment

Additional treatment to recurrent meningioma is similar to those used in initial surgery for grade I meningioma, namely, stereotactic radiosurgery or radiotherapy, particularly in the context of a surgically inaccessible lesion or following subtotal or partial resection [26]. Continued observation of higher rates of recurrence in incompletely resected tumors and significant morbidity in aggressive resections has driven interest in neoadjuvant therapy in an effort to maximize quality of life [27]. Other therapies are currently the subject of ongoing trials and are described including trials of grade II/III meningioma below.

Future Directions

The Status Quo

While surgery remains the most efficacious first-line treatment, it is clear to those who see patients with meningiomas that there is a real need to improve treatments for these patients [27]. The multidisciplinary team needs to balance their recommendations of the oncological treatment with the drive to preserve quality of life, weighing up surgery against alternative treatments to deliver the right overall treatment for each individual patient. While treatment strategy is agreed with the patient preoperatively, intraoperative judgment needs to be made regarding the relative benefits of more aggressive surgery versus employing other treatment modalities. Because the surgeon will de facto represent the patient at surgery, it is essential that a detailed discussion between the surgeon and the patient takes place preoperatively. Better preoperative visualization, understanding, and prediction of factors that determine intraoperative findings and incomplete resection will enhance the quality of such a discussion.

Radiotherapy

Although surgery remains the standard of care, there remains clinical uncertainty regarding the use of adjuvant external beam radiotherapy. A phase II clinical trial (NCT00895622) evaluating the delivery of 54Gy with radiation therapy, intensity-modulated (IMRT) or 3D conformal (3DCRT), reported initial findings relating to patients in their "intermediate-risk group" encompassing grade II meningioma or recurrent grade I meningioma irrespective of extent of resection. The study identified a 3-year progression-free survival of 93.8% [28]. A second phase II study investigated the delivery of 60Gy radiotherapy in patients with grade II meningioma (Simpson grades 1–3) reported 3-year progression-free survival rates of 93.8% [28, 29]. However, the median follow-up was only 3.7 years, and there was no neuropsychological evaluation. The Radiotherapy versus Observation following surgical resection of Atypical Meningioma (ROAM) trial is an ongoing randomized controlled trial comparing early adjuvant radiotherapy (60Gy in 30 fractions for 6 weeks) in patients following gross total resection of atypical meningioma with a primary endpoint of time to MRI evidence of tumor recurrence or death due to any cause (EORTC 1308, ISRCTN71502099) [30].

Other than external beam radiation, aggressive meningiomas in eloquent locations such as the skull base may be candidates for fractionated stereotactic radiosurgery. Despite reporting promising results in presumed and histologically confirmed grade I meningiomas, 5-year freedom from progression was poor for more aggressive tumors (56% for grade II and 47% for grade III tumors) [31]. More novel delivery methods for radiotherapy, including peptide receptor radionuclide therapy with ^{90}Y-DOTATOC in recurrent meningioma, have shown some results stabilizing disease in patients with tumors with high levels of somatostatin receptor expression. Further studies are required to demonstrate efficacy relative to the current standard of care [32, 33].

Chemotherapy

Although a number of compounds have been tried, currently there is no compelling evidence supporting the use of chemotherapy in aggressive meningioma, either in the up-front setting or at recurrence. There is no evidence of any efficacy of temozolomide in patients in meningioma [34]. Combination therapy of cyclophosphamide, adriamycin, and vincristine results in a survival benefit but at the cost of toxicity, while hydroxyurea failed to deliver clinical benefit in trials after promising in vitro results [35]. A phase II trial of trabectedin in recurrent grade II/III failed to deliver improvement in PFS and OS and was associated with significantly higher toxicity as compared to the local standard treatment (EORTC-1320-BTG) [36].

Hormonal Therapy

Meningiomas are known to express hormonal receptors, notably progesterone and estrogen receptors. Meningioma growth has been observed during pregnancy, and meningiomas are more common in women with breast cancer and obesity [37]. Furthermore, there is observed increased incidence of diagnosis of meningioma in transsexual patients receiving hormone replacement therapy [38]. Further observed case series have demonstrated a reduction in tumor volume following discontinuation of hormonal therapy [39]. Specifically, studies investigating the use of estrogen inhibitors have identified a clinical benefit in only a minority of patients, though this may be due to the fact only 10% of meningiomas express estrogen receptors. A significantly higher proportion of meningiomas express progesterone receptors. Unfortunately, the results of a phase III trial in the use of mifepristone, an antiprogestogen, did not show any statistical improvement compared to placebo control [40, 41]. A phase II study of the use of a somatostatin analog failed to demonstrate an improvement in survival for recurrent or progressive meningioma [42]. Further potential hormonal targets including androgen receptor inhibitors and growth hormone receptor inhibitors require investigation. Overall, there is currently no evidence supporting the routine use of hormonal therapy in patients with aggressive meningioma.

Molecular Therapy

Initial insights into the molecular mechanisms for the growth, proliferation, and angiogenesis of meningiomas led to the development and investigation of inhibitors to growth factor signaling including cell surface receptors (PDGFR, EGFR), the MAP kinase pathway, the PI3K/Akt pathway, and TGF-β-SMAD pathways [35]. Further inhibitors of angiogenesis have been investigated. A phase II study of the use of PDFGR inhibitor imatinib showed no benefit in patients with recurrent meningiomas [43], while a phase II trial of sunitinib did meet its primary endpoint with a PFS6 rate of 42% [44]. Trials in the use of EGFR inhibitors erlotinib and gefitinib have failed to show any significant activity as a treatment for recurrent meningioma [45]. No trials have yet been completed on the use of monoclonal antibodies against EGFR despite their successful systemic use in other malignancies. Activation of MAP kinase and Akt signaling pathways has been associated with grade II and III meningioma indicating possible targets [46], while TGF-β appears to have an inhibitory effect on meningioma proliferation [47]. Currently no known trials are underway to investigate modulators of these pathways in patients with aggressive meningioma.

In an era of next-generation sequencing, molecular agents are increasingly being developed to target identified mutation profiles. Following evidence of control of a metastatic meningioma with an AKT inhibitor AZD5563 [48], a phase II trial is underway to investigate SMO, AKT1, and FAK inhibitors in patients with recurrent meningioma (NCT02523014), while cyclin-dependent kinase inhibition is a potential target for atypical and anaplastic meningioma [49]. The results of a phase II study investigating the use of a dual mTORC1 and mTORC2 inhibitor vistusertib (NCT03071874) in recurrent grade II-III meningiomas are awaited. Additional molecular signatures including POLR2A [50], TRAF7 [51], KLF4 [51], FOXM1 [52], TERT [53, 54], and BAP1 [55] all represent potential targets for therapies where further preclinical investigation is required prior to trialing these in patients with aggressive meningioma. The suspected presence of a significant number of neoantigens leaves open the possibility of the use of immunotherapy to treat higher-grade meningiomas where except for NF2, few consistently significantly mutated genes have been identified [56]. This hypothesis forms the basis for two phase II trials investigating the efficacy of checkpoint inhibitors (NCT03279692, NCT02648997).

Work to define robust response assessment and endpoints in meningioma clinical trials is welcomed as more targeted therapies capitalizing on the greater understanding of the underlying biology of meningiomas are developed [57].

Other Modalities

Prospective phase II studies of small molecule antiangiogenic inhibitors such as vatalanib and sunitinib have demonstrated very limited efficacy [44, 58], while retrospective data of antibody therapy, namely, bevacizumab, demonstrate similarly modest results in recurrent or progressive meningiomas [59, 60].

There is currently no randomized controlled evidence to support the use of other local therapies such as brachytherapy. Although a single center study of 42 patients reported median survival of 3.5 years after re-resection and ^{125}I brachytherapy, the authors also identified a high rate of complications including radiation necrosis (16%) and wound breakdown (12%) [61].

The use of laser interstitial thermal therapy has only been used in limited case series without clear conclusions regarding efficacy in recurrent grade I meningioma [62].

Proton beam therapy is currently the subject of multiple ongoing phase II studies of grade I–III meningiomas (NCT01117844, NCT02693990).

In three studies investigating the use of interferon alpha in patients with recurrent grade I and grade II and III meningiomas, a reduction in tumor volume was measured in only one patient. For the remaining patients, the majority had stable disease, but nonetheless a significant proportion still demonstrated progression [63–65].

Conclusions

This chapter has explored the presentation and diagnosis of aggressive meningiomas incorporating recurrent WHO grade I and WHO grade II and grade III meningioma. Standard of care where possible remains gross total resection of the tumor with due consideration to optimize quality of life with subtotal resection or primary treatment with radiotherapy if necessary. Standard of care in WHO grade III meningioma includes adjuvant radiotherapy; its use in grade II meningioma is currently the subject of two large clinical trials. The era of next-generation sequencing is heralding a transformation in classification and, consequently, treatment stratification and introduction of biological therapies to improve outcomes for patients with these tumors.

References

1. Goldbrunner R, Minniti G, Preusser M, et al. EANO guidelines for the diagnosis and treatment of meningiomas. Lancet Oncol. 2016;17(9):e383–91. Available from: https://linkinghub. elsevier.com/retrieve/pii/S1470204516303217.
2. Louis DN, Perry A, Reifenberger G, et al. The 2016 World Health Organization classification of tumors of the central nervous system: a summary. Acta Neuropathol. 2016 [cited 2019 Jun 16];131(6):803–20. Available from: https://braintumor.org/wp-content/assets/WHO-Central-Nervous-System-Tumor-Classification.pdf.
3. Simpson D. The recurrence of intracranial meningiomas after surgical treatment. J Neurol Neurosurg Psychiatry. 1957;20(1):22–39. Available from: http://www.ncbi.nlm.nih.gov/pubmed/13406590.
4. Perry A, Stafford SL, Scheithauer BW, et al. Meningioma grading: an analysis of histologic parameters. Am J Surg Pathol. 1997;21(12):1455–65. Available from: http://www.ncbi.nlm.nih.gov/pubmed/9414189.
5. Sughrue ME, Sanai N, Shangari G, et al. Outcome and survival following primary and repeat surgery for World Health Organization Grade III meningiomas. J Neurosurg. 2010;113(2):202–9.
6. Gousias K, Schramm J, Simon M. The Simpson grading revisited: aggressive surgery and its place in modern meningioma management. J Neurosurg. 2016;125(3):551–60.
7. Oya S, Kawai K, Nakatomi H, et al. Significance of Simpson grading system in modern meningioma surgery: integration of the grade with MIB-1 labeling index as a key to predict the recurrence of WHO Grade I meningiomas. J Neurosurg. 2012;117(4):806. Available from: https://thejns.org/view/journals/j-neurosurg/117/1/article-p121.xml.
8. Mirimanoff RO, Dosoretz DE, Linggood RM, et al. Meningioma: analysis of recurrence and progression following neurosurgical resection. J Neurosurg. 2009;62(1):18–24.
9. van Alkemade H, de Leau M, Dieleman EMT, et al. Impaired survival and long-term neurological problems in benign meningioma. Neuro Oncol. 2012;14(5):658–66. Available from: http://www.ncbi.nlm.nih.gov/pubmed/22406926.
10. Kshettry VR, Ostrom QT, Kruchko C, et al. Descriptive epidemiology of World Health Organization grades II and III intracranial meningiomas in the United States. Neuro Oncol. 2015;17(8):1166–73. Available from: http://www.ncbi.nlm.nih.gov/pubmed/26008603.

11. Kallio M, Sankila R, Hakulinen T, et al. Factors affecting operative and excess long-term mortality in 935 patients with intracranial meningioma. Neurosurgery. 1992;31(1):2–12. Available from: http://www.ncbi.nlm.nih.gov/pubmed/1641106.
12. Pearson BE, Markert JM, Fisher WS, et al. Hitting a moving target: evolution of a treatment paradigm for atypical meningiomas amid changing diagnostic criteria. Neurosurg Focus. 2008;24(5):E3.
13. Backer-Grøndahl T, Moen BH, Torp SH. The histopathological spectrum of human meningiomas. Int J Clin Exp Pathol. 2012;5(3):231–42. Available from: http://www.ncbi.nlm.nih.gov/pubmed/22558478.
14. Rogers L, Barani I, Chamberlain M, et al. Meningiomas: knowledge base, treatment outcomes, and uncertainties. A RANO review. J Neurosurg. 2015;122(1):4–23. Available from: http://www.ncbi.nlm.nih.gov/pubmed/25343186.
15. Ostrom QT, Gittleman H, Truitt G, et al. CBTRUS statistical report: primary brain and other central nervous system tumors diagnosed in the United States in 2011–2015. Neuro Oncol. 2018;20(suppl_4):iv1–86. Available from: https://academic.oup.com/neuro-oncology/article/20/suppl_4/iv1/5090960.
16. Brodbelt A, Barclay M, Greenberg D, et al. The outcome of patients with surgically treated meningioma in England: 1999-2013. Br J Neurosurg. 2019;33:641–7.
17. Al-Mefty O, Topsakal C, Pravdenkova S, et al. Radiation-induced meningiomas: clinical, pathological, cytokinetic, and cytogenetic characteristics. J Neurosurg. 2009;100(6):1002–13.
18. Takeguchi T, Miki H, Shimizu T, et al. The dural tail of intracranial meningiomas on fluid-attenuated inversion-recovery images. Neuroradiology. 2004;46(2):130–5. Available from: http://link.springer.com/10.1007/s00234-003-1152-4.
19. Dalle Ore CL, Magill ST, Yen AJ, et al. Meningioma metastases: incidence and proposed screening paradigm. J Neurosurg. 2019;132:1447–55.
20. Zhang H, Rödiger LA, Shen T, et al. Preoperative subtyping of meningiomas by perfusion MR imaging. Neuroradiology. 2008;50(10):835–40. Available from: http://link.springer.com/10.1007/s00234-008-0417-3.
21. Fountain DM, Soon WC, Matys T, et al. Volumetric growth rates of meningioma and its correlation with histological diagnosis and clinical outcome: a systematic review. Acta Neurochir. 2017;159(3):435–45.
22. Soon WC, Fountain DM, Koczyk K, et al. Correlation of volumetric growth and histological grade in 50 meningiomas. Acta Neurochir. 2017;159(11):2169–77.
23. Magill ST, Dalle Ore CL, Diaz MA, et al. Surgical outcomes after reoperation for recurrent skull base meningiomas. J Neurosurg. 2018;130(3):876–83.
24. Magill ST, Dalle Ore CL, Diaz MA, et al. Surgical outcomes after reoperation for recurrent non–skull base meningiomas. J Neurosurg. 2019;131:1179–87.
25. di Bonaventura R, Young A, Zakaria R, et al. MNGI-07. The anaplastic meningioma international consortium (AMICo) retrospective study of treatment and outcome of patients with anaplastic meningiomas. Neuro Oncol. 2018;20(suppl_6):vi149. Available from: https://academic.oup.com/neuro-oncology/article/20/suppl_6/vi149/5154451.
26. Soyuer S, Chang EL, Selek U, et al. Radiotherapy after surgery for benign cerebral meningioma. Radiother Oncol. 2004;71(1):85–90. Available from: https://www.sciencedirect.com/science/article/pii/S0167814004000477.
27. Nassiri F, Price B, Shehab A, et al. Life after surgical resection of a meningioma: a prospective cross-sectional study evaluating health-related quality of life. Neuro Oncol. 2019;21(Supplement_1):i32–43. Available from: https://academic.oup.com/neuro-oncology/article/21/Supplement_1/i32/5289362.
28. Rogers L, Zhang P, Vogelbaum MA, et al. Intermediate-risk meningioma: initial outcomes from NRG Oncology RTOG 0539. J Neurosurg. 2018;129(1):35–47. Available from: http://www.ncbi.nlm.nih.gov/pubmed/28984517.
29. Weber DC, Ares C, Villa S, et al. Adjuvant postoperative high-dose radiotherapy for atypical and malignant meningioma: a phase-II parallel non-randomized and observation study

(EORTC 22042-26042). Radiother Oncol. 2018;128(2):260–5. Available from: https://www. sciencedirect.com/science/article/pii/S0167814018333334.

30. Jenkinson MD, Javadpour M, Haylock BJ, et al. The ROAM/EORTC-1308 trial: radiation versus observation following surgical resection of Atypical Meningioma: study protocol for a randomised controlled trial. Trials. 2015;16(1):519. Available from: http://trialsjournal. biomedcentral.com/articles/10.1186/s13063-015-1040-3.

31. Kaprealian T, Raleigh DR, Sneed PK, et al. Parameters influencing local control of meningiomas treated with radiosurgery. J Neuro-Oncol. 2016;128(2):357–64. Available from: http:// link.springer.com/10.1007/s11060-016-2121-1.

32. Bartolomei M, Bodei L, De Cicco C, et al. Peptide receptor radionuclide therapy with 90Y-DOTATOC in recurrent meningioma. Eur J Nucl Med Mol Imaging. 2009;36(9):1407–16. Available from: http://link.springer.com/10.1007/s00259-009-1115-z.

33. Seystahl K, Stoecklein V, Schüller U, et al. Somatostatin-receptor-targeted radionuclide therapy for progressive meningioma: benefit linked to ^{68}Ga-DOTATATE/-TOC uptake. Neuro Oncol. 2016;18(11):now060. Available from: https://academic.oup.com/neuro-oncology/ article-lookup/doi/10.1093/neuonc/now060.

34. Chamberlain MC, Tsao-Wei DD, Groshen S. Temozolomide for treatment-resistant recurrent meningioma. Neurology. 2004;62(7):1210–2. Available from: http://www.ncbi.nlm.nih.gov/ pubmed/15079029.

35. Wen PY, Quant E, Drappatz J, et al. Medical therapies for meningiomas. J Neuro-Oncol. 2010;99(3):365–78. Available from: http://link.springer.com/10.1007/s11060-010-0349-8.

36. Preusser M, Silvani A, Le Rhun E, et al. Trabectedin for recurrent WHO grade II or III meningioma: a randomized phase II study of the EORTC Brain Tumor Group (EORTC-1320-BTG). J Clin Oncol. 2019;37(15_suppl):2007. Available from: https://ascopubs.org/doi/10.1200/ JCO.2019.37.15_suppl.2007.

37. Schoenberg BS, Christine BW, Whisnant JP. Nervous system neoplasms and primary malignancies of other sites. The unique association between meningiomas and breast cancer. Neurology. 1975;25(8):705–12. Available from: http://www.ncbi.nlm.nih.gov/pubmed/1171403.

38. Raj R, Korja M, Koroknay-Pál P, et al. Multiple meningiomas in two male-to-female transsexual patients with hormone replacement therapy: a report of two cases and a brief literature review. Surg Neurol Int. 2018;9:109. Available from: http://www.ncbi.nlm.nih.gov/ pubmed/29930875.

39. Passeri T, Champagne P-O, Bernat A-L, et al. Spontaneous regression of meningiomas after interruption of nomegestrol acetate: a series of three patients. Acta Neurochir (Wien). 2019;161(4):761–5. Available from: http://www.ncbi.nlm.nih.gov/pubmed/30783806.

40. Grunberg SM, Weiss MH, Spitz IM, et al. Treatment of unresectable meningiomas with the antiprogesterone agent mifepristone. J Neurosurg. 2009;74(6):861–6.

41. Ji Y, Rankin C, Grunberg S, et al. Double-Blind Phase III Randomized Trial of the Antiprogestin Agent Mifepristone in the Treatment of Unresectable Meningioma: SWOG S9005 Listen to the podcast by Dr Maher at www.jco.org.podcasts. J Clin Oncol. 2015;33:4093–8. Available from: www.jco.orgon.

42. Norden AD, Ligon KL, Hammond SN, et al. Phase II study of monthly pasireotide LAR (SOM230C) for recurrent or progressive meningioma. Neurology. 2015;84(3):280–6. Available from: http://www.ncbi.nlm.nih.gov/pubmed/25527270.

43. Wen PY, Yung WKA, Lamborn KR, et al. Phase II study of imatinib mesylate for recurrent meningiomas (North American Brain Tumor Consortium study 01–08). Neuro Oncol. 2009;11(6):853–60. Available from: http://www.ncbi.nlm.nih.gov/pubmed/19293394.

44. Kaley TJ, Wen P, Schiff D, et al. Phase II trial of sunitinib for recurrent and progressive atypical and anaplastic meningioma. Neuro-Oncology. 2015;17(1):116–21. Available from: https:// academic.oup.com/neuro-oncology/article-lookup/doi/10.1093/neuonc/nou148.

45. Norden AD, Raizer JJ, Abrey LE, et al. Phase II trials of erlotinib or gefitinib in patients with recurrent meningioma. J Neurooncol. 2010;96(2):211–7. Available from: http://www.ncbi. nlm.nih.gov/pubmed/19562255.

46. Mawrin C, Sasse T, Kirches E, et al. Different activation of mitogen-activated protein kinase and Akt signaling is associated with aggressive phenotype of human meningiomas. Clin Cancer Res. 2005;11(11):4074–82. Available from: http://www.ncbi.nlm.nih.gov/pubmed/15930342.
47. Johnson MD, Okediji E, Woodard A. Transforming growth factor- effects on meningioma cell proliferation and signal transduction pathways. J Neuro-Oncol. 2004;66(1/2):9–16. Available from: http://link.springer.com/10.1023/B:NEON.0000013461.35120.8a.
48. Weller M, Roth P, Sahm F, et al. Durable control of metastatic AKT1-mutant WHO grade 1 meningothelial meningioma by the AKT inhibitor, AZD5363. J Natl Cancer Inst. 2017;109(3). Available from: https://academic.oup.com/jnci/article-lookup/doi/10.1093/jnci/djw320.
49. Boström J, Meyer-Puttlitz B, Wolter M, et al. Alterations of the tumor suppressor genes CDKN2A (p16INK4a), p14ARF, CDKN2B (p15INK4b), and CDKN2C (p18INK4c) in atypical and anaplastic meningiomas. Am J Pathol. 2001;159(2):661–9. Available from: https://www.sciencedirect.com/science/article/pii/S0002944010617373.
50. Clark VE, Harmancı AS, Bai H, et al. Recurrent somatic mutations in POLR2A define a distinct subset of meningiomas. Nat Genet. 2016;48(10):1253–9. Available from: http://www.nature.com/articles/ng.3651.
51. Clark VE, Erson-Omay EZ, Serin A, et al. Genomic analysis of non-NF2 meningiomas reveals mutations in TRAF7, KLF4, AKT1, and SMO. Science. 2013;339(6123):1077–80. Available from: http://www.ncbi.nlm.nih.gov/pubmed/23348505.
52. Vasudevan HN, Braunstein SE, Phillips JJ, et al. Comprehensive molecular profiling identifies FOXM1 as a key transcription factor for meningioma proliferation. Cell Rep. 2018;22(13):3672–83. Available from: http://www.ncbi.nlm.nih.gov/pubmed/29590631.
53. Sahm F, Schrimpf D, Olar A, et al. TERT promoter mutations and risk of recurrence in meningioma. J Natl Cancer Inst. 2016;108(5). Available from: http://www.ncbi.nlm.nih.gov/pubmed/26668184.
54. Goutagny S, Nault JC, Mallet M, et al. High incidence of activating TERT promoter mutations in meningiomas undergoing malignant progression. Brain Pathol. 2014;24(2):184–9. Available from: https://onlinelibrary.wiley.com/doi/pdf/10.1111/bpa.12110.
55. Shankar GM, Santagata S. BAP1 mutations in high-grade meningioma: implications for patient care. Neuro-Oncology. 2017;19(11):1447–56. Available from: http://academic.oup.com/neuro-oncology/article/19/11/1447/3803447.
56. Bi WL, Greenwald NF, Abedalthagafi M, et al. Genomic landscape of high-grade meningiomas. NPJ Genomic Med. 2017;2. Available from: http://www.ncbi.nlm.nih.gov/pubmed/28713588.
57. Huang RY, Bi WL, Weller M, et al. Proposed response assessment and endpoints for meningioma clinical trials: report from the Response Assessment in Neuro-Oncology Working Group. Neuro-Oncology. 2019;21(1):26–36. Available from: https://academic.oup.com/neuro-oncology/article/21/1/26/5076187.
58. Raizer JJ, Grimm SA, Rademaker A, et al. A phase II trial of PTK787/ZK 222584 in recurrent or progressive radiation and surgery refractory meningiomas. J Neuro-Oncol. 2014;117(1):93–101. Available from: http://link.springer.com/10.1007/s11060-014-1358-9.
59. Lou E, Sumrall AL, Turner S, et al. Bevacizumab therapy for adults with recurrent/progressive meningioma: a retrospective series. J Neuro-Oncol. 2012;109(1):63–70. Available from: http://link.springer.com/10.1007/s11060-012-0861-0.
60. Nunes FP, Merker VL, Jennings D, et al. Bevacizumab treatment for meningiomas in NF2: a retrospective analysis of 15 patients. O. Pieper R, editor. PLoS One. 2013;8(3):e59941. Available from: http://dx.plos.org/10.1371/journal.pone.0059941.
61. Magill ST, Lau D, Raleigh DR, et al. Surgical resection and interstitial Iodine-125 brachytherapy for high-grade meningiomas: a 25-year series. Neurosurgery. 2017;80(3):409–16. Available from: https://academic.oup.com/neurosurgery/article-abstract/80/3/409/2847230.
62. Ivan ME, Diaz RJ, Berger MH, et al. Magnetic resonance–guided laser ablation for the treatment of recurrent dural-based lesions: a series of five cases. World Neurosurg. 2017;98:162–70. Available from: https://www.sciencedirect.com/science/article/pii/S1878875016310257?via%3Dihub.

63. Kaba SE, DeMonte F, Bruner JM, et al. The treatment of recurrent unresectable and malignant meningiomas with interferon alpha-2B. Neurosurgery. 1997;40(2):271–5. Available from: http://www.ncbi.nlm.nih.gov/pubmed/9007858.

64. Muhr C, Gudjonsson O, Lilja A, et al. Meningioma treated with interferon-alpha, evaluated with [(11)C]-L-methionine positron emission tomography. Clin Cancer Res. 2001;7(8):2269–76. Available from: http://www.ncbi.nlm.nih.gov/pubmed/11489801.

65. Chamberlain MC, Glantz MJ. Interferon-α for recurrent World Health Organization grade 1 intracranial meningiomas. Cancer. 2008;113(8):2146–51. Available from: http://www.ncbi.nlm.nih.gov/pubmed/18756531.

Surgical Considerations for Recurrent Meningiomas

11

Amol Raheja and William T. Couldwell

Introduction

Meningiomas, which are among the most common intracranial tumors, account for 20–35% of all brain tumors and have an annual incidence of ~6 per 100,000 people [1–3]. Approximately 90% of meningiomas are classified as benign (World Health Organization (WHO) grade I), 5–7% are characterized as atypical (WHO grade II), and only 1–3% are considered malignant (WHO grade III) [3]. Tumor recurrence is an important long-term complication of meningioma surgery [4–7]. Recurrence rates can vary from 7 to 94% after 10 years, depending on the WHO grade of resected tumor [4–8]. High-grade meningiomas follow a more aggressive clinical course characterized by local recurrence and poor long-term survival [4–7]. Atypical meningiomas have recurrence rates up to 50% and 10-year survival rates less than 80% [9]. The median time to progression of atypical meningiomas is approximately 24 months [9]. Biologically aggressive tumors located in the parasagittal and posterior fossa tend to recur more frequently [4, 6, 7, 9]. Patient age, degree of major venous sinus invasion, extent of resection (EOR) (Simpson's grade of removal [10], Fig. 11.1), use of adjuvant therapy, and MIB index beyond other pathological features also govern the relapse patterns in these tumors [1, 3, 4, 6, 7, 9, 11–15].

Recurrent meningiomas challenge neurosurgeons at every step. Surgery and radiation therapy remain the treatments of choice for recurrent meningiomas [6, 7, 15–18]. At present, chemotherapy and molecular targeted therapy have limited

A. Raheja
Department of Neurosurgery, All India Institute of Medical Sciences, New Delhi, India

W. T. Couldwell (✉)
Department of Neurosurgery, Clinical Neurosciences Center, University of Utah, Salt Lake City, UT, USA
e-mail: william.couldwell@hsc.utah.edu; neuropub@hsc.utah.edu

© Springer Nature Switzerland AG 2020
J. Moliterno, A. Omuro (eds.), *Meningiomas*,
https://doi.org/10.1007/978-3-030-59558-6_11

Fig. 11.1 Simpson grade of meningioma removal and recurrence rate

Grade	Tumor Resection	Recurrence Rate
I	Macroscopically complete removal of dura, bone	9%
II	Macroscopically complete removal, dural coagulation	19%
III	Complete tumor resection dura not coagulated	29%
IV	Partial removal	44%
V	Simple decompression	

* Based on Simpson grade.

roles in management of these patients [19–21]. Resection for these lesions can be distinctly complicated owing to postoperative or radiogenic scars, tissue adhesions, and altered anatomy after the initial treatment. Major venous sinus invasion with the development of collateral draining veins is also an important consideration when planning surgical intervention, especially to aptly tailor the intended extent of resection and possibly venous sinus reconstruction for each patient [6, 7, 17, 18, 22–24]. A detailed evaluation of vascular anatomy via preoperative imaging is paramount in achieving optimal patient outcome. Planning and decision-making based on individualized case-based analysis is as important as execution of meticulous surgery for achieving good long-term outcomes in these patients [6, 7, 17, 18, 22–24]. In this chapter, we discuss relevant concepts, technical pearls, nuances, and current literature for surgical management of recurrent meningiomas.

Incidence of Meningioma Recurrence

Extent of resection is probably the most important factor, besides WHO grading, in governing the recurrence rates in meningiomas [10]. In Simpson's original series, grade I through grade IV tumor resections had recurrence rates at 10 years of 9%, 19%, 29%, and 44%, respectively [10]. The reported recurrence rates for malignant meningioma and atypical meningioma with complete resection are 58.3% and 27.3%, respectively, while reported incidences with subtotal resection are 88.9% and 66.7%, respectively [25]. Another study has reported higher recurrence rates after complete resection: 38% for atypical meningioma and 78% for malignant meningioma at 5 years and up to 100% eventual recurrence with complete or subtotal resection of malignant meningioma [26]. Atypical meningiomas carry a seven- to eightfold greater risk of recurrence and a twofold greater risk of death at 3–5 years after resection compared with WHO grade I meningiomas [4, 9, 25]. Recurrence rates for histologically benign meningioma also vary widely within the literature. Two studies with large sample size showed a 19% recurrence rate at 20 years after complete removal and 32% at 15 years after complete removal, respectively [27, 28]. Other studies have shown lower recurrence rates, with a 7.6% recurrence after complete resection but 34.4% after subtotal resection [25]. Some subgroups of histologically benign meningioma tumors behave aggressively clinically even though they do not meet the criteria for atypical or malignant variants. Included in this subgroup are those with elevated MIB index.

Natural History and Pathogenesis

Recurrent meningioma is clinically, histologically, and biologically more aggressive than primary meningioma [6, 7, 29, 30]. Furthermore, meningiomas that recur are prone to further recurrence at progressively shorter intervals, and patients can experience significant adverse events from serial salvage therapies, as well as a significant risk of death from progressive disease (Fig. 11.2) [6, 7, 29, 30]. Recurrent meningiomas are usually associated with higher MIB-1 index labeling on serial pathological analysis. Approximately 8% of recurrent atypical meningiomas eventually transform into malignant meningiomas over time, and 5% tend to metastasize [2]. Hypotheses to explain this distant metastasis include multicentric foci, spread along cerebrospinal fluid (CSF) pathways, and venous transmission [2, 29]. The increasingly rapid progression of recurrent tumors may be driven by clonal outgrowth of biologically more aggressive meningioma cells over time. Furthermore, recurrent tumors may accumulate genetic mutations and epigenetic changes related either to the natural history of disease or to DNA damage from prior radiotherapy (RT) that promotes meningioma cell growth [1, 2, 4, 29]. Peritumoral edema is yet

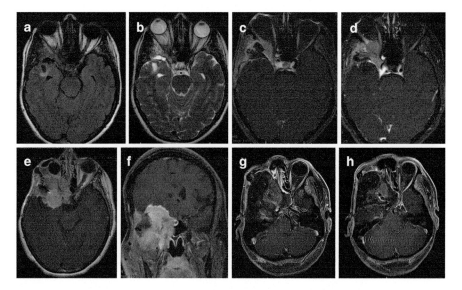

Fig. 11.2 Imaging obtained from a 41-year-old woman who presented with progressive proptosis (**a**, **b**). She had undergone resection of a WHO grade I meningioma 9 years earlier. (**c**, **d**) Four years after her presentation with proptosis, she underwent three orbital surgeries to address orbital and cavernous sinus invasion. (**e**, **f**) After 2 years, there was again orbital, ethmoidal, and sphenoid sinus invasion and further cavernous sinus invasion. (**g**, **h**) She underwent exenteration of the orbit and facial and sinus tumor with free flap placement for closure

another clinically and radiologically underestimated finding that has been demonstrated to be significantly associated with early aggressive behavior and meningioma recurrence at 24 months [9]. Tumor size, growth rate, leptomeningeal invasion, development of pial blood supply, as well as specific histological types have all been implicated in the development of peritumoral edema [9].

Risk factors for serial recurrence include multifocal primary recurrence within the resection cavity, prior subtotal resection with or without RT, parafalcine/parasagittal location, brain invasion, absence of epidermal growth factor receptor, bone involvement, peritumoral edema on preoperative magnetic resonance (MR) imaging scan, progression from WHO grade I, as well as a high mitotic index (MI) >7/10 high-powered field and high proliferation index (MIB-1/Ki-67). These risk factors have all been implicated in prognosis [1, 2, 4, 8, 9, 29, 31].

Surgical Planning and Strategizing

The principal question is whether to operate on a patient with recurrent meningioma or to subject them directly to adjuvant RT [15, 22, 24, 32]. This can be a complex problem and requires an individualized approach for each patient. As a general principle, the authors choose a surgical resection of the tumor if the patient is of sufficient health to undergo the procedure, and the procedure can be performed with acceptable risk [22, 32]. This may forestall the relentless progression of inadequate surgical resection and adjuvant treatments for progression demonstrated in the clinical case in Fig. 11.3. Adjuvant RT as the primary treatment is typically reserved for

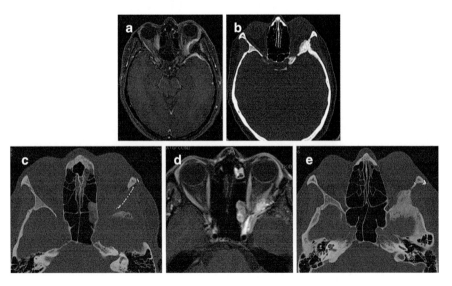

Fig. 11.3 The natural history of meningioma recurrence. (**a, b**) A 57-year-old woman presented with spheno-orbital meningioma and proptosis. The tumor was removed by a frontotemporal approach with drilling of the lateral sphenoid wing. (**c–e**) Three years later, she developed progressive disease with tumor within the nasal sinus requiring an endoscopic resection

patients with appropriately sized asymptomatic recurrent meningiomas not amenable to complete resection and partially resected high-grade meningiomas [2, 5, 13, 16, 33–35]. On the other hand, resection is clearly indicated for symptomatic tumor recurrences and asymptomatic large recurrences [2, 5, 13, 33]. Furthermore, surgery can be helpful in the diagnosis of any change in tumor grade, which would otherwise go unnoticed and might have prognostic implications.

Surgery for recurrent meningiomas is generally associated with similar risk of postoperative complications compared with resection of primary tumors. It is imperative to understand, however, that Simpson's grade and EOR do not have similar correlation with tumor recurrence in recurrent meningiomas as in primary surgery, except recurrent falx/parasagittal meningiomas [5, 8]. In other words, maximal safe resection should be the goal in repeat surgery, and, while aiming for complete resection should be the goal in all meningioma surgery, aiming for radical resection in aggressive (WHO grade II and III tumor) does not alter the overall prognosis in the biologically aggressive recurrent meningiomas as in WHO grade I lesions [5, 22]. The patient's neurological function and quality of life should be prioritized rather than radiological perfection. Thus, the treatment strategy needs to be tailored based on the individual patient's neurological status and wishes/expectations; the surgeons' expertise, experience, and preferences; and the radiographic characteristics of the tumor (location, extent, size, and regrowth pattern).

In general, patients who decline treatment have poor overall survival compared with patients receiving treatment, whether surgery or RT. Therefore, a proactive attitude toward treatment is important for recurrent/progressive meningiomas because conservative observation can lead to disastrous prognosis in some cases. The goal of repeat surgery is to maintain or improve the patient's neurological function and to prolong subsequent progression-free survival time and life span [6, 7, 13, 17, 18, 22, 32]. Besides the tumor characteristics and surgeons' experience, the prior surgical approach needs to be considered while selecting the surgical corridor for reoperation. The relative aggressiveness and surgical strategy may alter depending on the anatomical location of the recurrent tumor [6, 7, 13, 17, 18, 22, 32]. For convexity meningiomas and others (olfactory groove, anterior third of the sagittal sinus, and some tentorial and posterior fossa tumors) that may be completely resectable, the challenge is to leave the patient functionally intact and able to return expeditiously to his or her previous occupation. Deliberate incomplete resection may be the goal for some tumors of the skull base in which the risk of resection is associated with increasing neurological deficit. Even today, it may be best for the patient to live with some tumors, such as those of the optic nerve sheath, to undergo a biopsy, or simply to be monitored [1]. Choosing the appropriate surgical approach, deciding how far to go with the resection, and deciding whether to attempt to take tumor away from vital and sensitive structures such as the cavernous sinus, brainstem, and lower cranial nerves are continuing problems [6, 7, 13, 17, 18, 22, 32]. Meticulous surgical technique is necessary to achieve optimal patient outcome. Invasion of a major venous sinus is yet another enigmatic issue with no global consensus in the neurosurgical literature for planning aggressiveness of tumor resection and sinus reconstruction, especially in recurrent meningiomas [6, 7, 13, 17, 18, 22, 24, 32].

Major Venous Sinus Invasion and Sinus Reconstruction Techniques

Venous meningiomas arise in close proximity to major venous sinuses and are often analyzed separately as parasagittal, tentorial, and torcular meningiomas [17, 18, 22–24, 36–39]. Their potential for invading the sinus walls and affecting bridging veins is a common denominator that complicates radical surgery and poses a substantial risk to safe resection of offending lesions. Although the risk of recurrence is associated with EOR, complete removal of meningiomas in these locations must be weighed against the iatrogenic venous outflow obstruction, which can lead to venous infarction and significant neurological consequences [17, 18, 22–24, 36–39]. When a meningioma occludes a venous sinus completely, complete resection of the intravascular portion can be safely performed. On the contrary, when the tumor invades but does not completely obliterate a major venous sinus, opinions vary on whether to accept a partial resection or to open up the sinus, perform a complete resection, and reconstruct the venous outflow tract [17, 18, 22–24, 36–39].

Careful preoperative assessment using imaging tools such as MR or computed tomography (CT) venogram usually suffices for initial evaluation of venous occlusion by tumors. To get a more detailed understanding of the collateral circulation, aberrant drainage, vascular anatomy, and degree of sinus occlusion, late-phase digital subtraction angiography is still the gold standard [17, 18, 22–24, 36–39]. One of the most widely accepted classification schemes for venous sinus occlusion is Sindou's classification [23, 24, 38], which is simpler than the Krause and Merrem [40] or Bonnal and Brotchil [36] classifications. Sindou [38] described six types (Type I–VI) of progressively increasing venous sinus occlusion by meningeal tumors and recommended progressively aggressive tumor removal along with sinus wall repair and reconstruction techniques for optimal long-term patient outcomes. The sinus wall can be repaired either primarily using 6-0 or 7-0 Prolene monofilament suture (to reduce thrombogenicity) or via patch grafting with autologous pericranium, fascia lata, etc. [17, 22, 24]. If the sinus wall cannot be repaired, then a venous bypass across the sinus defect is contemplated using autologous saphenous vein graft [17, 22, 24]. Use of Gore-Tex tubes for conduit has fallen out of practice because of its high failure rates [17, 22, 24]. If the torcula is completely involved and sacrificed, venous bypass from the sagittal sinus to the external jugular vein is required to maintain venous outflow, at least until the alternative venous collaterals take up the bulk of the cerebral venous drainage [17, 22, 24]. Mantovani et al. [17] have proposed another clinically relevant classification scheme for sinus involvement, which considers the degree of sinus patency as total occlusion, subtotal with 50–95% occlusion, and partial with less than 50% occlusion. This classification assigns different risk profiles to managing patients with complete and incomplete sinus occlusion, which influences decision-making regarding venous reconstruction [17].

Besides counseling patients with recurrent meningioma about possible sinus exploration and the risks involved, patient safety can be further augmented by the use of perioperative aspirin/heparin, judicious use of preoperative embolization, placement of precordial Doppler probe and central venous catheter for detecting and managing possible air embolism, use of intraoperative electrophysiological neuromonitoring via motor evoked potentials and somatosensory evoked potentials, and optimal patient positioning [17, 18, 22, 24]. Grossly, the management of recurrent meningiomas invading the sinuses can be divided into conservative or aggressive strategies based on the extent of sinus manipulation [22]. The decision-making factors for choosing the radicality of surgical approach include the patient's age, informed consent, and known/anticipated tumor WHO grade [22]. Lastly, in patients with meningiomatosis, an aggressive approach has no theoretical advantage because of the propensity of these lesions to develop new sporadic tumors despite radical tumor resection [22]. We choose a general approach with these patients to address symptomatic lesions as they arise and make no effort to provide surgical treatment for incidental lesions given the burden of surgery that patients will endure during their lifetime.

Conservative Management

This surgical approach generally aims at near-total/subtotal tumor resection and leaving a small intraluminal sinus component of tumor in situ, which can be managed either expectantly via radiological surveillance or more actively via upfront radiosurgery/RT to contain tumor growth [12, 17, 18, 22, 39]. This approach carries a lower risk of postoperative venous infarct and its sequelae as compared with an aggressive surgical approach, although the risk of tumor recurrence is higher using these conservative approaches. Because of the risks associated with an aggressive surgical approach, several authors consider the presence of sinus patency to be a contraindication to aggressive management [12, 17, 18, 22, 39]. A Swedish study evaluating long-term outcomes after a 25-year follow-up noted a 47% recurrence rate and found that subtotal resection was correlated with increased tumor-related morbidity and mortality in the long run [12]. In a review of the literature on meningiomas involving the superior sagittal sinus, Tomasello et al. [39] stratified study populations by treatment strategy from conservative to most radical. The authors found that the recurrence rate was 6%–29% when a conservative strategy was adopted; 14%–19% when an intrasinus tumor was resected, requiring sinus repair but not reconstruction; and 4% when sinus outflow was restored after tumor resection.

Aggressive Management

As the name suggests, a more radical surgical approach is taken to resect maximal tumor and reconstruct the venous outflow channels [17, 18, 22–24, 38]. Appropriate care is taken to preserve any normal, tumor-free sinus walls, as well as the ostia of affluent veins. Despite adequate precautions, the risk of immediate postoperative venous infarction and even death is higher than with the conservative surgical approach, although the risk of tumor recurrence is lower using this surgical strategy [17, 18, 22–24, 38]. Brisk bleeding from normal sinus ends is expected after radical tumor excision, and it can be managed using the technique described by Sindou and Alvernia [24], which includes insertion of Surgicel (Johnson Medical) pledgets into the vessel orifice for temporary hemostasis until the sinus wall reconstruction is completed. Alternative options of using balloons/shunts and vascular clamps/aneurysm clips for temporary hemostasis are limited by the presence of septations in the sinus lumen and the risk of endothelium damage, respectively [17, 18, 22–24, 38]. Intraoperatively, reconstitution of venous flow can be confirmed using a micro-Doppler probe or indocyanine green fluorescence angiography. In cases in which complete sinus exclusion from circulation is planned, test clamping of the sinus should be performed to rule out any unusual brain swelling, before finally ligating the sinuses A more objective assessment method is to perform manometric measurements in upstream sinus channels before and after test clamping [41]. Any increase in sinus pressure of more than 10 mm Hg is a contraindication for sinus occlusion without venous bypass [41]. If the sinus is only partially occluded, preserving its patency is important. Normal vessel walls should be kept intact whenever feasible. Resection of occluded sinus can be disastrous, with a reported mortality of 50% after the resection of occluded portions of major dural sinuses without reconstruction [17, 18, 22–24, 38]. Once the intraluminal portion of tumor is resected, the sinus wall can be repaired via primary resuturing, patching, or venous bypass [17, 18, 22–24, 38]. Stent placement preoperatively may also facilitate safe tumor removal without compromising the existing sinus lumen and venous outflow. On the contrary, if the sinus is already completely obliterated/occluded by the intraluminal tumor, complete tumor removal can be done without any need for sinus reconstruction, as there is generally an adequate collateral circulation, which has been naturally formed to suffice venous outflow [17, 18, 22–24, 38]. Those collateral venous pathways need to be carefully preserved intraoperatively to alleviate the risk of iatrogenic venous infarct and poor neurological sequelae. Even in the situation of complete sinus occlusion, some surgeons still favor flow restoration with a prophylactic venous bypass to allow time for any circulatory deficiencies in venous outflow to correct themselves and tolerate alterations in the venous circulations that may occur after resection [23, 24]. In many cases, an angiographically occluded sinus is found to be patent during surgery, so final decision-making should be done intraoperatively. In a study by Sindou and Alvernia [24] of attempted radical resection of 100 meningiomas involving any major dural sinus, the tumor recurrence rate was 4%. However, the authors also reported a 3% mortality rate and an 8% venous-related morbidity rate for their aggressive approach. In a series of 108 patients with meningiomas invading the superior sagittal sinus, DiMeco et al. [37] advocated radical resection and sinus entry with primary suture repair in the setting of partial sinus occlusion and complete excision in cases of complete occlusion. They reported severe brain swelling in 9 of 108 patients (8.3%) and postoperative hematoma in 2 (1.85%) patients. Although their 5-year recurrence-free survival was similar across Simpson grade I–IV resections, the 10-year recurrence-free survival rate was 86.5% in patients with Simpson grade I removal compared with 76% and 51% for Simpson grade II and IV resections, respectively ($p = 0.03$). In other series, recurrence rates have been demonstrated to vary from 4% to 24% [17, 18, 22, 24, 37].

Adjuvant Therapies

Recurrent meningiomas are often not amenable to radical resection because of the frequent involvement of the cavernous sinus, other major venous sinuses, and vital neurovascular structures. In addition, many of these tumors have transformed into aggressive higher-grade lesions, which often have infiltrative margins not amenable to complete resection. Hence, adjuvant treatment with either stereotactic radiosurgery (SRS) or fractionated RT is required to control the disease progression and ensure long-term remission [2, 5, 11, 16, 18, 22, 33–35]. The primary candidates for adjuvant SRS include patients with poor neurological status or who refuse surgery because of surgical risk or older age and patients with asymptomatic recurrent tumors less than 3 cm in size, those with lesions mainly involving the cavernous sinus, or those with lesions presenting with multiple recurrent sites or en plaque regrowth pattern along the skull base dura but without compressing the brainstem [2, 5, 11, 16, 18, 22, 33–35]. However, the use of SRS may be limited by large tumor size, irregular tumor contour, the lesion's proximity to vital neurovascular structures, poor long-term remission rates, and the increased risk of radiation necrosis in patients who have received prior radiation. Chemotherapy and hormonal and targeted molecular therapy are additional options but have limited effectiveness in routine clinical practice [19–21]. Lastly, recurrent tumors that have been subjected to comprehensive radiation therapy can be managed with permanent seed (I-125) brachytherapy [2]. A close collaboration among microneurosurgeons, medical oncologists, and radiation oncologists is a prerequisite for this treatment option to decrease the potential morbidity from each of the individual techniques and plan a comprehensive multimodality management.

Treatment Outcome

There is limited available literature on long-term outcomes for surgical management of purely recurrent meningiomas [6, 7]. Since the natural history, surgical challenges, and overall/progression-free survival of skull base meningiomas is different from that of non-skull base lesions, it is quite natural to dichotomize the outcome description accordingly.

Recurrent Skull Base Meningiomas

Skull base meningiomas are surgically challenging because of the intricate skull base anatomy and the proximity of cranial nerves and critical cerebral vasculature. Approximately 1/3 of meningiomas arise from the skull base [7]. There is a propensity toward more residual/recurrent tumors in the skull base region compared with non-skull base anatomical locations [7]. Recurrence rates as high as 26%–29% for skull base meningiomas have been reported; yet, there are limited data to counsel patients and neurosurgeons regarding the management of these tumors [7].

Interestingly, the relative growth rates of tumors in the skull base region are lower than in their non-skull base counterparts [30]. Hence, in some instances, especially residual lesions in the cavernous sinus, skull base meningiomas can be monitored conservatively without upfront adjuvant therapy [13, 32]. In a series of 78 patients undergoing 100 reoperations for recurrent skull base meningiomas, Magill et al. [7] demonstrated that the median time from initial resection to first reoperation was 4.4 years, and the median time from first to second reoperation was 4.1 years. The sphenoid wing was the most common location (31%), followed by the cerebello-pontine angle (14%), cavernous sinus (13%), olfactory groove (12%), tuberculum sellae (12%), and middle fossa floor (5%) [7]. Overall, 72% of tumors were WHO grade I, 22% were WHO grade II, and 6% were WHO grade III. In 100 reoperations, 60 complications were recorded in 30 patients. Twenty of the 60 complications required surgical intervention (33%). The most common complication was hydro-cephalus (12 cases), followed by CSF leak/pseudomeningocele (11 cases), wound infection (9 cases), postoperative hematoma (4 cases), venous infarction (1 case), and pneumocephalus (1 case) [7]. Postoperative neurological deficits included new or worsened cranial nerve deficits (10 cases) and hemiparesis (3 cases). On multi-variate analysis, a posterior fossa location was significantly associated with a higher complication profile (OR 3.45, $p = 0.0472$). The 1-, 2-, 5-, and 10-year overall sur-vival rates after the first reoperation were 94%, 92%, 88%, and 76%, respectively. The median survival after the first reoperation was 17 years [7].

In another study, Li et al.[31] analyzed their cohort of 39 patients with recur-rent/progressive petroclival meningioma who were monitored for an average of 70.4 months. There was a second recurrence/progression-free survival rate of 88%, 67%, and 40% for gross-total, subtotal, and partial resection, respectively. The over-all survival after the first recurrence/progression of gross-total, subtotal, and par-tial resection was 88%, 63%, and 33%, respectively. Patients rejecting treatment experienced significantly poorer overall survival (7%; $p = 0.001$) and shorter sur-vival duration (42.0 months; $p = 0.016$) compared with patients receiving treatment (67% and 86.9 months, respectively). Li et al. [31] also reviewed the literature on recurrent petroclival meningiomas. In the 21 included studies with 98 patients with recurrent/progressive petroclival meningiomas, 17 patients presented with a second recurrence/progression and 10 died as a result; patients undergoing observation had a significantly poorer tumor regrowth control rate compared with patients undergo-ing surgery ($p = 0.004$) or radiotherapy alone ($p < 0.001$). Li et al. [31] concluded that proactive treatment should be performed for patients with recurrent/progressive petroclival meningiomas. Gross-total or maximal safe resection is a preferential therapeutic strategy and should be pursued as far as possible while ensuring mini-mal iatrogenic neurological morbidity. Recurrent skull base meningiomas are surgi-cally challenging tumors, and repeat surgery is associated with high morbidity and complication rates. Despite the risks involved, reoperation for these difficult-to-treat lesions in carefully selected patients can provide excellent overall and progression-free survival [7, 31].

In the case of recurrent tumor involving the cavernous sinus, the options include surgical resection or radiosurgery or stereotactic radiation therapy. These options have been extensively discussed by the authors in other publications [13, 32]. Our general philosophy regarding management has been that while the patient has functional binocular vision, we try to preserve it as long as possible. Thus, tailored surgical resection with adjuvant radiation therapy is recommended [13, 32]. When or if such time comes that the patient loses functional binocular vision, or there is visual loss, we will recommend cavernous sinus exenteration in younger healthy patients as salvage treatment to prolong life (Fig. 11.2) [13, 32].

Recurrent Non-skull Base Meningiomas

Approximately 2/3 of meningiomas arise from the non-skull base anatomical regions [6]. There is a propensity toward more biologically aggressive and invasive meningeal tumors, with higher WHO grade at recurrence in non-skull base region compared with their skull base counterparts [6, 30]. Innate tumor biology and skin-related complications from prior RT/SRS often lead to a higher risk of complications in non-skull base lesions as compared with recurrent skull base meningiomas. Magill et al. [6] analyzed their patient cohort of 67 non-skull base supratentorial meningiomas (111 reoperations) with a median follow-up of 9.8 years. The most common involved location was the convexity (52%), followed by parasagittal (33%), falx (31%), and multifocal (19%) locations. The WHO grade after the last reoperation was grade I in 22% of cases, grade II in 51%, and grade III in 27%. The tumor grade increased at redo surgery in 22% of cases, suggesting a high rate of transformation in this subset of patients. Overall, in the 111 reoperations, 48 complications occurred in 32 patients (48%). There were 26 (54%) complications requiring surgical intervention. Complications included neurological deficits (14% total, 8% permanent), wound dehiscence/infection (14%), and CSF leak/pseudo-meningocele/hydrocephalus (9%). On multivariate analysis, tumors that involved the middle third of the sagittal plane (OR 6.97, 95% CI 1.5–32.0, $p = 0.006$) and presentation with cognitive changes (possibly an epiphenomenon reflecting a combination of symptomatic elderly patient and tumor-related factors) (OR 20.7, 95% CI 2.3–182.7, $p = 0.001$) were significantly associated with complication occurrence.[6] The median survival after the first reoperation was 11.5 years, and the 2-, 5-, and 10-year overall survival rates were 91.0%, 68.8%, and 50.0%, respectively [6].

Conclusions

Recurrent meningiomas remain an enigmatic problem in the modern neurosurgical era. Careful patient selection, rationalizing the decision-making process, balancing the aggressiveness of resection between tumor biology and chance of recurrence along with tumor-related morbidity, maintenance/reconstruction of venous drainage pathways invaded by tumor, judicious use of adjuvant therapeutic options, and tailoring them to the individual patient's requirement can lead to favorable long-term overall and progression-free survival with acceptable complication profile in patients with recurrent meningioma despite the potentially aggressive nature of these lesions. Future efforts aimed at identifying histologic, molecular, and genetic factors associated with aggressive and recurrent meningioma are warranted.

References

1. Black PM. Meningiomas. Neurosurgery. 1993;32(4):643–57.
2. Chen WC, Hara J, Magill ST, et al. Salvage therapy outcomes for atypical meningioma. J Neuro-Oncol. 2018;138(2):425–33.
3. Louis DN, Ohgaki H, Wiestler OD, et al. The 2007 WHO classification of tumours of the central nervous system. Acta Neuropathol. 2007;114(2):97–109.
4. Buster WP, Rodas RA, Fenstermaker RA, Kattner KA. Major venous sinus resection in the surgical treatment of recurrent aggressive dural based tumors. Surg Neurol. 2004;62(6):522–9; discussion 529–530.
5. Chohan MO, Ryan CT, Singh R, et al. Predictors of treatment response and survival outcomes in meningioma recurrence with atypical or anaplastic histology. Neurosurgery. 2018;82(6):824–32.
6. Magill ST, Dalle Ore CL, Diaz MA, et al. Surgical outcomes after reoperation for recurrent non-skull base meningiomas. J Neurosurg. 2018;130(3):876–83.
7. Magill ST, Lee DS, Yen AJ, et al. Surgical outcomes after reoperation for recurrent skull base meningiomas. J Neurosurg. 2018;130(3):876–83.
8. Schipmann S, Schwake M, Sporns PB, et al. Is the Simpson grading system applicable to estimate the risk of tumor progression after microsurgery for recurrent intracranial meningioma? World Neurosurg. 2018;119:e589–97.
9. Budohoski KP, Clerkin J, Millward CP, et al. Predictors of early progression of surgically treated atypical meningiomas. Acta Neurochir. 2018;160(9):1813–22.
10. Simpson D. The recurrence of intracranial meningiomas after surgical treatment. J Neurol Neurosurg Psychiatry. 1957;20(1):22–39.
11. Aghi MK, Carter BS, Cosgrove GR, et al. Long-term recurrence rates of atypical meningiomas after gross total resection with or without postoperative adjuvant radiation. Neurosurgery. 2009;64(1):56–60; discussion 60.
12. Pettersson-Segerlind J, Orrego A, Lonn S, Mathiesen T. Long-term 25-year follow-up of surgically treated parasagittal meningiomas. World Neurosurg. 2011;76(6):564–71.
13. Raheja A, Couldwell WT. Cavernous sinus meningiomas. Handb Clin Neurol 2020;170:69–85.
14. Rogers L, Gilbert M, Vogelbaum MA. Intracranial meningiomas of atypical (WHO grade II) histology. J Neuro-Oncol. 2010;99(3):393–405.
15. Wang YC, Chuang CC, Wei KC, et al. Long term surgical outcome and prognostic factors of atypical and malignant meningiomas. Sci Rep. 2016;6:35743.
16. Kondziolka D, Mathieu D, Lunsford LD, et al. Radiosurgery as definitive management of intracranial meningiomas. Neurosurgery. 2008;62(1):53–8; discussion 58–60.
17. Mantovani A, Di Maio S, Ferreira MJ, Sekhar LN. Management of meningiomas invading the major dural venous sinuses: operative technique, results, and potential benefit for higher grade tumors. World Neurosurg. 2014;82(3–4):455–67.
18. Mathiesen T, Pettersson-Segerlind J, Kihlstrom L, Ulfarsson E. Meningiomas engaging major venous sinuses. World Neurosurg. 2014;81(1):116–24.
19. Kyritsis AP. Chemotherapy for meningiomas. J Neuro-Oncol. 1996;29(3):269–72.
20. Newton HB, Slivka MA, Stevens C. Hydroxyurea chemotherapy for unresectable or residual meningioma. J Neuro-Oncol. 2000;49(2):165–70.

21. Raheja A, Colman H, Palmer CA, Couldwell WT. Dramatic radiographic response resulting in cerebrospinal fluid rhinorrhea associated with sunitinib therapy in recurrent atypical meningioma: case report. J Neurosurg. 2017;127(5):965–70.
22. Mazur MD, Cutler A, Couldwell WT, Taussky P. Management of meningiomas involving the transverse or sigmoid sinus. Neurosurg Focus. 2013;35(6):E9.
23. Sindou M, Hallacq P. Venous reconstruction in surgery of meningiomas invading the sagittal and transverse sinuses. Skull Base Surg. 1998;8(2):57–64.
24. Sindou MP, Alvernia JE. Results of attempted radical tumor removal and venous repair in 100 consecutive meningiomas involving the major dural sinuses. J Neurosurg. 2006;105(4):514–25.
25. Maier H, Ofner D, Hittmair A, Kitz K, Budka H. Classic, atypical, and anaplastic meningioma: three histopathological subtypes of clinical relevance. J Neurosurg. 1992;77(4):616–23.
26. Jaaskelainen J, Haltia M, Servo A. Atypical and anaplastic meningiomas: radiology, surgery, radiotherapy, and outcome. Surg Neurol. 1986;25(3):233–42.
27. Jaaskelainen J. Seemingly complete removal of histologically benign intracranial meningioma: late recurrence rate and factors predicting recurrence in 657 patients. A multivariate analysis. Surg Neurol. 1986;26(5):461–9.
28. Mirimanoff RO, Dosoretz DE, Linggood RM, Ojemann RG, Martuza RL. Meningioma: analysis of recurrence and progression following neurosurgical resection. J Neurosurg. 1985;62(1):18–24.
29. Boylan SE, McCunniff AJ. Recurrent meningioma. Cancer. 1988;61(7):1447–52.
30. Chamoun R, Krisht KM, Couldwell WT. Incidental meningiomas. Neurosurg Focus. 2011;31(6):E19.
31. Li D, Hao SY, Wang L, et al. Recurrent petroclival meningiomas: clinical characteristics, management, and outcomes. Neurosurg Rev. 2015;38(1):71–86; discussion 86–87.
32. Gozal YM, Alzhrani G, Abou-Al-Shaar H, Azab MA, Walsh MT, Couldwell WT. Outcomes of decompressive surgery for cavernous sinus meningiomas: long-term follow-up in 50 patients. J Neurosurg. 2019;132(2):380–7.
33. Cao X, Hao S, Wu Z, et al. Treatment response and prognosis after recurrence of atypical meningiomas. World Neurosurg. 2015;84(4):1014–9.
34. Ojemann SG, Sneed PK, Larson DA, et al. Radiosurgery for malignant meningioma: results in 22 patients. J Neurosurg. 2000;93(Suppl 3):62–7.
35. Stafford SL, Pollock BE, Foote RL, et al. Meningioma radiosurgery: tumor control, outcomes, and complications among 190 consecutive patients. Neurosurgery. 2001;49(5):1029–37; discussion 1037–1038.
36. Bonnal J, Brotchi J. Surgery of the superior sagittal sinus in parasagittal meningiomas. J Neurosurg. 1978;48(6):935–45.
37. DiMeco F, Li KW, Casali C, et al. Meningiomas invading the superior sagittal sinus: surgical experience in 108 cases. Neurosurgery. 2004;55(6):1263–72; discussion 1272–1274.
38. Sindou M. Meningiomas invading the sagittal or transverse sinuses, resection with venous reconstruction. J Clin Neurosci. 2001;8(Suppl 1):8–11.
39. Tomasello F, Conti A, Cardali S, Angileri FF. Venous preservation-guided resection: a changing paradigm in parasagittal meningioma surgery. J Neurosurg. 2013;119(1):74–81.
40. Merrem G. Parasagittal meningiomas. Fedor Krause memorial lecture. Acta Neurochir. 1970;23(2):203–16.
41. Spetzler RF, Daspit CP, Pappas CT. The combined supra- and infratentorial approach for lesions of the petrous and clival regions: experience with 46 cases. J Neurosurg. 1992;76(4):588–99.

Radiotherapy for Aggressive Meningiomas and Recurrent Low Grade Tumors

12

Diana A. Roth O'Brien, Swathi Chidambaram,
Sean S. Mahase, Jana Ivanidze, and Susan C. Pannullo

Introduction

Meningiomas are predominantly benign intracranial lesions, thought to arise from the arachnoid cap cells in the dura [1, 2]. However, in approximately 20–35% of cases, meningiomas display more aggressive behavior, conferring increased recurrence risk and reducing overall survival (OS) [1, 3, 4]. Such meningiomas are histopathologically categorized as World Health Organization (WHO) Grade II or III. While overall, meningioma incidence is higher among women, Grade III meningiomas occur more commonly in men [4–9]. For Grade II–III meningiomas, surgical resection and adjuvant radiotherapy (RT) are commonly considered standard of care. Other treatment modalities, such as chemotherapy, hormonal therapy, immune therapy, or other targeted agents, are under investigation but remain experimental at present. This chapter will discuss the histopathologic classification, management, and outcomes for Grade II–III meningiomas, with an emphasis on the role

D. A. Roth O'Brien · S. S. Mahase
Department of Radiation Oncology, NewYork Presbyterian and Weill Cornell Medicine, New York, NY, USA
e-mail: sem9050@nyp.org

S. Chidambaram · S. C. Pannullo (✉)
Department of Neurological Surgery, Weill Cornell Medicine, New York, NY, USA
e-mail: sc1240@georgetown.edu; scp2002@med.cornell.edu

J. Ivanidze
Department of Radiology, Weill Cornell Medicine, New York, NY, USA
e-mail: jai9018@med.cornell.edu

© Springer Nature Switzerland AG 2020
J. Moliterno, A. Omuro (eds.), *Meningiomas*,
https://doi.org/10.1007/978-3-030-59558-6_12

of RT. Specifically, RT delivery techniques and planning considerations, as well as treatment-related adverse effects (AEs), will be addressed.

Histopathology

There is no staging system for meningiomas, but rather a grading system is utilized, based upon lesion pathology. Historically, a major obstacle in the appropriate treatment of meningiomas was the use of varied histopathologic classification systems and lack of universally adopted grading criteria. Fortunately, this issue is gradually being resolved in contemporary and ongoing trials, through the increasing adoption of the WHO grading system. The WHO criteria were initially established in 1993 and then refined in 2000, in 2007, and most recently again in 2016 [10]. Details of the current pathologic criteria for characterization of meningioma grade can be found in Chap. 9, Table 9.1. Factors contributing to grade classification include mitotic activity, sheetlike growth, hypercellularity, nucleolar prominence, nuclear-to-cytoplasmic ratio, and spontaneous necrosis. Since 2007, brain invasion has been a sufficient diagnostic criterion for Grade II classification [1]. WHO Grade II, or atypical, meningiomas display 4–9 mitoses per ten high-power fields, brain invasion, or three out of five atypical features, which can include sheeting architecture, hypercellularity, prominent nucleoli, high nuclear-to-cytoplasmic ratio, or necrosis. Choroidal and clear cell histologies are also considered WHO Grade II. In a secondary analysis of central pathology review for the landmark Phase II RTOG 0539 trial, 88% concordance for diagnosis of Grade II meningiomas was found, supporting the reproducibility of the WHO criteria and congruence among separate pathologists [11].

Historical series prior to 2000 reported that approximately 5% of meningiomas were Grade II, but by updated criteria, this has increased to as many as 20–35% [1, 2]. As standardized WHO grading criteria are increasingly adopted, the literature has reflected increasing incidence of WHO Grade II disease, as well as improving correlation between pathologic grade and treatment outcomes [12–14]. Willis et al. retrospectively evaluated 300 meningioma cases utilizing WHO 2000 criteria and observed a 20% incidence of Grade II disease, four times the rate with initial classification [15]. Similarly, in modern series, Pearson et al. noted that 32.7–35.5% of meningioma cases managed at their institution from 2004–2006 were atypical, and Backer-Grondahl et al. reported a rate of 30% of Grade II meningiomas [16, 17].

WHO Grade III, malignant or anaplastic, meningiomas display yet more aggressive behavior compared to lower grade disease. Histopathologically, they are characterized by at least 20 mitoses per ten high-power fields, or frank anaplasia; papillary and rhabdoid histologies are also considered Grade III. Based upon WHO 2016 criteria, the incidence of Grade III meningiomas is 1–3% [1, 2, 4].

Along with extent of surgical resection, histopathologic grading is among the strongest prognostic predictors for meningioma patients, as WHO histologic grade correlates with local recurrence-free survival (LRFS) and even

OS [12, 14, 18–20]. Compared to Grade I disease, atypical meningiomas carry a seven- to eightfold increase in recurrence risk and a slightly increased risk of mortality. A diagnosis of WHO Grade III meningioma is associated with a mean OS of less than 2 years [13]. Although WHO grading is the most widely utilized system, numerous other classification schemas exist. Given the variety of criteria used, and the significant changes in WHO criteria over the preceding decades, it is of utmost importance to be aware of the precise diagnostic criteria being utilized when reviewing the literature. Additionally, this variety limits meaningful comparisons across studies [1, 4].

Management and Outcomes

Management of patients with Grade II and III or recurrent meningiomas is based upon suboptimal publications, provider preference, or institutional practices, as there is a dearth of Level 1 evidence or consensus guidelines. Much of the evidence guiding management decisions for this patient population derives from retrospective studies, with heterogeneous diagnostic criteria and treatment strategies. As will be discussed at length, standard of care for high-grade meningiomas generally includes resection and adjuvant RT [1, 2, 4, 11].

General Principles of Surgical Resection

Microsurgery is the primary diagnostic and therapeutic modality in the management of Grade II–III meningiomas [21–23]. Maximal safe resection is attempted, and ideally, the meningioma, involved dura, and any involved bone or soft tissue are resected [4, 24]. The Simpson grading system is used to categorize the extent of surgical resection, as detailed in Chap. 9 [4, 25]. Briefly, Simpson Grade I resection entails removal of the entire meningioma, as well as dural attachments. Grade II consists of gross total resection (GTR) and dural cautery. Grade III describes resection of the meningioma only, Grade IV is subtotal resection (STR), and Grade V consists of decompression or biopsy only [25]. Together, Simpson Grade I–III resections are considered GTR, whereas Grade IV and V are classified as STR, and there is robust evidence that Simpson grade corresponds to local recurrence (LR) rate [21–23, 26–28]. Ability to achieve Simpson Grade I–III resection is sometimes limited, secondary to risk of damage to nearby vascular or neurological structures [22, 28–33]. GTR is most commonly attainable for meningiomas of the convexity and tentorium, but most challenging for the base of the skull [33]. Overall, GTR cannot be achieved in approximately one-third of patients [28]. Clinically, the surgical literature indicates that significant sequelae of surgery are observed in 15–26% of patients [34–38].

Radiotherapy for WHO Grade II Meningiomas

LR rates for patients with Grade II disease are significantly higher than for those with Grade I lesions, so surgical excision, as a single modality of treatment, may be inadequate [21, 23, 28]. Highlighting this point, in a cohort of 100 WHO Grade II meningioma patients receiving GTR alone, Aghi et al. reported a 5-year LR rate of 41% [39]. Likewise, Perry et al. evaluated 108 Grade II patients who underwent GTR and found a 5-year LR rate of 40% [12]. As a result of these unacceptably high LR rates, many authors recommend postoperative RT (PORT) for all WHO Grade II meningioma patients, regardless of extent of resection [4, 21, 40]. However, the role of adjuvant RT following GTR of WHO Grade II meningiomas remains the area of greatest controversy in meningioma management. Disappointingly, the evidence regarding PORT for Grade II–III meningiomas is largely Level IV or V, and the studies conducted have reached conflicting conclusions, as will be outlined [41].

Several studies have explored PORT for WHO Grade II patients following GTR and have concluded that adjuvant RT does not improve local control (LC) of disease [42–46]. In a large retrospective study of non-benign meningioma patients, Jaaskelainen et al. found a 5-year LR rate of 38% for Grade II disease, not significantly improved with PORT [42]. Goyal et al. evaluated 22 patients, 15 with GTR of their disease, with the remainder receiving STR, or unknown extent of resection. Of this cohort, a small subset of eight patients completed PORT, to a median dose of 54 Gy, two adjuvantly, and six as salvage for recurrent disease. They reported a 5- and 10-year LC rate of 87%, with no influence of PORT on OS or LR [43]. Hardesty et al. managed over 200 WHO Grade II meningiomas with GTR, with or without adjuvant RT, and were unable to demonstrate a statistically significant difference in recurrence risk with the addition of PORT. However, none of the patients who received adjuvant RT, which was 54 Gy in 27–30 fractions, experienced LR [41]. British investigators evaluated 79 Grade II meningioma patients managed with surgery, where approximately half of patient received PORT. Only Simpson grade correlated with LR risk, but not receipt of PORT [46]. Of note, in this retrospective study, the patients receiving adjuvant RT were more likely to have undergone STR, confounding interpretation of the results. In a recent study of 69 Grade II meningioma patients managed at the Mayo Clinic, eight of whom received PORT, the authors did not find a correlation between receipt of RT and LR, progression-free survival (PFS), or OS [47]. A historical SEER database study assessed 657 patients with non-Grade I meningiomas from 1988 to 2007, as defined by contemporaneous WHO classification. In this cohort, 37% of patients underwent adjuvant RT. External beam radiotherapy (EBRT) did not significantly improve OS or disease-free survival (DFS), after controlling for grade, lesion size, extent of resection, or year of diagnosis. Indeed, a detriment in OS was noted for subjects managed with adjuvant RT, likely resulting from the selection bias inherent in a database study [45].

Despite these studies that have failed to demonstrate a benefit to PORT for WHO Grade II meningiomas following GTR, treatment recommendations are complicated by a compelling body of literature that does suggest improved outcomes with adjuvant RT. In these studies, with surgery only, 5-year PFS ranges from 32% to

90%, while with adjuvant EBRT, 5-year PFS ranges from 52% to 100% [39, 41, 47–53]. As cited above, in a study of 108 Grade II meningioma patients conducted by Aghi et al., following Simpson Grade I resection and observation, half of patients recurred by 10 years postoperatively. In a small subset of eight patients who did receive adjuvant RT to a mean dose of 60.2 Gy, 100% LC was observed [39]. For 45 patients with atypical meningiomas and Simpson Grade I and II resection, Komotar et al. found a 65% rate of LR at 6 years without PORT, compared to 20% with. In this study, adjuvant RT was 59.4 Gy to the resection cavity with a 5–10 mm margin [49]. Park et al. reported on outcomes of 82 Grade II meningioma patients, 56 managed with surgery alone, and 27 with the addition of adjuvant RT, to a median dose of 61.2 Gy. For the whole cohort, PORT significantly lengthened PFS, though on subset analysis, adjuvant RT did not significantly improve PFS following GTR [50]. This lack of benefit has been attributed to the definition of GTR based upon the neurosurgeon's assessment, rather than postoperative imaging, and upon the use of older RT techniques. Bagshaw et al. evaluated 63 Grade II meningiomas among 59 patients, following either GTR or STR. The median interval to LR when PORT was given was 180 months, compared to only 46 months following resection alone. When the GTR subset was analyzed, there remained a statistically significant improvement in LC for the addition of adjuvant RT [52]. In a recent Canadian retrospective study of 70 patients with Grade II meningiomas, GTR and receipt of PORT correlated with decreased progression risk. After STR, the 5-year PFS with PORT was 75%, compared to 0% without PORT. Even after GTR, adjuvant RT was significantly associated with improved PFS, 100% versus 54% [53].

In reviewing this conflicting literature on the role of adjuvant RT for WHO Grade II meningioma patients, it is important to note that these studies are retrospective and encompass a wide variety of extents of resection; of RT dose, fractionation, and treatment planning; as well as of the use of salvage versus truly adjuvant RT. These inconsistencies make it difficult to reach definitive conclusions regarding optimal postoperative management of WHO Grade II patients. Until recently, prospective studies addressing the role of adjuvant RT in this clinical scenario have been lacking. Fortunately, two Phase II trials, RTOG 0539 and EORTC 22042-26042, have completed accrual, with some results available. Additionally, two Phase III studies exploring the role of adjuvant RT following GTR are currently underway, the ROAM trial and NRG BN-003.

The Phase II RTOG 0539 trial stratified postoperative meningioma patients into three categories, which then dictated adjuvant care. Low-risk patients had WHO Grade I disease following GTR or STR and were managed with observation. Intermediate-risk patients had GTR of WHO Grade II disease, or recurrent WHO Grade I disease, and received adjuvant RT, 54 Gy in 1.8 Gy per fraction. The high-risk cohort included all WHO Grade IIII patients, and WHO Grade II patients with STR or recurrence, and was managed with 60 Gy in 2 Gy per fraction PORT [2]. RTOG 0539 has published results of their intermediate-risk cohort, comprised 52 patients, 69% with WHO Grade II meningiomas and GTR, and 31% with recurrent WHO Grade I disease, regardless of extent of surgery. 3-year LC was 95.9%, 3-year PFS was 93.8%, and 3-year OS was 96% [11]. In the results available to date of the

Phase II observational trial EORTC 22042-26042, 56 WHO Grade II meningiomas and GTR were managed with PORT to 60 Gy. The investigators report local failure (LF) of 14%, 3-year PFS of 89%, and 3-year OS of 98% [54]. While these studies did not have a control cohort without PORT, the excellent outcomes highlight the potential benefit of adjuvant RT. The Phase III trial NRG BN003 enrolled WHO Grade II meningioma patients following GTR and randomized to observation or adjuvant RT to 59.4 Gy in 1.8 Gy per fraction. ROAM/EORTC 1308 is very similar in study design. The much-anticipated results of these two trials will provide guidance in the management of Grade II meningiomas following GTR.

In the context of low-level existing data, and conflicting outcomes in the literature, it is worthwhile to consider how meningioma patients are treated outside of the setting of clinical trials. With regard to practice patterns, in Germany, researchers found that 84% of surveyed medical centers recommended resection with no adjuvant RT for WHO Grade II meningiomas following GTR, while a rate of 80% was found in the UK [55, 56].

Obviously, controversy remains regarding optimal postoperative management of WHO Grade II meningiomas following GTR. Some patients would likely obtain durable disease control from resection alone and are overtreated or placed at unnecessary risk of adverse events (AEs) with the addition of PORT. In contrast, among other patients, omission of adjuvant RT results in LR and compromised long-term outcomes. Further research is required to more thoroughly risk stratify patients and to offer the optimal management strategy. Further, the conflicting data regarding the benefit of adjuvant RT in this population suggests that details of RT delivery, such as dose and fractionation, the techniques employed, and target delineation, may be of importance.

Compared to lower grade disease, Grade II meningiomas tend to experience more rapid progression with STR, so adjuvant RT is generally, though not universally, considered to provide LC benefit [1, 2, 4, 23, 40, 43]. Though the evidence supporting this practice is not consistent, and prospective evidence is lacking, several studies have demonstrated significant improvements in outcomes conferred by adjuvant RT for WHO Grade II patients following STR. Goldsmith et al. reported that Grade II patients managed with STR and EBRT experienced 5-year relapse-free survival of 48%. Of note, in this study, similarly treated Grade I lesions had significantly improved outcomes, with RFS of 89% [57]. In a study by Mair et al., the authors demonstrated improved PFS in patients managed with STR and adjuvant EBRT, compared to STR only, 72% versus 13%, respectively [48]. Of note, the RT dose employed in this study, 51.8 Gy in 28 fractions, was lower than what is now recommended.

With regard to practice patterns, PORT is not uniformly offered to WHO Grade II meningioma patients following STR. For example, a recent study reported that only 13% of WHO Grade II meningioma patients received adjuvant RT following STR [53]. Two European studies surveyed neurosurgeons and found that approximately 30–40% do not routinely recommend PORT in this clinical situation [55, 56].

Stereotactic Radiosurgery

There is robust retrospective data regarding the efficacy and safety of stereotactic radiosurgery (SRS), or fractionated SRS (fSRS), for benign meningiomas, but such literature is lacking for higher grade lesions [1, 4, 58, 59]. SRS or fSRS can be deployed for WHO Grade II disease following resection, though often it is reserved for recurrent disease or salvage treatment [1, 4, 60–62]. Widely variable outcomes are reported in the literature following SRS for WHO Grade II disease, with LC rates of 16–95% and PFS of 48–84%. Hakim et al. reported on the treatment of 155 meningiomas, including Grade II–III lesions, with linear accelerator-based SRS to a marginal dose of 15 Gy. With a median follow-up time of almost 2 years, freedom from progression was 84% [63]. Stafford et al. reported on a subset of their WHO Grade II meningiomas managed with SRS. In this cohort of 13 patients, the median marginal dose was 16 Gy, and the investigators reported a 5-year LC rate of 68%, compared to 93% for WHO Grade I patients [64]. Among 30 patients with Grade II and III meningiomas treated with SRS, Harris et al. reported 5-year PFS of 83% [65]. A large series of resected meningioma patients managed with postoperative SRS or fSRS from UCLA included 21 patients with atypical histology. The median treatment dose was 15.6 Gy for SRS and 48.4 Gy for fSRS. The authors report that control of tumor growth was observed in 31% of patients managed with SRS and 60% for patients managed with fRS [66]. Milker-Zabel et al. managed 26 patients with Grade II meningiomas with fSRS and observed LRFS at 3, 5, and 10 years of 96%, 89%, and 67%, respectively [67]. Huffman et al. observed 1-, 3-, and 5-year LC of 74%, 39%, and 16% for 22 WHO Grade II meningioma patients treated with Gamma Knife SRS with median dose of 18 Gy [68]. Kano et al. evaluated 12 patients with WHO Grade II and III meningiomas managed with SRS, with a median dose of 18 Gy, and reported 5-year PFS of 48% [69]. Attia et al. reported LC of 44% at 5 years with SRS to a median dose of 14 Gy [70]. In a retrospective cohort of 13 patients with WHO Grade II and III meningiomas, Williams et al. reported PFS of 92% and 31% at 1 and 4 years, respectively [60]. More recently, Acker et al. reported PFS of 59% at 60 months for Grade II lesions and 46% at 24 months for Grade III lesions in a mixed cohort of 35 patients who were treated with surgery and adjuvant SRS [61]. Pollock et al. noted that negative predictive factors for tumor control and OS for patients undergoing SRS for WHO II and III meningiomas from 1990 to 2008 were tumor progression despite prior EBRT and larger tumor volumes, based on results from a cohort of 50 patients [62]. There is also a growing area of inquiry evaluating parameters that affect LC of Grade II–III meningiomas treated with SRS. Based upon univariate analysis of 264 patients, Kaprealian et al. report that higher grade, larger target volume (median diameter 2.4 cm) and SRS were associated with poorer LC and that larger target volume and SRS remained significant predictors of poor LC on multivariate analysis [71].

Radiotherapy for WHO Grade III Meningiomas

As discussed, only 1–2% of meningiomas are categorized as Grade III; the annual incidence of Grade III meningioma in the USA is a mere 500 patients. As a result, the literature regarding optimal management for this disease population is relatively scant. WHO Grade III meningiomas are locally aggressive, conferring significantly worse LC and OS, when compared with lower grade disease [1]. 5-year OS for Grade III disease is estimated at 32–64%, compared to 90–100% for Grade I [72, 73]. As with lower grade disease, surgical resection is the primary treatment for Grade III meningiomas, and the extent of residual disease following resection is predictive of recurrence [1, 13, 74, 75]. However, only maximal safe resection should be pursued. Sughrue et al. noted that in their cohort of WHO Grade III patients managed with excision and adjuvant RT, near-total resection (removal of >90% of tumor) resulted in reduced neurological sequelae and improved OS compared to GTR [76]. Following surgery alone, outcomes for WHO Grade III disease are poor. In a study by Jaaskelainen et al., 78% of patients had recurred at 5 years following GTR [42]. Similarly, among WHO Grade III patients, Dziuk et al. observed a 5-year PFS of only 28% following GTR and 0% after STR [75]. Therefore, there is a broad consensus that Grade III meningiomas be managed aggressively, with maximal safe resection, and PORT in all cases, including following GTR [1, 40, 42]. Prospective randomized literature regarding the benefit of PORT in this population is lacking [1]. As with Grade II disease, the evidence underpinning treatment recommendations for WHO Grade III meningiomas is derived from retrospective studies. Additionally, these studies use variable and outdated histological classifications, varying extent of resection, and heterogeneous RT techniques. However, taken together, the literature appears to indicate a benefit of PORT for WHO Grade III disease [73, 75, 77]. Milosevic et al. evaluated 59 high-grade meningioma patients, of whom 30 (51%) were Grade III. For these malignant meningioma patients, they reported a 5-year cause-specific survival (CSS) of 27%. There was a trend toward statistically significant reduced CSS with Grade III disease, 27% compared to 51% with Grade II disease [77]. Dziuk et al. evaluated 38 patients diagnosed with malignant meningioma, though by modern criteria, 11 patients had hemangiopericytoma. 5-year PFS was 28% for patients who did not receive PORT, compared to 80% for those who did, with extent of resection and receipt of adjuvant RT predictive of LR [75]. Coke et al. found a rate of disease progression of 65% with surgery only, compared to only 18% with PORT [72]. Investigators from the Cleveland Clinic reported on 22 Grade III primary or recurrent meningioma patients, seven of whom were managed with adjuvant RT to a median dose of 59.4 Gy in 1.8 Gy per fraction. They reported median survival following RT was 5.4 years, compared to only 2.5 years following surgery only. Due to the small sample size, this difference was not statistically significant [73]. Comprehensive results of RTOG 0539, which includes WHO Grade III patients in the high-risk arm, will provide some prospective evidence for optimal EBRT management [2].

Stereotactic Radiosurgery

There is some limited literature supporting the use of SRS for WHO Grade III disease. Reported rates of OS range from 0 to 59% and of PFS from 26% to 72%. Ojemann et al. treated 22 patients with malignant meningioma in the primary or recurrent setting with Gamma Knife SRS. They reported 5-year OS of 40%, and PFS of 26%, and found that outcomes were significantly worse in patients 50 or older and in tumors of volume 8 cm^3 or larger [78]. Stafford et al. treated 22 patients with Grade II or III meningiomas with Gamma Knife SRS and observed 5-year LC and OS of 0% for Grade III lesions [64]. Likewise, Harris et al. reported on outcomes for 30 patients with Grade II–III meningiomas managed with Gamma Knife SRS. For malignant cases, 5-year OS was 59%, and PFS was 72% [65]. Another study by Balasubramanian et al. retrospectively studied outcomes from a cohort of 18 patients with WHO Grade III meningiomas and reported that surgical resection followed by RT and salvage SRS and/or chemotherapy can lead to extended OS in some cases, highlighting the potential value of a multimodal treatment plan in these patients [79].

Recurrent Disease

Unfortunately, recurrent meningiomas behave more aggressively than primary disease of the same grade. For patients with recurrent meningiomas, durable disease control is difficult to attain, regardless of adjuvant treatment employed and even if histologic grade is unchanged [1, 2, 7, 80, 81]. Though the literature indicates that in 82–96% of meningioma recurrences, histologic grade is stable, increase in grade with subsequent recurrences, known as dedifferentiation, can occur [1, 4, 40, 42, 74, 82, 83]. When meningiomas increase in grade, architecture is lost, epithelial membrane antigen expression is decreased, expression of vimentin is increased, and abnormal intermediate filament proteins are expressed [84].

Compared to newly diagnosed disease, meningiomas recurrent after primary treatment, whether surgical or RT, have poor rates of durable LC, with reported mean disease-free interval of 4 years [7, 21, 28, 80]. Of note, failure rates for recurrent Grade I meningiomas are similar to those for primary Grade II disease [2]. Numerous studies have reported high rates of progression of disease for WHO Grade I meningiomas after salvage treatment, especially with resection alone [7, 23, 80, 85]. For recurrent WHO Grade I disease, 3-year rates of LF of 55–60% are reported following resection [7, 80]. Stafford et al. reported that at 10 years, LF was 25% for primary Grade I meningiomas, but that this approximate LR risk was reached after only 2 years for first recurrence [23]. Similarly, when evaluating patients with STR of sphenoid wing meningioma involving the optic apparatus, Peele et al. reported time to first LR of 4.4 years, compared to only 14 months following first recurrence [85]. Among 463 meningioma patients, Mehdorn et al. observed first recurrences after a mean 65 months, compared to only 34 months for second recurrence of the disease [86].

Aghi et al. reported that for WHO Grade II meningioma patients with recurrent disease, 10-year CSS was only 69%, even with aggressive management [39]. In the previously referenced study by Sughure et al., salvage surgery at the time of recurrence conferred a survival benefit, with median OS of 53 months for resected patients, compared to 25 months for unresected patients [76]. Similarly, Komotar et al. found that for WHO Grade II meningioma patients, OS was decreased following recurrence of disease [49]. Talacchi et al. demonstrated that for atypical meningiomas, with each successive recurrence, disease-free interval was reduced. At first recurrence, disease-free interval was 33 months, but was only 5–10 months for the fourth or fifth recurrence [87]. For a large cohort of WHO Grade II patients, Kessel et al. reported that 64% of patients without recurrence were alive at 15 years, compared to no survivors among those with recurrent disease [88]. Overall, these comparatively poor outcomes for meningioma patients with recurrent disease underscore the importance of appropriate upfront management.

Radiotherapy for Recurrent Disease

For recurrent disease, re-resection should be attempted if deemed safe. If RT has not been previously given, it should utilized postoperatively, even following GTR. If there is progression of disease outside of the previous target volume, RT can be considered. Additionally, re-irradiation, whether via EBRT or SRS, can be considered if dose constraints to critical normal tissues can be respected and there has been a sufficient interval since prior RT [1]. Existing evidence suggests that outcomes are improved when recurrent disease is managed with surgical resection and adjuvant RT, rather than surgery alone [2, 7, 80, 81]. Of note, the literature regarding management of recurrent meningioma is based upon retrospective studies, and the caveats regarding varied diagnostic criteria and treatment regimens apply here as well. Taylor et al. reported 10-year LC of 30% for recurrent meningioma patients managed with surgery alone, compared to 89% for salvage PORT, with or without surgical intervention. Patients managed with RT also had improved OS, 89% at 10 years, compared to only 43% for surgery alone. In this study, RT consisted of 54–59.4 Gy in 1.8–2 Gy per fraction [80]. Likewise, in a study of patients with recurrent meningioma managed with resection and PORT, Miralbell et al. found 78% PFS at 8 years, but only 11% when surgery alone was utilized [7]. These promising LC and OS results emphasize the importance of aggressive management of recurrent meningioma and highlight the efficacy of this EBRT dose scheme. However, here too, the literature regarding the benefit of PORT is not uniform. Dziuk et al. reported that EBRT in the management of recurrent meningioma improved DFS at 2 years, but this benefit was lost at 5 years [75]. In a population of patients with recurrent WHO Grade II meningioma, Mair et al. observed that no salvage treatment, whether surgery or RT, correlated with outcome [48].

Radiotherapy Planning

Grade II: Intermediate Risk

In the past several decades, RT techniques have improved significantly, allowing for treatment to be delivered more precisely, more conformally, and with reduced risk of treatment-related sequelae. These advances have further translated into improvements in LC of disease [32, 57, 77]. Goldsmith et al. demonstrated that when RT targets were identified using computed tomography (CT) or magnetic resonance imaging (MRI), and appropriate immobilization was utilized, a 22% improvement in PFS resulted [32, 57]. Indeed, a longitudinal evaluation of publications reporting on clinical outcomes for meningioma patients following EBRT reveals significant improvements after 2000, once MRI-based target delineation and image-guided RT were commonly employed [4].

Whenever possible, for all meningioma patients managed with adjuvant RT, postoperative MRI with contrast enhancement is utilized for delineation of the target, as well as adjacent organs at risk (OARs). Preoperative imaging can also be helpful in distinguishing between true extent of disease and reactive postoperative changes [4]. The definition of the volume to be irradiated, or planning target volume (PTV), employed in the literature has varied considerably, from gross tumor volume (GTV) plus a 2 mm margin to GTV plus a 20 mm margin [2, 13, 89]. For resected Grade II meningiomas, the GTV is comprised of the resection cavity, as well as any residual nodular enhancement seen on T1 postcontrast MRI. Any surrounding edema or dural tail is generally not included. The clinical target volume (CTV) is created with a variable uniform expansion upon the GTV, respecting anatomical boundaries to disease spread. For WHO Grade II disease with brain invasion, a rim of brain tissue must also be included in the CTV. The PTV is created as a uniform expansion upon the CTV, and is dependent upon reproducibility of the set up, but is generally at least 3 mm [1].

Based upon the completed Phase II RTOG 0539, and the ongoing Phase III NRG/BN-003 trial, the standard EBRT dose utilized for WHO Grade II patients is 54–59.4 Gy in 1.8 Gy per fraction following GTR and 59.4–60 Gy in 1.8–2 Gy per fraction following STR [2]. Doses as high as 66–70 Gy can be employed if clinically indicated and if dose constraints for OARs are met [1, 39, 40, 49, 90]. The Phase II trial EORTC 22042-26042 of WHO Grade II–III meningiomas is treated postoperatively to 60 Gy in 2 Gy per fraction following GTR. A boost was used in the setting of STR, to a total dose of 70 Gy [54]. However, more robust data is required to establish the optimal RT dose in this patient population.

There is some evidence of improved outcomes with higher doses of EBRT for Grade II–III meningiomas, especially following STR [90]. Aghi et al. reported no LR in WHO Grade II meningioma patients when doses of 59.4–61.2 Gy were delivered [39]. Komatar et al. found significantly improved outcomes for patients with median dose of at least 59.4 Gy [49]. Park et al. reported significantly improved PFS with median dose of 61.2 Gy or higher [50]. Boskos et al. reported outcomes for 24 high-grade meningioma patients (79% WHO Grade II) following predominantly STR and combined photon and proton RT. For patients receiving PORT of >60 Gy, CSS at 5 years was significantly improved, 80% compared to only 24%. Further, there was a trend toward improved outcomes with doses >65 Gy [91]. Employing protons, Hug et al. reported improved LC with doses of at least 60 cobalt gray equivalent (CGE). Of note, the majority of their subjects had STR or recurrent disease [40].

While EBRT has been employed for meningiomas for many years, SRS is a more recently introduced treatment modality that is increasingly utilized in the management of meningiomas [1, 4, 92]. As with any SRS, immobilization and stereotactic target localization is required. For SRS to be safely delivered, setup should be reproducible within 1 mm. The GTV is determined as for EBRT, based upon the T1 postcontrast MRI. For SRS, no CTV is created, and PTV is often GTV with an expansion of 0–2 mm [1, 4]. Though there are fewer publications regarding SRS for meningiomas, with shorter follow-up, the two treatment modalities appear comparable, both conferring good LC and safety profiles if SRS is appropriately planned, as will be discussed. However, the majority of studies regarding SRS for meningiomas have been conducted on Grade I or presumed Grade I disease [2].

Robust evidence guiding dosing for WHO Grade II meningioma SRS is lacking. Generally, marginal doses of 14–20 Gy are used in a single fraction. For larger lesions, often those greater than 2 cm, or 20 cm^3, or for lesions within 2–4 mm of critical OARs, fSRS can be employed, for example, 27.5–30 Gy in 5 fractions [1, 93, 94]. Of note, Kano et al. found that PFS was significantly improved when SRS doses of 20 Gy or higher were utilized for Grade II–III patients [69]. Attia et al. reported that for WHO Grade II meningioma patients managed with SRS, lower conformality index, defined as prescription dose volume divided by tumor volume, was predictive of increased LF [70]. Given rapid dose drop-off outside of the PTV when SRS is used, appropriate and comprehensive PTV delineation is key. Some publications suggest that WHO Grade II meningiomas fail outside of the SRS target, but within the extent of the initial lesion or resection bed, if this entire volume is not adequately treated. For example, in patients with WHO Grade II–III meningiomas, Pollock et al. reported that a majority of recurrences were marginal or adjacent to the PTV. Recurrences occurred separate from the original PTV in only 30% of patients [62]. Huffmann et al. evaluated 15 patients treated with a median of 16 Gy in a single fraction of SRS. Forty percent of patients recurred, with only one in-field LR, but with all failures within the surgical tract or tumor bed [68]. Likewise, Mattozo et al. assessed patterns of failure following SRS or fSRS and reported that more than three quarters of failures occurred within the tumor bed [95]. Similarly, Choi et al. investigated 25 WHO Grade II meningioma patients irradiated to a median dose of 22 Gy in 1–4 fractions. They reported a LR of 41%, with one-third of failures occurring within the SRS target; more than half within the resection bed, but outside the target; and one (11%) in both areas [96]. These findings are corroborated by Zhang et al., who evaluated WHO Grade II meningiomas managed with SRS and reported locoregional control of 36% at 5 years [97]. Valery et al., investigating a similar patient population, found PFS of 23% at 3 years [98]. The authors of both of these studies reported that many recurrences were regional [97, 98]. Taken together, this body of literature suggests that a region beyond the radiographically apparent recurrent or residual disease is at risk for recurrence, including the entire resection bed, and should be treated with SRS. If the PTV becomes prohibitively large, EBRT or fSRS can be employed.

Grade III

As discussed, PORT is always recommended for Grade III patients, even following GTR. As with Grade II cases, the GTV consists of the resection bed, as well as any residual nodular enhancement. As with lower grade disease, any dural tail or surrounding edema need not be encompassed. The appropriate PTV for PORT of WHO Grade III meningiomas requires further research. In the high-risk arm of RTOG 0539, two CTVs were created. The CTV 54 Gy consists of the GTV with a 20 mm uniform expansion, respecting anatomic boundaries to spread. CTV 60 Gy consists of a 1 cm margin on the GTV, again respecting anatomic boundaries. Using intensity-modulated RT (IMRT), these two volumes can be treated concurrently in daily fractions, employing a simultaneous integrated boost technique [4]. PTV considerations are similar to those for Grade II disease and generally range from 3 to 5 mm [1].

In the management of WHO Grade III disease, doses of approximately 60 Gy are employed. The high-risk arm of RTOG 0539 was treated with 60 Gy in 30 fractions and included those with WHO Grade III disease, any grade of resection, WHO Grade II lesions following STR, and recurrent WHO Grade II disease [2]. There is evidence that the RT doses typically employed for low-grade disease are inadequate and that higher adjuvant RT dose confers improved LC. Among the patients evaluated by Milosevic et al., those who received <50 Gy adjuvant RT had worse CSS, 0% compared to 42% [77]. Similarly, Goldsmith et al. found 5-year PFS for WHO Grade III patients receiving >53 Gy adjuvant RT of 63%, compared to only 17% for those managed with lower dose [57]. In this patient population, Dziuk et al. recommended a dose of 60 Gy adjuvantly [75]. Employing protons, DeVries et al. and Hug et al. both reported significantly improved LC and OS when doses >60 Gy were utilized [40, 90]. Hug et al. evaluated 13 Grade III patients managed with resection and RT, two-thirds with conventional photon RT, and the remaining one-third with combined photons and protons. The six patients treated with equivalent doses above 60 Gy had 5-year LC of 100%, compared to 0% for those managed with lower dose [40].

Recurrence

For recurrent disease, as with primary lesions, the GTV encompasses the resection cavity on postcontrast T1 MR, as well as any radiographically evident persistent nodular enhancement. Generally, the dural tail and any associated edema need not be included in the target volume. Given the aggressive nature of recurrent disease, and the associated poor LC, recurrent WHO Grade I meningioma should be managed with EBRT to at least 54 Gy in 27–30 fractions. If SRS is employed, a dose of at least 14 Gy in a single fraction is recommended [4, 99, 100]. The CTV is created with a 1 cm uniform margin around the GTV, respecting natural anatomic barriers to spread. As with other cases, a uniform margin of 3–5 mm from the CTV creates the PTV [4].

Advanced Imaging Techniques

As discussed, the sobering LR rates following surgical resection of meningiomas prompted implementation of PORT to improve outcomes. However, adaption of PORT as standard practice is highly heterogeneous, owing to concerns over weighing its putative benefits with potential AEs. These concerns can be considered as three points: (1) accurate delineation of residual disease, (2) delivering adequate dose to the residual disease, and (3) minimizing irradiation of surrounding normal tissues. The transition to CT and MRI-based RT planning improved conformality with newer linear accelerator-based technology, contemporary interfraction motion management, and innovative planning software translated to incrementally improved LR rates and improved toxicity profiles [4, 11, 32, 57, 77]. Nevertheless, continued uncertainty regarding disease delineation has warranted the investigation of novel imaging biomarkers.

A recent study by Chidambaram et al. demonstrated a potential role for dynamic contrast-enhanced (DCE) MRI in the preoperative characterization and stratification of meningiomas, laying the foundation for future prospective studies incorporating DCE as a biomarker in meningioma treatment planning [101].

Meningiomas express an abundance of somatostatin receptors (SSTR), enabling the utilization of octreotide-based imaging to aid in delineating the extent of disease. Silva et al. investigated the immunohistochemical expression of five SSTR subtypes (SSTR1–SSTR5) in tumor tissue sections from 60 patients with meningioma following surgical resection. Forty-seven (78.3%) meningiomas were Grade I, 11 (18.3%) were Grade II, and 2 (3.3%) were Grade III. All five SSTRs were expressed, at frequencies ranging from 61.6 to 100%, with a predominance of SSTR2 [102]. Menke et al. elaborated on these findings, performing a histopathological study using tissue microarrays on 176 meningiomas to determine SSTR2A was the most reliable biomarker in distinguishing meningiomas [103]. In a cohort of 50 patients with meningiomas, Nathoo et al. reported (111)indium-octreotide brain scintigraphy had a sensitivity, specificity, positive, and negative predictive values of 100, 50, 75, and 100, respectively, in cases where a definitive diagnosis could be made. Furthermore, the use of (111)indium-octreotide brain scintigraphy with MRI to differentiate meningiomas from other lesions was highly significant ($p < 0.001$) [104].

SSTR2 imaging is particularly useful in delineating disease located at the base of the skull, as well as differentiating postoperative changes from residual disease. In 26 patients with skull base meningiomas, Gehler and colleagues complemented MRI and CT datasets with (68)Ga-DOTA-D Phe(1)-Tyr(3)-Octreotide (DOTATOC)-PET/CT. The initial GTV was defined on MRI only and was secondarily refined with DOTATOC-PET information. The integration of the DOTATOC data led to additional information concerning tumor extension in 17 of 26 patients, with major CTV changes in 14 patients. The GTV-MRI/CT was larger than the GTV-DOTATOC-assisted plans in 10 patients (38%), smaller in 13 patients (50%), and almost the same in 3 patients (12%). Most of adaptations were performed in close vicinity to bony skull base structures or after complex surgery [105]. Another study evaluated the value of (68)Ga-DOTATOC in 48 patients with 54 skull-based meningiomas previously treated with fSRS. The GTVs were first delineated with MRI and CT data, and then by PET, with the addition of (68)Ga-DOTATOC, resulting in more than 10% modification of the size of the GTV in 32 (67%) of the subjects [106]. Afshar-Oromieh et al. evaluated 134 patients with CE-MRI and (68) Ga-DOTATOC PET/CT. 190 meningiomas were detected by (68)Ga-DOTATOC PET/CT and 171 by CE-MRI. The MRI scans were reinvestigated following PET/ CT, leading to detection of 4 of the 19 incidental meningiomas, thus detecting 92% of the meningioma found by PET/CT. The authors noted SSTR2 imaging was particularly valuable in detecting tumors adjacent to the falx cerebri, located at the skull base, or obscured by imaging artifacts or calcifications [107].

(68)Ga-DOTATATE PET/CT has been shown to be far superior to other SSTR-based imaging, with improved specificity owing to a higher affinity for SSTR2A [108, 109]. However, there is a dearth of literature evaluating this emerging modality. Rachinger et al. prospectively evaluated 12 patients with primary meningiomas and 9 with recurrent disease in whom preoperative MRI and (68)Ga-DOTATATE PET were used for a spatially precise, neuronavigated tissue sampling procedure during tumor resection. At each individual sampling site, the maximum standardized uptake value (SUVmax) of (68)Ga-DOTATATE was correlated with MR imaging findings, histology, and SSTR2 expression. There was a significant positive correlation between SUVmax and SSTR2 expression, with (68)Ga-DOTATATE PET imaging showing higher sensitivity (90% vs. 79%; $p = 0.049$), and similar specificity and positive predictive values relative to MRI, for both de novo and recurrent tumors [110]. Another group investigated the utility of (68)Ga-DOTATATE PET/CT and contrast-enhanced MRI (CE-MRI) in detecting osseous infiltration in 82 patients with pathologically confirmed meningiomas. (68)Ga-DOTATATE PET/CT in comparison to CE-MRI conferred higher sensitivity (98.5% vs. 53.7%) while maintaining high specificity (86.7% vs. 93.3%) in the detection of osseous involvement ($p < 0.001$). (68) Ga-DOTATATE PET/CT- and CE-MRI-based volume estimation was performed similarly for extraosseous meningiomas ($p = 0.132$), whereas the volume of the intraosseous part was assessed as significantly larger using (68)Ga -DOTATATE PET/CT ($p < 0.001$) [109]. In 20 patients with clinically suspected or pathology-proven meningiomas, Ivanidze and colleagues used (68)Ga-DOTATATE PET/MRI to confirm the diagnosis or determine tumor recurrence/progression, in order to guide surgical and/ or RT management in cases in which MRI findings were indeterminate or equivocal. (68)Ga-DOTATATE confirmed recurrent meningioma in 17 patients, with excellent differentiation between meningioma and posttreatment changes, ultimately aiding in subsequent management [111].

Thus, SSTR2-based imaging can guide a number of clinical decisions in the multidisciplinary management of meningiomas. Given its high specificity and sensitivity, postoperative beds without any discernable SSTR2 uptake may be safely observed, identifying a subset of patients who would likely not benefit from PORT. This can be especially helpful for lesions along the base of skull and dural reflections, where MRI-based imaging may be unable to discern residual disease from postoperative changes. This imaging modality has the additional benefit of guiding RT planning volumes to accurately encompass residual disease while sparing nearby normal tissues. SSTR2-based imaging can accurately assess the volume of the remaining disease, aiding in the determination of whether a particular patient is a candidate for SRS, fSRS, or conventional EBRT. This is especially important for patients who may have difficulties attending daily treatment over several weeks, or who may require anxiolytic medications during RT. The ability to accurately delineate residual disease obviates the need for large GTV to CTV expansions, which will also reduce excess dose to surrounding OARs [1, 11]. Another corollary of reducing the treatment volume is the ability to dose escalate residual disease, supported by literature suggesting PFS is improved with higher biological equivalent doses in higher grade meningiomas [1, 40, 57, 69, 75, 77, 90].

Figures 12.1 and 12.2 demonstrate the postsurgical DOTATATE PET/ T1-weighted postcontrast MRI fusion image and RT plan for a patient planned with conventional EBRT to 59.4 Gy and an SRS plan generated using DOTATATE PET/ MRI to guide target volume. With use of DOTATATE PET/MRI, the target volume is significantly decreased as shown in Fig. 12.3, reducing dose to surrounding tissues and allowing for the utilization of SRS. Nevertheless, further investigation is necessitated to validate this promising imaging modality.

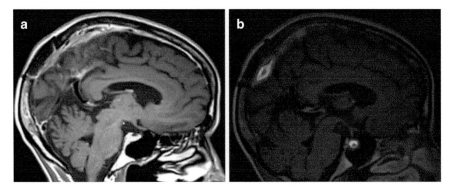

Fig. 12.1 Postsurgical MRI brain, T1-weighted postcontrast, of a 50-year-old female presenting with a left parietal convexity WHO Grade II meningioma status-post Simpson Grade II resection (**a**). Postsurgical DOTATATE PET/T1-weighted postcontrast MRI fusion image (windowed SUV 0-15) demonstrated intense DOTATATE avidity along the left aspect of the posterior third of the superior sagittal sinus, compatible with residual meningioma (**b**)

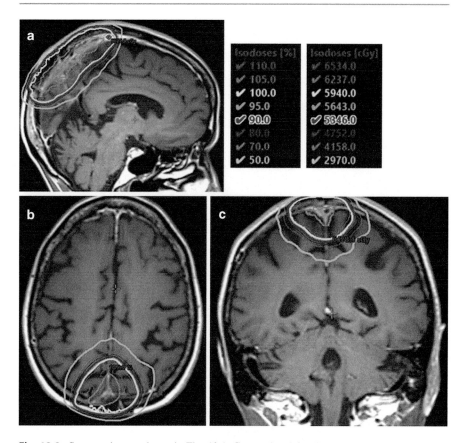

Isodoses [%]	Isodoses [cGy]
✔ 110.0	✔ 6534.0
✔ 105.0	✔ 6237.0
✔ 100.0	✔ 5940.0
✔ 95.0	✔ 5643.0
✔ 90.0	✔ 5346.0
✔ 80.0	✔ 4752.0
✔ 70.0	✔ 4158.0
✔ 50.0	✔ 2970.0

Fig. 12.2 Same patient as shown in Fig. 12.1. Conventional fractionated EBRT plan generated based upon MRI, 59.4 Gy in 33 fractions, demonstrated in the sagittal (**a**), axial (**b**), and coronal (**c**) plane

Adverse Effects

Since the vast majority of treated meningiomas are benign, much of the data regarding toxicities associated with treatment come from this patient population. Also of note, much of the published information regarding treatment-related toxicities derives from retrospective work. Treatment-related sequelae would be most robustly documented and graded in a prospective manner, but such data is lacking.

External Beam Radiation Therapy

In historical series, employing older RT techniques, Al-Mefty et al. reported a 38% rate of clinically significant AEs among irradiated benign meningioma patients [112]. Meyers et al. conducted a study of cognitive function from 20 months to

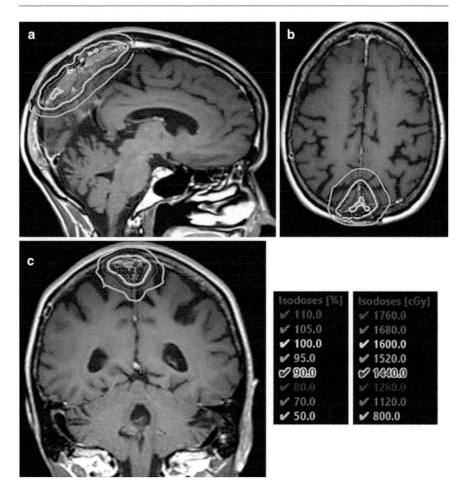

Fig. 12.3 Same patient as shown in Fig. 12.1. SRS plan generated using DOTATATE PET/MRI to guide target volume, 16 Gy in 1 fraction, demonstrated in the sagittal (**a**), axial (**b**), and coronal (**c**) plane. With use of DOTATATE PET/MRI, the target volume is significantly decreased, reducing dose to surrounding tissues and allowing for the utilization of SRS

20 years following EBRT for skull base meningiomas. The 19 patients in this historical series were treated to a dose of 60 Gy in 30 fractions, most using three-field technique. Four-fifths of patients experienced memory deficits, and one-third experienced impairments in visual-motor speed, executive functions, and fine motor skills. The authors reported that deficits correlated with total dose, but not with volume of normal brain irradiated, and postulated that their findings were attributable to irradiation of the subcortical white matter [113].

More contemporary series report that EBRT is well-tolerated, with minimal treatment-related toxicities at doses below 60 Gy [1, 4, 114–116]. Of course, care must be taken that hot spots within the treatment plan are reasonable, and fall within the

PTV, away from critical OARs. With modern, conformal techniques, such as IMRT, integral dose to uninvolved brain parenchyma is greatly reduced compared to older treatments [113]. IMRT has specifically been shown to confer low complication rates [115, 116]. Additionally, advances in RT image guidance ensure accurate targeting, and allow for smaller setup error, such that smaller PTVs can be safely used [4]. With modern treatment planning, the literature indicates that approximately 5% of meningioma patients undergoing EBRT experience clinically significant AEs beyond temporary neurologic deficits and reported rates in the literature range from 0 to 8% in modern series. In particular, optic pathway structures, such as the chiasm and optic nerves, are at risk, as are other cranial nerves.

The results of EORTC 22042-26042 available thus far indicate a 14% incidence of Grade III or higher toxicity [54]. In the intermediate-risk arm of RTOG 0539, where patients were treated postoperatively to 54 Gy in 1.8 Gy per fraction, treatment was very well-tolerated, with no Common Terminology Criteria for Adverse Events (CTCAE) Grade III or higher toxicities. The Grade II AEs of highest incidence were seizure, speech disorder, depression, trigeminal nerve impairment, olfactory nerve impairment, peripheral sensory neuropathy, memory deficits, and dizziness. The Grade I AEs most commonly encountered were dermatologic, visual (including blurry vision, flashing vision, dry eye, and diplopia), and neurological (including dizziness, memory deficits, peripheral sensory neuropathy, peripheral motor neuropathy). Of note, use of IMRT reduced toxicity compared to 3D RT planning [11]. Debus et al. managed 189 patients with conventional EBRT to a mean total dose of 56.8 Gy in 1.8 Gy per fraction. At 3 years of median follow-up, only 2.2% of patients experienced Grade III or higher toxicity. Furthermore, for patients with no baseline deficits, the rate was only 1.7%. Visual deficits and trigeminal neuropathy were the most commonly encountered AEs [89]. Similarly, of 140 meningioma patients managed with EBRT following STR, Goldsmith et al. noted a toxicity rate of 3.6%. The AEs noted included retinopathy, optic neuropathy, and cerebellar necrosis. AEs were uncommon when each daily fraction was <2 Gy, and the total dose administered was <54 Gy [57]. Based upon modeling, Goldsmith et al. suggested a dose constraint of 54 Gy in 30 fractions maximum dose to the optic nerves [117]. Beyond deficits of the visual pathway, other toxicities related to EBRT for meningiomas are rare. Selch et al. did not encounter any cranial neuropathy in 45 patients with cavernous sinus meningioma managed with EBRT to 50.4 Gy in 1.7–1.8 Gy per fraction [118]. Necrosis is also rare, but possible, following EBRT for meningiomas [7, 112, 116]. Other rare, but documented, AEs include pituitary dysfunction, cerebrovascular events, radiation-induced malignancies, edema, orbital fibrosis, personality changes, and memory loss [7, 21, 112, 115–117, 119, 120]. It is important to note that with EBRT, extra care must be taken when dose escalating above 60 Gy, as may be employed for high-risk disease. Such doses confer increased risk of neurologic AEs [121]. A thorough discussion of RT treatment-related sequelae can be found in Chap. 9.

Stereotactic Radiosurgery

Debus et al. reported on patients managed with fSRS for meningioma and found only a 2.2% rate of clinically significant AEs. None of their cohort experienced Grade IV toxicities [89]. Likewise, Selch et al. have reported that fSRS is very well-tolerated, with minimal significant toxicity [118]. In a prospective study, Steinvorth et al. followed patients with skull base meningiomas managed with fSRS with comprehensive neurocognitive testing. They documented a decline in memory function and improved attention following the first fraction of treatment, but at completion of treatment and 1 year after RT, no cognitive deficits were documented [122].

Conclusion

WHO Grade II and III meningiomas, as well as recurrent lesions, represent a small subset of all meningiomas, and confer poor LC and OS, even with aggressive upfront management. Maximal safe resection is standard of care for WHO Grade II and III and recurrent meningiomas. The role of adjuvant RT in the management of WHO Grade II meningiomas following GTR represents the greatest area of ongoing controversy in meningioma management. WHO Grade II lesions following STR and all Grade III lesions should be managed with PORT. Both EBRT and SRS can be used in this clinical setting, though more robust evidence supports the use of EBRT to date. Despite the considerable published evidence supporting this aggressive treatment approach, studies of practice patterns reveal suboptimal utilization of adjuvant RT. Several currently ongoing trials should provide further guidance in evidence-based management of high-grade meningiomas. For recurrent disease, a combination of maximal safe resection and PORT can be used, dependent upon prior use of RT and the ability to protect surrounding brain parenchyma and OARs. Several radiographic modalities are currently under investigation, which may improve meningioma identification and radiotherapy targeting.

References

1. Harris TJ, Chao ST, Rogers CL. Meningioma. In: Chang EL, Brown PD, Lo SS, Sahgal A, Suh JH, editors. Adult CNS radiation oncology. Cham: Springer International Publishing AG; 2018. p. 3–18.
2. Rogers CL, Vogelbaum MA, Perry A, et al. Phase II trial of observation for low-risk meningiomas and of radiotherapy for intermediate- and high-risk meningiomas (RTOG 0539). http://www.rtog.org. Published 2014. Accessed 14 Jan 2020.
3. Perry A. Meningiomas. In: Rosenblum M, McLendon R, Bigner DD, editors. Russell & Rubinstein's pathology of tumors of the nervous system. London: Hodder Arnold; 2006. p. 427–74.
4. Barani IJ, Perry A, Rogers CL. Meningioma—viewpoint: fractionated radiotherapy. In: Chin LS, Regine WF, editors. Principles and practice of stereotactic radiosurgery. 2nd ed. New York: Springer New York; 2015.

5. Ostrom QT, Gittleman H, Xu J, et al. CBTRUS statistical report: primary brain and other central nervous system tumors diagnosed in the United States in 2009–2013. Neuro-Oncology. 2016;18:v1–v75.
6. Longstreth WT Jr, Dennis LK, McGuire VM, et al. Epidemiology of intracranial meningioma. Cancer. 1993;72:639–48.
7. Miralbell R, Linggood RM, de la Monte S, et al. The role of radiotherapy in the treatment of subtotally resected benign meningiomas. J Neuro-Oncol. 1992;13:157–64.
8. Kuratsu J, Kochi M, Ushio Y. Incidence and clinical features of asymptomatic meningiomas. J Neurosurg. 2000;92:766–70.
9. Louis DN, Ohgaki H, Wiestler OD, et al. The 2007 WHO classification of tumours of the central nervous system. Acta Neuropathol. 2007;114:97–109.
10. Varlotto JM, Flickinger JC, Pavelic MT, et al. Distinguishing grade I meningioma from higher grade meningiomas without biopsy. Oncotarget. 2015;6(35):3842–8.
11. Rogers L, Zhang P, Vogelbaum MA, et al. Intermediate-risk meningioma: initial outcomes from NRG Oncology RTOG 0539. J Neurosurg. 2018;129(1):35–47.
12. Perry A, Stafford SL, Scheithauer BW, Suman VJ, Lohse CM. Meningioma grading: an analysis of histologic parameters. Am J Surg Pathol. 1997;21:1455.
13. Perry A, Scheithauer BW, Stafford SL, Lohse CM, Wollan PC. Malignancy. In meningiomas: a clinicopathologic study of 116 patients, with grading implications. Cancer. 1999;85:2046–56.
14. Durand A, Labrousse F, Jouvet A, et al. WHO grade II and III meningiomas: a study of prognostic factors. J Neuro-Oncol. 2009;95:367–75.
15. Willis J, Smith C, Ironside JW, et al. The accuracy of meningioma grading: a 10-year retrospective audit. Neuropathol Appl Neurobiol. 2005;31:141–9.
16. Pearson BE, Markert JM, Fisher WS, et al. Hitting a moving target: evolution of a treatment paradigm for atypical meningiomas amid changing diagnostic criteria. Neurosurg Focus. 2008;24(5):E3.
17. Backer-Grondahl T, Moen BH, Torp SH. The histopathological spectrum of human meningiomas. Int J Clin Exp Pathol. 2012;5(3):231–42.
18. Combs SE, Schulz-Ertner D, Debus J, et al. Improved correlation of the neuropathologic classification according to adapted world health organization classification and outcome after radiotherapy in patients with atypical and anaplastic meningiomas. Int J Radiat Oncol Biol Phys. 2011;81:1415–21.
19. Domingues PH, Sousa P, Otero Á, et al. Proposal for a new risk stratification classification for meningioma based on patient age, WHO tumor grade, size, localization, and karyotype. Neuro-Oncology. 2014;16:735–47.
20. Olar A, Wani KM, Sulman EP, et al. Mitotic index is an independent predictor of recurrence-free survival in meningioma. Brain Pathol. 2015;25:266–75.
21. Condra KS, Buatti JM, Mendenhall WM, Friedman WA, Marcus RBJ, Rhoton AL. Benign meningiomas: primary treatment selection affects survival. Int J Radiat Oncol Biol Phys. 1997;39:427–36.
22. DeMonte F, Al-Mefty O. Meningiomas. In: Kaye A, Edward Laws E, editors. Brain tumors. Edinburgh: Churchill Livingstone; 1995. p. 675–704.
23. Stafford S, Perry A, Suman V, et al. Primarily resected meningiomas: outcome and prognostic factors in 581 Mayo Clinic patients, 1978 through 1988. Mayo Clin Proc. 1998;73:936–42.
24. Perry A, Giannini C, Raghavan R, et al. Aggressive phenotypic and genotypic features in pediatric and NF2- associated meningiomas: a clinicopathologic study of 53 cases. J Neuropathol Exp Neurol. 2001;60:994–1003.
25. Simpson D. The recurrence of intracranial meningiomas after surgical treatment. J Neurol Neurosurg Psychiatry. 1957;20:22–39.
26. Adegbite AB, Kahn MI, Paine KWE, Tan LK. The recurrence of intracranial meningiomas after surgical treatment. J Neurosurg. 1983;58:51–6.
27. Marks LB, Spencer DP. The influence of volume on the tolerance of the brain to radiosurgery. J Neurosurg. 1991;75:177–80.

28. Mirimanoff RO, Dosoretz DE, Linggood RM, et al. meningioma: analysis of recurrence and progression following neurosurgical resection. J Neurosurg. 1985;62:18–24.
29. Sekhar LN, Patel S, Cusimano M, et al. Surgical treatment of meningiomas involving the cavernous sinus: evolving ideas based on a ten year experience. Acta Neurochir. 1996;65 Suppl:58–62.
30. Sen C, Hague K. Meningiomas involving the cavernous sinus: histological factors affecting the degree of resection. J Neurosurg. 1997;87:535–43.
31. Sindou MP, Alaywan M. Most intracranial meningiomas are not cleavable tumors: anatomic-surgical evidence and angiographic predictability. Neurosurgery. 1998;42:476–80.
32. Goldsmith B. Meningioma. In: Leibel S, Phillips T, editors. Textbook of radiation oncology. Philadelphia: WB Saunders; 1998. p. 324–40.
33. Pollock BE, Stafford SL, Link MJ. Gamma knife radiosurgery for skull base meningiomas. Neurosurg Clin North Am. 2000;11:659–66.
34. O'Sullivan MG, van Loveren HR, Tew JM Jr. The surgical resectability of meningiomas of the cavernous sinus. Neurosurgery. 1997;40:238–44. discussion 245–37.
35. De Jesus O, Sekhar LN, Parikh HK, et al. Long-term follow-up of patients with meningiomas involving the cavernous sinus: recurrence, progression, and quality of life. Neurosurgery. 1996;39:915–9. discussion 919–20.
36. Little KM, Friedman AH, Sampson JH, et al. Surgical management of petroclival meningiomas: defining resection goals based on risk of neurological morbidity and tumor recurrence rates in 137 patients. Neurosurgery. 2005;56:546–59.
37. Nanda A, Jawahar A, Sathyanarayana S. Microsurgery for potential radiosurgical skull base lesions: a retrospective analysis and comparison of results. Skull Base. 2003;13:131–8.
38. Soyuer S, Chang EL, Selek U, et al. Radiotherapy after surgery for benign cerebral meningioma. Radiother Oncol. 2004;71:85–90.
39. Aghi MK, Carter BS, Cosgrove GR, et al. Long-term recurrence rates of atypical meningiomas after gross total resection with or without postoperative adjuvant radiation. Neurosurgery. 2009;64:56–60.
40. Hug EB, Devries A, Thornton AF, et al. Management of atypical and malignant meningiomas: role of high-dose, 3D-conformal radiation therapy. J Neuro-Oncol. 2000;48:151–60.
41. Hardesty DA, Wolf AB, Brachman DG, et al. The impact of adjuvant stereotactic radiosurgery on atypical meningioma recurrence following aggressive microsurgical resection. J Neurosurg. 2013;119:475–81.
42. Jaaskelainen J, Haltia M, Servo A. Atypical and anaplastic meningiomas: radiology, surgery, radiotherapy, and outcome. Surg Neurol. 1986;25:233–42.
43. Goyal LK, Suh JH, Mohan DS, Prayson RA, Lee J, Barnett GH. Local control and overall survival in atypical meningioma: a retrospective study. Int J Radiat Oncol Biol Phys. 2000;46:57–61.
44. Jenkinson MD, Waqar M, Farah JO, et al. Early adjuvant radiotherapy in the treatment of atypical meningioma. J Clin Neurosci. 2016;28:87–92.
45. Stessin AM, Schwartz A, Judanin G, et al. Does adjuvant external-beam radiotherapy improve outcomes for nonbenign meningiomas? A Surveillance, Epidemiology, and End Results (SEER)-based analysis. J Neurosurg. 2012;117(4):669–75.
46. Hammouche S, Clark S, Wong AH, Eldridge P, Farah JO. Long-term survival analysis of atypical meningiomas: survival rates, prognostic factors, operative and radiotherapy treatment. Acta Neurochir. 2014;156(8):1475–81.
47. Graffeo CS, Leeper HE, Perry A, et al. Revisiting adjuvant radiotherapy after gross total resection of World Health Organization Grade II meningioma. World Neurosurg. 2017;103:655–63.
48. Mair R, Morris K, Scott I, Carroll TA. Radiotherapy for atypical meningiomas. J Neurosurg. 2011;115(4):811–9.
49. Komotar RJ, Iorgulescu JB, Raper DM, et al. The role of radio- therapy following gross-total resection of atypical meningiomas. J Neurosurg. 2012;117:679–86.
50. Park HJ, Kang HC, Kim IH, et al. The role of adjuvant radiotherapy in atypical meningiomas. J Neuro-Oncol. 2013;115(2):241–7.

51. Klinger DR, Flores BC, Lewis JJ, et al. Atypical meningiomas: recurrence, reoperation, and radiotherapy. World Neurosurg. 2015;84(3):839–45.
52. Bagshaw HP, Burt LM, Jensen RL, et al. Adjuvant radiotherapy for atypical meningiomas. J Neurosurg. 2017;126(6):1822–8.
53. Shakir SI, Souhami L, Petrecca K, et al. Prognostic factors for progression in atypical meningioma. J Neurosurg. 2018;129:1240–8.
54. Weber DC, Area C, Villa S, et al. Adjuvant postoperative high-dose radiotherapy for atypical and malignant meningioma: a phase-II parallel non-randomized and observation study (EORTC 22042-26042). Radiother Oncol. 2018;128(2):260–5.
55. Simon M, Boström J, Koch P, Schramm J. Interinstitutional variance of postoperative radiotherapy and follow up for meningiomas in Germany: impact of changes of the WHO classification. J Neurol Neurosurg Psychiatry. 2006;77:767–73.
56. Marcus HJ, Price SJ, Wilby M, Santarius T, Kirollos RW. Radiotherapy as an adjuvant in the management of intracranial meningiomas: are we practising evidence-based medicine? Br J Neurosurg. 2008;22:520–8.
57. Goldsmith BJ, Wara WM, Wilson CB, Larson DA. Postoperative irradiation for subtotally resected meningiomas. A retrospective analysis of 140 patients treated from 1967 to 1990. J Neurosurg. 1994;80:195–201.
58. Sun SQ, Hawasli AH, Huang J, Chicoine MR, Kim AH. An evidence-based treatment algorithm for the management of WHO Grade II and III meningiomas. Neurosurg Focus. 2015;38(3):E3.
59. Ding D, Starke RM, Hantzmon J, Yen CP, Williams BJ, Sheehan JP. The role of radiosurgery in the management of WHO Grade II and III intracranial meningiomas. Neurosurg Focus. 2013;35(6):E16.
60. Williams BJ, Salvetti DJ, Starke RM, Yen CP, Sheehan JP. Stereotactic radiosurgery for WHO II and III meningiomas: analysis of long-term clinical and radiographic outcomes. J Radiosurg SBRT. 2013;2(3):183–91.
61. Acker G, Meinert F, Conti A, et al. Image-guided robotic radiosurgery for treatment of recurrent grade II and III meningiomas. A Single-Center Study. World Neurosurg. 2019;131:e96–107.
62. Pollock BE, Stafford SL, Link MJ, Garces YI, Foote RL. Stereotactic radiosurgery of World Health Organization grade II and III intracranial meningiomas: treatment results on the basis of a 22-year experience. Cancer. 2012;118(4):1048–54.
63. Hakim R, Alexander E III, Loeffler JS, et al. Results of linear accelerator based radiosurgery for intracranial meningiomas. Neurosurgery. 1998;42:446–53.
64. Stafford SL, Pollock BE, Foote RL, et al. Meningioma radiosurgery: tumor control, outcomes, and complications among 190 consecutive patients. Neurosurgery. 2001;49(5):1. –29–37.
65. Harris AE, Lee JY, Omalu B, et al. The effect of radiosurgery during management of aggressive meningiomas. Surg Neurol. 2003;60:298–305.
66. Torres RC, De Salles AAF, Frighetto L, et al. Long-term follow-up using linac radiosurgery and stereotactic radiotherapy as a minimally invasive treatment for intracranial meningiomas. In: Kondziolka D, editor. Radiosurgery, vol 5. Basel: Krager; 2004. p. 115–23.
67. Milker-Zabel S, Zabel A, Schulz-Ertner D, Schlegel W, Wannenmacher M, Debus J. Fractionated stereotactic radiotherapy in patients with benign or atypical intracranial meningioma: Long-term experience and prognostic factors. Int J Radiat Oncol Biol Phys. 2005;61(3):809–16.
68. Huffmann BC, Reinacher PC, Gilsbach JM. Gamma knife surgery for atypical meningiomas. J Neurosurg. 2005;102(Suppl):283–6.
69. Kano H, Takahashi JA, Katsuki T, et al. Stereotactic radiosurgery for atypical and anaplastic meningiomas. J Neuro-Oncol. 2007;84:41–7.
70. Attia A, Chan MD, Mott RT, et al. Patterns of failure after treatment of atypical meningioma with gamma knife radiosurgery. J Neuro-Oncol. 2012;108:179–85.
71. Kaprealian T, Raleigh DR, Sneed PK, Nabavizadeh N, Nakamura JL, McDermott MW. Parameters influencing local control of meningiomas treated with radiosurgery. J Neuro-Oncol. 2016;128(2):357–64.
72. Coke CC, Corn BW, Werner-Wasik M, et al. Atypical and malignant meningiomas: an outcome report of seventeen cases. J Neuro-Oncol. 1998;39:65–70.

73. Rosenberg LA, Prayson RA, Lee J, et al. Long term experience with WHO Grade III meningiomas at the Cleveland Clinic Foundation. Int J Radiat Oncol Biol Phys. 2007;69(3):S256.
74. Palma L, Celli P, Franco C, Cervoni L, Cantore G. Long-term prognosis for atypical and malignant meningiomas: a study of 71 surgical cases. J Neurosurg. 1997;86:793–800.
75. Dziuk TW, Woo S, Butler EB, et al. Malignant meningioma: an indication for initial aggressive surgery and adjuvant radiotherapy. J Neuro-Oncol. 1998;37:177–88.
76. Sughrue ME, Sanai N, Shangari G, et al. Outcome and survival following primary and repeat surgery for World Health Organization Grade III meningiomas. J Neurosurg. 2010;113(2):202–9.
77. Milosevic M, Frost P, Laperriere N, et al. Radiotherapy for atypical or malignant intracranial meningioma. Int J Radiat Oncol Biol Phys. 1996;34:817–22.
78. Ojemann SG, Sneed PK, Larson DA, et al. Radiosurgery for malignant meningioma: results in 22 patients. J Neurosurg. 2000;93(Suppl 3):62–7.
79. Balasubramanian SK, Sharma M, Silva D, Karivedu V, Schmitt P, Stevens GH, et al. Longitudinal experience with WHO Grade III (anaplastic) meningiomas at a single institution. J Neuro-Oncol. 2017;131(3):555–63.
80. Taylor BWJ, Marcus RBJ, Friedman WA, Ballinger WEJ, Million RR. The meningioma controversy: postoperative radiation therapy. Int J Radiat Oncol Biol Phys. 1988;15:299–304.
81. Wara W, Sheline G, Newman H, et al. Radiation therapy of meningiomas. Am J Roentgenol Ther Nucl Med. 1975;123:453–8.
82. McGovern SL, Aldape KD, Munsell MF, et al. A comparison of World Health Organization tumor grades at recurrence in patients with non-skull base and skull base meningiomas. J Neurosurg. 2010;112:925–33.
83. Pourel N, Auque J, Bracard S, et al. Efficacy of external fractionated radiation therapy in the treatment of meningiomas: a 20-year experience. Radiother Oncol. 2001;61:65–70.
84. Ikeda H, Yoshimoto T. Immunohistochemical study of anaplastic meningioma with special reference to the phenotypic change of intermediate filament protein. Ann Diagn Pathol. 2003;7:214–22.
85. Peele KA, Kennerdell JS, Maroon JC, et al. The role of postoperative irradiation in the management of sphenoid wing meningiomas. A preliminary report. Ophthalmology. 1996;103:1761–6.
86. Mehdorn HM. Intracranial meningiomas: A 30-year experience and literature review. Adv Tech Stand Neurosurg. 2016;43:139–84.
87. Talacchi A, Muggiolu F, De Carlo A, et al. Recurrent atypical meningiomas: combining surgery and radiosurgery in one effective multimodal treatment. World Neurosurg. 2016;87:565–72.
88. Kessel KA, Fischer H, Oechsner M, et al. High-precision radiotherapy for meningiomas: long-term results and patient- reported outcome (PRO). Strahlenther Onkol. 2017;193:921–30.
89. Debus J, Wuendrich M, Pirzkall A, et al. High efficacy of fractionated stereotactic radiotherapy of large base-of-skull meningiomas: long-term results. J Clin Oncol. 2001;19:3547–53.
90. DeVries A, Munzenrider JE, Hedley-Whyte T, et al. The role of radiotherapy in the treatment of malignant meningiomas. Strahlenther Onkol. 1999;175:62–7.
91. Boskos C, Feuvret L, Noel G, et al. Combined proton and photon conformal radiotherapy for intracranial atypical and malignant meningioma. Int J Radiat Oncol Biol Phys. 2009;75(2):399–406.
92. McDermott M, Quinones-Hinojosa A, Bollen A, et al. Meningiomas. In: Steele G, Phillips T, Chabner B, editors. American cancer society atlas of clinical oncology: brain cancer. Hamilton: BC Decker Inc; 2002. p. 333–64.
93. Jensen R, Lee J. Predicting outcomes of patients with intracranial meningiomas using molecular markers of hypoxia, vascularity, and proliferation. Neurosurgery. 2012;71:146–56.
94. Glaholm J, Bloom HJ, Crow JH. The role of radiotherapy in the management of intracranial meningiomas: the Royal Marsden Hospital experience with 186 patients. Int J Radiat Oncol Biol Phys. 1990;18:755–61.
95. Mattozo CA, De Salles AA, Klement IA, et al. Stereotactic radiation treatment for recurrent nonbenign meningiomas. J Neurosurg. 2007;106(5):846–54.
96. Choi CY, Soltys SG, Gibbs IC, et al. Cyberknife stereotactic radio- surgery for treatment of atypical (WHO grade II) cranial meningiomas. Neurosurgery. 2010;67:1180–8.

97. Zhang M, Ho AL, D'Astous M, et al. CyberKnife stereotactic radiosurgery for atypical and malignant meningiomas. World Neurosurg. 2016;91:574–81 e571.
98. Valery CA, Faillot M, Lamproglou I, et al. Grade II meningiomas and Gamma Knife radiosurgery: analysis of success and failure to improve treatment paradigm. J Neurosurg. 2016;125:89–96.
99. Rogers L, Jensen R, Perry A. Chasing your dural tail. Re: factors predicting local tumor control after Gamma Knife stereotactic radiosurgery for benign intracranial meningiomas. Int J Radiat Oncol Biol Phys. 2005;2:616–8.
100. Qi ST, Liu Y, Pan J, Chotai S, Fang LX. A radiopathological classification of dural tail sign of meningiomas. J Neurosurg. 2012;117:645–53.
101. Chidambaram S, Pannullo SC, Roytman M, et al. Dynamic contrast-enhanced magnetic resonance imaging perfusion characteristics in meningiomas treated with resection and adjuvant radiosurgery. Neurosurg Focus. 2019;46(6):E10.
102. Silva CB, Ongaratti BR, Trott G, et al. Expression of somatostatin receptors (SSTR1-SSTR5) in meningiomas and its clinicopathological significance. Int J Clin Exp Pathol. 2015;8:13185–92.
103. Menke JR, Raleigh DR, Gown AM, et al. Somatostatin receptor 2a is a more sensitive diagnostic marker of meningioma than epithelial membrane antigen. Acta Neuropathol. 2015;130:441–3.
104. Nathoo N, Ugokwe K, Chang AS, et al. The role of 111indium-octreotide brain scintigraphy in the diagnosis of cranial, dural-based meningiomas. J Neuro-Oncol. 2007;81(2):167–74.
105. Gehler B, Paulsen F, Oksüz MO, et al. [68Ga]-DOTATOC-PET/CT for meningioma IMRT treatment planning. Radiat Oncol. 2009;4:56.
106. Graf R, Nyuyki F, Steffen IG, et al. Contribution of 68Ga-DOTATOC PET/CT to target volume delineation of skull base meningiomas treated with stereotactic radiation therapy. Int J Radiat Oncol Biol Phys. 2013;85(1):68–73.
107. Afshar-Oromieh A, Giesel FL, Linhart HG, et al. Detection of cranial meningiomas: comparison of (6)(8)Ga-DOTATOC PET/CT and contrast-enhanced MRI. Eur J Nucl Med Mol Imaging. 2012;39:1409–15.
108. Reubi JC, Schar JC, Waser B, et al. Affinity profiles for human somatostatin receptor subtypes SST1-SST5 of somatostatin radiotracers selected for scintigraphic and radiotherapeutic use. Eur J Nucl Med. 2000;27:273–82.
109. Kunz WG, Jungblut LM, Kazmierczak PM, et al. Improved detection of transosseous meningiomas using (68)Ga-DOTATATE PET/CT compared with contrast-enhanced MRI. J Nucl Med. 2017;58:1580–7.
110. Rachinger W, Stoecklein VM, Terpolilli NA, et al. Increased 68Ga-DOTATATE uptake in PET imaging discriminates meningioma and tumor-free tissue. J Nucl Med. 2015;56:347–53.
111. Ivanidze J, Roytman M, Lin E. Gallium-68 DOTATATE PET in the Evaluation of Intracranial Meningiomas. J Neuroimaging. 2019;29(5):650–6.
112. Al-Mefty O, Kersh JE, Routh A, Smith RR. The long-term side effects of radiation therapy for benign brain tumors in adults. J Neurosurg. 1990;73:502–12.
113. Meyers CA, Geara F, Wong PF, Morrison WH. Neurocognitive effects of therapeutic irradiation for base of skull tumors. Int J Radiat Oncol Biol Phys. 2000;46(1):51–5.
114. Urie MM, Fullerton B, Tatsuzaki H, et al. A dose response analysis of injury to cranial nerves and/or nuclei following proton beam radiation therapy. Int J Radiat Oncol Biol Phys. 1992;23(1):27–39.
115. Pirzkall A, Debus J, Haering P, et al. Intensity modulated radiotherapy (IMRT) for recurrent, residual, or untreated skull-base meningiomas: preliminary clinical experience. Int J Radiat Oncol Biol Phys. 2003;55(2):362–72.
116. Uy NW, Woo SY, Teh BS, et al. Intensity-modulated radiation therapy (IMRT) for meningioma. Int J Radiat Oncol Biol Phys. 2002;53:1265–70.
117. Goldsmith BJ, Rosenthal SA, Wara WM, Larson DA. Optic neuropathy after irradiation of meningioma. Radiology. 1992;185:71–6.

118. Selch MT, Ahn E, Laskari A, et al. Stereotactic radiotherapy for treatment of cavernous sinus meningiomas. Int J Radiat Oncol Biol Phys. 2004;59(1):101–11.
119. Nutting C, Brada M, Brazil L, et al. Radiotherapy in the treatment of benign meningioma of the skull base. J Neurosurg. 1999;90(5):823–7.
120. Maguire PD, Clough R, Friedman AH, Halperin EC. Fractionated external-beam radiation therapy for meningiomas of the cavernous sinus. Int J Radiat Oncol Biol Phys. 1999;44(1):75–9.
121. Katz TS, Amdur RJ, Yachnis AT, Mendenhall WM, Morris CG. Pushing the limits of radiotherapy for atypical and malignant meningioma. Am J Clin Oncol. 2005;28:70–4.
122. Steinvorth S, Welzel G, Fuss M, et al. Neuropsychological outcome after fractionated stereotactic radiotherapy (FSRT) for base of skull meningiomas: a prospective 1-year follow-up. Radiother Oncol. 2003;69(2):177–82.

The Role of Medical Therapy for Menigniomas

Ashley M. Roque and Antonio Omuro

Introduction and General Treatment Strategies

As described in previous chapters, the current standard of care for meningiomas that are symptomatic or progressively enlarging is maximum surgical resection. Subsequent treatment is based on degree of resection achieved and tumor grade. Meningiomas are classified as WHO Grade I ("benign"), II ("atypical"), or III ("malignant"). Grade I tumors generally have a benign course, with a recurrence rate of 5–10% at 5 years. As such, these can be followed with surveillance imaging after complete resection, with re-resection or radiation initiated at recurrence. Partially resected tumors may also be followed depending on patient characteristics. Grade II and III tumors have a higher rate of recurrence, exceeding 50% of atypical tumors and 80% for anaplastic tumors. Postoperative radiation is generally recommended in patients with Grade III meningioma and partially resected Grade II meningioma. The role of postoperative radiation in completely resected atypical tumors is controversial. There is currently no defined role for chemotherapy for newly diagnosed meningiomas. Chemotherapy can be considered in patients with recurrent disease with no further surgical or therapeutic radiation options; however, there is no consistent evidence that it prolongs survival, and no drug has ever received FDA approval for this indication. Evaluation of systemic treatments in

A. M. Roque
Department of Neuro-Oncology, Mount Sinai Hospital, New York, NY, USA
e-mail: ashley.roque@mssm.edu

A. Omuro (✉)
Yale New Haven Hospital and Smilow Cancer Hospital, New Haven, CT, USA

Yale Brain Tumor Center at Smilow Cancer Hospital, New Haven, CT, USA

Department of Neurology, Yale School of Medicine, Yale University, New Haven, CT, USA
e-mail: antonio.omuro@yale.edu

© Springer Nature Switzerland AG 2020
J. Moliterno, A. Omuro (eds.), *Meningiomas*,
https://doi.org/10.1007/978-3-030-59558-6_13

these tumors has been challenging as studies often have small treatment groups, varying inclusion criteria, no control arms, and variable outcome measures. Given the lack of control arms in studies, there is limited data on the natural history of the disease if left untreated, making it difficult to interpret trial results. To address this issue, a recent meta-analysis of 47 publications on medical treatment of meningioma was performed to determine benchmarks for clinically meaningful responses for future trials. The study found that the most consistently reported outcome in meningioma trials was progression-free survival at 6 months (PFS-6). They determined the weighted PFS-6 average for WHO I meningiomas was 26% and the average for WHO Grade II/II meningiomas was 29% [1]. These numbers confirmed the poor outcomes for medical therapy in recurrent/progressive meningiomas. Based on this analysis and overall experience with meningiomas thus far, the Revised Assessment in Neuro-Oncology (RANO) working group recommends that rate of interest for single arm or phase II studies in meningioma be PFS-6 > 50% in WHO Grade 1 tumors and PFS-6 > 35% in Grade II and III tumors. While optimal endpoints and inclusion criteria remain uncertain, such numbers can serve as a starting point when evaluating medical therapies in recurrent/progressive meningiomas. Adding to the difficulties of cross-trial comparisons and interpretation of the literature is the fact that criteria for tumor progression leading to the trial also vary; patients with very slow growth could potentially be enrolled along with highly aggressive and rapid-growing tumors and at varying frequencies. Likewise, trials differ in terms of required previous surgical and radiation therapies, with some studies enrolling more heavily pre-treated patients than others.

Based on available literature and expert consensus, the most recent NCCN Guidelines for Central Nervous System Tumors recommend consideration of three systemic agents for recurrent meningiomas not amenable to surgery or radiation: interferon-alpha-2 beta, somatostatin analogues, and sunitinib. Providers should nevertheless be aware that there is no evidence that these agents affect the natural history of the disease. If possible, enrollment on a clinical trial should be considered first. Here we will review the existing evidence on chemotherapy and hormonal therapy in recurrent meningiomas and outline the various treatment strategies that have been evaluated (see Tables 13.1 and 13.2). Emerging therapies, such as molecularly targeted therapies from genomic analyses and newer immunotherapies, will be described in subsequent chapters.

Cytotoxic Therapy

Hydroxyurea

Multiple studies have evaluated the use of traditional cytotoxic chemotherapy agents in meningioma. Hydroxyurea, an oral ribonucleotide reductase inhibitor, has been the most extensively studied agent. In an early report, three out of four patients treated with hydroxyurea had significant reduction in tumor size, and the fourth patient had stable disease for 24 months [2]. However, in later prospective phase II and retrospective studies [3–9], patients did not show similar responses. Response

Table 13.1 Medical therapies studied in meningioma

Cytotoxic therapy
Hydroxyurea
Other traditional chemotherapies (dacarbazine, Adriamycin, ifosfamide, mesna, temozolomide, and irinotecan)
Hormonal agents
Estrogen receptor inhibitors
Progesterone receptor inhibitors
Somatostatin analogues
Octreotide[a]
Sandostatin LAR[a]
Immunologic agents
Interferon alpha-2b[a]
Molecularly targeted agents
PDGFR inhibitors: imatinib
EGFR inhibitors: gefitinib, erlotinib
VEGF inhibitors: sunitinib[a], Avastin

[a]Agents recommended by NCCN guidelines

rates were generally less than 5% [10]. About 60% of patients had stable disease as their best response, and median progression-free survival has ranged from 2 months to 27 months. In vivo and vitro studies suggested promising results with the combination of hydroxyurea and calcium channel blockers; however a small patient cohort produced similarly disappointing results to prior studies [11]. It should be noted that these studies are difficult to interpret as many patients who received hydroxyurea also received RT. It is also unclear whether these responses represent an improvement over the natural history of the disease.

Other Chemotherapy Agents (Dacarbazine, Doxorubicin, Ifosfamide, Mesna, Temozolomide, and Irinotecan)

Treatment with other traditional agents such as dacarbazine, doxorubicin, ifosfamide, mesna, and temozolomide has also produced disappointing results. In a prospective phase II trial of 14 patients, the combination of doxorubicin, cyclophosphamide, and vincristine given as adjuvant therapy 2–4 weeks after the completion of surgery and radiation for Grade III meningiomas resulted in a median PFS of 4.6 years and an overall survival of 5.3 years. Three patients had partial response and 11 had stable disease. There was considerable toxicity of this regimen and only modest survival advantage; thus the agents are not recommended in current practice [12]. In a phase II study of 16 patients with refractory Grade I meningioma treated with temozolomide, median progression-free survival was 5 months, median overall survival was 7 months, and PF-6 was 0%. No patient showed a radiographic response, and 13 showed stable disease [13]. Irinotecan was similarly ineffective in a phase II trial, which resulted in a median PFS of 4.5 months and PFS-6 of 6% [14].

Table 13.2 Results of selected studies for systemic therapies in meningioma

Agent	Author	Year	Protocol type	N	WHO grade				Best radiographic response				PFS-6 (%)	PFS	OS
					Unknown	I	II	III	PR or MR (%)	SD (%)	PD (%)	Not assessed (%)			
Hydroxyurea	Schrell [2]	1997	Single arm, prospective	4		3	0	1	75	25	0	0			
Hydroxyurea	Newton [7]	2000	Single arm, prospective	17	4	12	1	0		82	12	6		20 weeks	
Hydroxyurea	Mason [6]	2002	Single arm, prospective	20		16	3	1	5	80	15	0			
Hydroxyurea	Rosenthal [8]	2002	Single arm, prospective	15		10	5	0		85	15	0			
Hydroxyurea	Loven [5]	2004	Single arm, prospective	12		8	4	0	8	75	0	17		13 months	
Hydroxyurea	Swinnen [9]	2009	Phase II, single arm, prospective	29		0	0	0						27 months	
Hydroxyurea	Chamberlain [4]	2011	Retrospective case series	60		60	0	0		35	65	0	10	4 months	
Hydroxyurea	Chamberlain [3]	2012	Retrospective case series	35		0	22	13	10	90		0	3	2 months	8 months
RT + adjuvant cyclophosphamide, Adriamycin, vincristine	Chamberlain [12]	1996	Single arm, prospective	14		0	0	14	21	79		0		4.6 years	5.3 years
Temozolomide	Chamberlain [13]	2004	Single arm, prospective	16		16	0	0		82	18	0	0	5 months	7.5 months

Drug	Author	Year	Study type	N											
Irinotecan	Chamberlain [14]	2006	Single arm, prospective	16		16	0	0	6	75	19	0	6	4.5 months	7 months
Tamoxifen	Markwalder [18]	1985	Single arm, prospective	6	6	0	0	0	17	83		0			
Tamoxifen	Goodwin [19]	1993	Single arm, prospective	21	21	0	0	0	14	28	47	10		15.1 months	
Mifepristone	Grunberg [20]	1991	Single arm, prospective	14	2	7	3	2	36	36	21	7			
Mifepristone	Ji [21]	2015	Phase 3, RCT	80 (84 placebo)	72	0	8	0	3	55	31	11		10 months (placebo, 11 months)	
Sandostatin LAR	Chamberlain [23]	2007	Single arm, prospective	16		8	3	5	31	31	38	0	44	5 months	7.5 months
Octreotide	Johnson [25]	2011	Phase II, prospective	11		3	3	5	0	73	27	0		17 weeks	2.7 years
Octreotide	Simó [26]	2014	Phase II, prospective	8		0	5	4	0	33	67	0	44	4 months	18.7 months
Pasireotide LAR	Norden [24]	2015	Phase II, prospective	34		16	12	6	0	71	24	6	32	18 weeks	
IFN-α-2B	Kaba [32]	1997	Retrospective case series	6		2	1	3	16.5	67	16.5	0			
IFN-α-2B	Chamberlain [33]	2008	Phase II, prospective	35		35	0	0	0	74	26	0	54	7 months	8 months
Imatinib	Wen [37]	2009	Phase II, prospective	23		13	5	5	0	39	43	17	29.4	2 months	
Imatinib + hydroxyurea	Reardon [38]	2012	Phase II, prospective	21		8	9	4	0	67	33	0	61.9	7 months	
Erlotinib or gefitinib	Norden [43]	2010	Phase II, prospective	25		8	9	8	0	32	68	0	28	10 weeks	

(continued)

Table 13.2 (continued)

Agent	Author	Year	Protocol type	N	WHO grade				Best radiographic response				PFS-6 (%)	PFS	OS
					Unknown	I	II	III	PR or MR (%)	SD (%)	PD (%)	Not assessed (%)			
Bevacizumab	Lou [55]	2012	Retrospective case series	14	1	5	5	3	7	79	14	0	85.7	17.9 months	
Bevacizumab	Nayak [56]	2012	Retrospective case series	15		0	6	9	13	87	0	0	43.8	26 weeks	
Bevacizumab + everolimus	Shi [57]	2016	Phase II prospective	17	1	4	7	5	0	88	6	6	69	22 months	23.8 months
Sunitinib	Kaley [58]	2014	Phase II, prospective	36		0	30	6	6	69	22	3	42	5.2 months	24.6 months
Vatalanib (PTK787)	Raizer [59]	2010	Phase II, prospective	25		2	14	8	0	60	28	12	54.6	7 months	26 months

Key: *PR* partial response, *MR* minor response, *SD* stable disease, *PD* progressive disease, *PFS-6* progression-free survival at 6 months, *PFS* progression-free survival (median), *OS* overall survival (median)

Current Agents Under Investigation

There is currently one chemotherapeutic agent, trabectedin, being investigated in a randomized, multicenter phase II trial for patients with recurrent WHO Grade II/III meningiomas (EORTC-1320-RTG). Trabectedin is a DNA-binding agent which inhibits transcription factor binding and has shown activity in vitro in meningioma [15, 16].

Hormonal Therapy

Meningiomas are almost twice as likely to occur in women, are found more often in patients with breast cancer, and may show increased growth during pregnancy. Tissue analysis has shown progesterone receptors are expressed on approximately 65% of meningiomas and estrogen receptors on 10% [10, 17]. As a result, there has been significant interest in the use of hormonal therapies in the treatment of meningiomas.

Estrogen Receptor Inhibitors

Tamoxifen, a selective estrogen receptor modulator (SERM) that competitively binds to estrogen receptors, is effective in treating estrogen receptor-positive breast cancer. In an early report, six patients with inoperable or recurrent meningioma received 8–12 months of tamoxifen. At the end of the treatment period, five out of the six patients showed no response, and one patient showed partial response [18]. In a later study of 19 patients with unresectable refractory meningioma treated with tamoxifen, 3 (15.7%) patients showed partial or minor responses, 6 patients (32%) were stable, and 10 (53%) demonstrated progression. The median progression-free survival was 15.1 months, and PFS-6 was not reported [19]. The authors felt that based on these results, they could not make a definite recommendation for tamoxifen use in refractory or unresectable meningiomas.

Progesterone Receptor Inhibitors

In an early trial of mifepristone for unresectable meningiomas, results were encouraging, with 4 of 14 patients showing a response on imaging [20]. However, subsequent studies were disappointing. The largest was a multicenter phase III study conducted by SWOG which randomized 164 patients with meningiomas (primary, recurrent, or residual) to receive mifepristone or placebo for 2 years (if they had not progressed). One patient in the mifepristone arm had partial response, and neither failure-free survival (10 months in placebo vs. 11 months in mifepristone) nor overall survival was significantly different between groups [21].

Somatostatin Analogues

Molecular analyses have revealed that almost 90% of meningiomas express somatostatin receptors [22]. Octreotide SPECT scanning is used to confirm receptor status in patients in the clinical setting. A pilot study of 16 patients with recurrent meningioma (8 Grade I, 3 Grade II, and 5 Grade III) treated with Sandostatin LAR showed encouraging results in terms of response rates. After 3 months, five patients had achieved partial response, five had achieved stable disease, and six had progressed. The median PFS was 5 months and the PFS 6 was 44% [23]. A subsequent phase II study of 26 patients with recurrent meningioma treated with a different somatostatin analogue, pasireotide LAR, did not show significant activity. 0 patients showed response, 16 showed stable disease, and 6 showed progressive disease. Median PFS was 20 weeks and PFS-6 was 29% [24]. In another study, 11 patients with recurrent Grade II or III meningioma were treated with subcutaneous octreotide; 0 patients showed radiographic response, and median PFS was 17 weeks [25]. Another phase II trial using octreotide in recurrent high-grade meningioma was terminated early after enrolling nine patients. In this study there were no responses and median PFS was 4.23 months, and stable disease was the best response in one third of patients [26]. The drug was well tolerated in all of these studies. While most of these studies have been disappointing, the response rate in the Sandostatin LAR study (31%) mentioned above is higher than that of any previously reported study. Therefore, this agent can be considered in treatment of refractory tumors with positive octreotide scans. An example of a patient treated with Sandostatin LAR can be seen in Fig. 13.1.

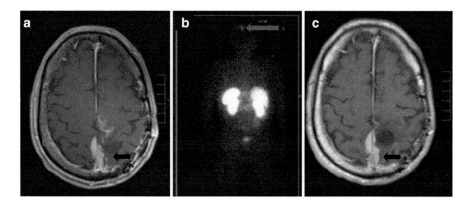

Fig. 13.1 Imaging shows an atypical meningioma (WHO Grade II) after treatment with 6 months of monthly Sandostatin injections. The patient previously underwent three surgical resections, GKRS, and fractionated XRT. (**a**) T1 post contrast MRI revealing meningioma along the posterior falx cerebri (black arrow). (**b**) shows octreotide scan with uptake within the region of the meningioma. (blue arrow). (**c**) shows stable size of meningioma along posterior falx on T1 post contrast imaging after 6 months (black arrow)

Immunologic Agents

Interferon-Alpha-2b

Interferon-alpha-2b is an endogenous agent produced by leukocytes that has anti-proliferative and immunomodulatory effects. Activity of this agent in other solid cancers such as hemangiomas, renal cell carcinomas, and melanomas prompted investigation into its use in meningiomas [27–30]. In vitro studies suggested that interferon-alpha-2b had inhibitory effect on meningioma cell cultures [31]. An early case series on six patients with unresectable meningioma (2 Grade I, 1 Grade II, 3 Grade III) treated with various doses (though majority treated with subcutaneous interferon-alpha-2b 4 million unit/m² days per week) showed that four out of six patients remained stable while on therapy, one patient had a minor response, and one patient had progressive disease [32]. Later, a phase II study of 35 patients with recurrent/progressive Grade I meningiomas used interferon-alpha-2b at 10 million units/m² subcutaneously every other day. After 3 months of treatment, 26 patients demonstrated stable disease, 9 patients had progressive disease, and no patients demonstrated partial or complete response. The progression-free survival rate was 54% at 6 months and 31% at 12 months. The median time to tumor progression was 7 months (range, 2–24 months). The median survival was 8 months (range, 3–28 months). Patients in this study experienced moderate toxicities, with fatigue, anemia, and thrombocytopenia being the most common Grade 3 or 4 toxicities [33].

Other immunotherapies, such as checkpoint blockade agents, are currently being evaluated in meningiomas and are discussed elsewhere in this book.

Molecularly Targeted Agents

PDGFR Inhibitors: Imatinib

Models of meningioma cells have demonstrated that platelet-derived growth factor (PDGF) signaling is involved in the growth of meningiomas. PDGF and PDGF receptors are co-expressed on the surface of most meningiomas [34]. Treatment of meningioma cells in culture with PDGF-BB activates promitotic signals via the MAPK pathway [35], and antibodies against PDGF inhibit meningioma growth in vitro [36]. Imatinib mesylate inhibits the PDGFR-a and b, c-Kit, and Bcr-Abl kinases and has shown antitumor activity in gastrointestinal stromal tumors and in chronic myelogenous leukemia, making it an attractive agent in refractory meningioma. It was studied in a phase II trial of 23 patients (13 Grade I, 5 Grade II, and 5 Grade 3) with disappointing results. 19 patients were evaluated for response, and of these 9 remained stable, and 10 progressed at the first scan. There were no complete or partial responses. Overall median PFS was 2 months and PFS-6 was 29.4% [37]. A subsequent study evaluated the combination of imatinib with hydroxyurea and also showed modest results. 21 patients were evaluated (8 Grade I, 13 Grade II or III), no patients had radiographic response, and the best response was stable disease in 14 patients. Median progression-free survival for all patients was 7 months. PFS-6 for all patients, those with Grade I tumors, and those with Grade II or III tumors were 61.9% (CI 38.1–78.8), 87.5% (CI 38.7–98.1), and 46.2% (CI 19.2–69.6), respectively [38].Though these PFS-6 values numbers reach the rate of interest specified earlier in the chapter, the confidence intervals are quite broad. The authors also note that prolonged stable disease was seen mainly in patients with Grade I tumors, which should be interpreted with caution.

Sunitinib has activity against both VEGF and PDGF-R and will be discussed in the section focusing on VEGF inhibitors.

EGFR Inhibitors: Erlotinib and Gefitinib

Over 60% of meningiomas overexpress epidermal growth factor receptor (EGFR) on their membranes [39–41]. Epidermal growth factor, the ligand for EGFR, is a polypeptide hormone that stimulates proliferation in many types of cells in vitro and in vivo. Studies have shown that EGFRs are activated in meningiomas and capable of initiating the promitotic Ras signaling pathway [42]. This pathway is thus felt to be involved in promoting the growth of meningiomas and represents a potential target for treatment. In a phase II NABTC trial, 25 patients (all grades) were treated with gefitinib 500 mg/day or erlotinib 150 mg/day until tumor progression [43]. For Grade I tumors, the PFS-6 was 25%, and for Grade II and III tumors, the PFS-6 was 29%. For total study enrollment, the median PFS was 10 weeks. There were no radiographic responses, and nine patients had stable disease. The treatment was well tolerated, but given these results, there is no evidence that single agent EGFR TKIs have activity in meningiomas.

VEGF Inhibitors

There has been significant interest in inhibition of angiogenesis to treat many different tumor types. Vascular endothelial growth factor (VEGF) is the most potent known activator of angiogenesis and plays a key role in the vascular proliferation involved in tumorigenesis [44–46]. Many studies have shown that blocking VEGF with a monoclonal antibody inhibits angiogenesis and tumor growth [47–49]. Treatment with bevacizumab, a humanized monoclonal antibody against VEGF, has led to improvement in outcomes in patients with colorectal cancer, non-small cell lung cancer, renal cell carcinoma, breast cancer, ovarian cancer, and glioblastoma [50–53]. Meningiomas are highly vascular tumors that express both VEGF-R and VEGF, with expression level increasing with increasing grade of tumor, making angiogenesis inhibition an attractive treatment strategy [54].

There are retrospective case series of patients treated with bevacizumab, but no prospective studies using single agent bevacizumab. One retrospective review included 14 patients (with WHO Grade I, II, and III tumors), treated with both bevacizumab monotherapy and combination therapy with other agents. The median PFS for Grade I tumors was 15.8 months and PFS-6 was 80%. For Grade II/III tumors, median overall survival was 15.8 months and PFS-6 was 87.5% [55]. In another retrospective study including patients from multiple sites, 15 patients with WHO Grade II and III meningiomas were examined [56]. All patients had stable disease, the median PFS was 26 weeks, and PFS-6 was 43.8%. In this study, rate of intralesional hemorrhage was 20%, which is higher than that seen in glioblastoma. While these trials suggest that bevacizumab may have potential therapeutic use in meningioma, they should be interpreted with caution given retrospective nature. A recently published phase II study evaluated bevacizumab combined with everolimus (mTOR inhibitor) for patients with recurrent/refractory meningioma. A total of 17 patients with WHO Grade I, II, and III recurrent meningiomas were included in the study and treated with bevacizumab 10 mg/kg on days 1 and 15 and everolimus (10 mg po) for 28-day cycles. No patient had a radiographic response, and 15 (88%) had stable disease as their best imaging response. PFS in the entire treatment cohort was 22 months, with PFS of 17.5 months in Grade I tumors and 22 months in Grade II and III tumors. Median overall survival was 23.8 months, and the median duration of disease stabilization was 10 months. PFS at 6, 12, and 18 months were 69, 57, and 57%, respectively [57]. This was a small cohort of patients, but results suggest that this combination of therapy may have some activity in higher-grade tumors and deserves further evaluation. mTOR inhibition is an active area of study in recurrent meningioma and is addressed elsewhere in this book.

Other inhibitors of angiogenesis, sunitinib and valatinib, have been evaluated as single agents in prospective trials. A multicenter, single arm phase II study evaluating sunitinib enrolled 36 patients with surgery and radiation refractory recurrent WHO Grade II and III meningiomas [58]. Patients were treated with sunitinib at 50 mg/day for days 1–28 of a 42-day cycle. The PFS-6 rate was 42%, median PFS was 5.2 months, and overall survival was 24.6 months. The PFS-6 met the primary endpoint for efficacy; however there was significant toxicity. The overall rate of CNS hemorrhage was 8%, which is as expected in angiogenesis inhibitors, but there was one fatal and three serious CNS hemorrhages. About 1/3 of patients required dose reduction, and 1/5 of patients were removed from the study for toxicity. Overall, results suggested that sunitinib demonstrates activity in recurrent meningioma. While this remains one of the best studied agents in this disease, further evaluation in a randomized setting is warranted. It's use may be considered in patients who have exhausted all surgical and radiation options; however potential benefits should be weighed against toxicities. Vatalanib (i.e., PTK787) is another agent used to target angiogenesis and functions an oral inhibitor of VEGFR1, 2, and 3. A phase II trial investigated the use of vatalanib in 25 patients with recurrent WHO Grade I, II, and III meningiomas [59]. No patient showed radiographic response, and 15 patients (68.2%) had stable disease as the best response. PFS-6 was 64.3% and 37.5% in Grade II and III tumors, respectively. Median progression-free survival was 6.5 months, and overall survival was 26 months in patients with Grade II tumors. In patients with Grade III tumors, progression-free survival was

3.6 months, and overall survival was 23 months. Outcomes with this agent are modest and, however, suggest that further studies with VEGF inhibitors in this population are warranted. Table 13.2 shows the results from some studies for systemic therapies in meningioma.

Summary and Conclusions

As evidenced by the protocols reviewed in this chapter, studies in this population are difficult to interpret given the lack of standardized inclusion criteria, outcome measures, and the absence of historical controls. Within the context of these limitations, there are no systemic treatments that have been definitively shown to cause tumor regression or improve survival in this patient population. As such, there is no defined role for systemic treatment in patients with newly diagnosed meningioma. Therapies can be considered in patients with relapse or refractory disease with no other options; however, lack of data showing significant activity and toxicity of the therapy should be taken into account. Clearly, developing effective treatments for patients with recurrent or refractory meningioma who have exhausted all surgical and radiation options is an area of unmet need in neuro-oncology. Recent genomic studies have led to an improvement in our understanding of the molecular basis of meningioma formation and growth. In the current era of precision medicine, research efforts have focused largely on developing effective targeted therapies based on genetic and epigenetic analyses. Such ongoing work and other emerging therapies are discussed in the next chapter.

References

1. Kaley T, Barani I, Chamberlain M, McDermott M, Panageas K, Raizer J, et al. Historical benchmarks for medical therapy trials in surgery- and radiation-refractory meningioma: a RANO review. Neuro-Oncology. 2014;16(6):829–40.
2. Schrell UM, Rittig MG, Anders M, Koch UH, Marschalek R, Kiesewetter F, et al. Hydroxyurea for treatment of unresectable and recurrent meningiomas. II. Decrease in the size of meningiomas in patients treated with hydroxyurea. J Neurosurg. 1997;86(5):840–4.
3. Chamberlain MC. Hydroxyurea for recurrent surgery and radiation refractory high-grade meningioma. J Neuro-Oncol. 2012;107(2):315–21.
4. Chamberlain MC, Johnston SK. Hydroxyurea for recurrent surgery and radiation refractory meningioma: a retrospective case series. J Neuro-Oncol. 2011;104(3):765–71.
5. Loven D, Hardoff R, Sever ZB, Steinmetz AP, Gornish M, Rappaport ZH, et al. Non-resectable slow-growing meningiomas treated by hydroxyurea. J Neuro-Oncol. 2004;67(1–2): 221–6.
6. Mason WP, Gentili F, Macdonald DR, Hariharan S, Cruz CR, Abrey LE. Stabilization of disease progression by hydroxyurea in patients with recurrent or unresectable meningiomas. J Neurosurg. 2002;97(2):341–6.
7. Newton HB, Slivka MA, Stevens C. Hydroxyurea chemotherapy for unresectable or residual meningioma. J Neuro-Oncol. 2000;49(2):165–70.
8. Rosenthal MA, Ashley DL, Cher L. Treatment of high risk or recurrent meningiomas with hydroxyurea. J Clin Neurosci. 2002;9(2):156–8.

9. Swinnen L, Rankin C, Rushing E, Laura H, Damek D, Barger G. Southwest oncology group s9811: a phase II study of hydroxyurea for unresectable meningioma. J Clin Oncol. 2009;27:15s.
10. Wen PY, Quant E, Drappatz J, Beroukhim R, Norden AD. Medical therapies for meningiomas. J Neuro-Oncol. 2010;99(3):365–78.
11. Karsy M, Hoang N, Barth T, Burt L, Dunson W, Gillespie DL, et al. Combined hydroxyurea and verapamil in the clinical treatment of refractory meningioma: human and orthotopic xenograft studies. World Neurosurg. 2016;86:210–9.
12. Chamberlain MC. Adjuvant combined modality therapy for malignant meningiomas. J Neurosurg. 1996;84(5):733–6.
13. Chamberlain MC, Tsao-Wei DD, Groshen S. Temozolomide for treatment-resistant recurrent meningioma. Neurology. 2004;62(7):1210–2.
14. Chamberlain MC, Tsao-Wei DD, Groshen S. Salvage chemotherapy with CPT-11 for recurrent meningioma. J Neuro-Oncol. 2006;78(3):271–6.
15. Brastianos PK, Galanis E, Butowski N, Chan JW, Dunn IF, Goldbrunner R, et al. Advances in multidisciplinary therapy for meningiomas. Neuro Oncol. 2019;21(Supplement_1):i18–31.
16. Karsy M, Guan J, Cohen A, Colman H, Jensen RL. Medical management of meningiomas: current status, failed treatments, and promising horizons. Neurosurg Clin. 2016;27(2):249–60.
17. Grunberg SM, Daniels AM, Muensch H, Daniels JR, Bernstein L, Kortes V, et al. Correlation of meningioma hormone receptor status with hormone sensitivity in a tumor stem-cell assay. J Neurosurg. 1987;66(3):405.
18. Markwalder T-M, Seiler RW, Zava DT. Antiestrogenic therapy of meningiomas—a pilot study. Surg Neurol. 1985;24(3):245–9.
19. Goodwin JW, Crowley J, Eyre HJ, Stafford B, Jaeckle KA, Townsend JJ. A phase II evaluation of tamoxifen in unresectable or refractory meningiomas: a Southwest Oncology Group study. J Neuro-Oncol. 1993;15(1):75–7.
20. Grunberg SM, Weiss MH, Spitz IM, Ahmadi J, Sadun A, Russell CA, et al. Treatment of unresectable meningiomas with the antiprogesterone agent mifepristone. J Neurosurg. 1991;74(6):861.
21. Ji Y, Rankin C, Grunberg S, Sherrod AE, Ahmadi J, Townsend JJ, et al. Double-blind phase III randomized trial of the antiprogestin agent mifepristone in the treatment of unresectable meningioma: SWOG S9005. J Clin Oncol. 2015;33(34):4093–8.
22. Arena S, Barbieri F, Thellung S, Pirani P, Corsaro A, Villa V, et al. Expression of somatostatin receptor mRNA in human meningiomas and their implication in in vitro antiproliferative activity. J Neuro-Oncol. 2004;66(1–2):155–66.
23. Chamberlain MC, Glantz MJ, Fadul CE. Recurrent meningioma. Salvage therapy with long-acting somatostatin analogue. Neurology. 2007;69(10):969–73.
24. Norden AD, Ligon KL, Hammond SN, Muzikansky A, Reardon DA, Kaley TJ, et al. Phase II study of monthly pasireotide LAR (SOM230C) for recurrent or progressive meningioma. Neurology. 2015;84(3):280–6.
25. Johnson DR, Kimmel DW, Burch PA, Cascino TL, Giannini C, Wu W, et al. Phase II study of subcutaneous octreotide in adults with recurrent or progressive meningioma and meningeal hemangiopericytoma. Neuro-Oncology. 2011;13(5):530–5.
26. Simó M, Argyriou AA, Macià M, Plans G, Majós C, Vidal N, et al. Recurrent high-grade meningioma: a phase II trial with somatostatin analogue therapy. Cancer Chemother Pharmacol. 2014;73(5):919–23.
27. Kirkwood JM, Ibrahim JG, Sosman JA, Sondak VK, Agarwala SS, Ernstoff MS, et al. High-dose interferon alfa-2b significantly prolongs relapse-free and overall survival compared with the GM2-KLH/QS-21 vaccine in patients with resected stage IIB-III melanoma: results of intergroup trial E1694/S9512/C509801. J Clin Oncol. 2001;19(9):2370–80.
28. Kirkwood JM, Strawderman MH, Ernstoff MS, Smith TJ, Borden EC, Blum RH. Interferon alfa-2b adjuvant therapy of high-risk resected cutaneous melanoma: the Eastern Cooperative Oncology Group Trial EST 1684. J Clin Oncol. 1996;14(1):7–17.
29. Neidhart JA. Interferon therapy for the treatment of renal cancer. Cancer. 1986;57(S8):1696–9.

30. Ricketts RR, Hatley RM, Corden BJ, Sabio H, Howell CG. Interferon-alpha-2a for the treatment of complex hemangiomas of infancy and childhood. Ann Surg. 1994;219(6):605.
31. Koper JW, Zwarthoff EC, Hagemeijer A, Braakman R, Avezaat CJ, Bergström M, et al. Inhibition of the growth of cultured human meningioma cells by recombinant interferon-α. Eur J Cancer Clin Oncol. 1991;27(4):416–9.
32. Kyritsis AP, Jaeckle KA, Victor L, Kaba SE, Yung WKA, DeMonte F, et al. The treatment of recurrent unresectable and malignant meningiomas with interferon alpha-2B. Neurosurgery. 1997;40(2):271–5.
33. Chamberlain MC, Glantz MJ. Interferon-α for recurrent World Health Organization grade 1 intracranial meningiomas. Cancer. 2008;113(8):2146–51.
34. Black PM, Carroll R, Glowacka D, Riley K, Dashner K. Platelet-derived growth factor expression and stimulation in human meningiomas. J Neurosurg. 1994;81(3):388–93.
35. Johnson MD, Woodard A, Kim P, Frexes-Steed M. Evidence for mitogen-associated protein kinase activation and transduction of mitogenic signals by platelet-derived growth factor in human meningioma cells. J Neurosurg. 2001;94(2):293–300.
36. Todo T, Adams EF, Fahlbusch R, Dingermann T, Werner H. Autocrine growth stimulation of human meningioma cells by platelet-derived growth factor. J Neurosurg. 1996;84(5):852–8.
37. Wen PY, Yung WA, Lamborn KR, Norden AD, Cloughesy TF, Abrey LE, et al. Phase II study of imatinib mesylate for recurrent meningiomas (North American Brain Tumor Consortium study 01-08). Neuro-Oncology. 2009;11(6):853–60.
38. Reardon DA, Norden AD, Desjardins A, Vredenburgh JJ, Herndon JE 2nd, Coan A, et al. Phase II study of Gleevec® plus hydroxyurea (HU) in adults with progressive or recurrent meningioma. J Neuro-Oncol. 2012;106(2):409–15.
39. Andersson U, Guo D, Malmer B, Bergenheim AT, Brännström T, Hedman H, et al. Epidermal growth factor receptor family (EGFR, ErbB2–4) in gliomas and meningiomas. Acta Neuropathol. 2004;108(2):135–42.
40. Johnson MD, Horiba M, Winnier AR, Arteaga CL. The epidermal growth factor receptor is associated with phospholipase C-γ1 in meningiomas. Human Pathol. 1994;25(2):146–53.
41. Jones NR, Rossi ML, Gregoriou M, Hughes JT. Epidermal growth factor receptor expression in 72 meningiomas. Cancer. 1990;66(1):152–5.
42. Carroll RS, Black PM, Zhang J, Kirsch M, Percec I, Lau N, et al. Expression and activation of epidermal growth factor receptors in meningiomas. J Neurosurg. 1997;87(2):315–23.
43. Norden AD, Raizer JJ, Abrey LE, Lamborn KR, Lassman AB, Chang SM, et al. Phase II trials of erlotinib or gefitinib in patients with recurrent meningioma. J Neuro-Oncol. 2010;96(2):211–7.
44. Ferrara N, Gerber H-P, LeCouter J. The biology of VEGF and its receptors. Nat Med. 2003;9(6):669.
45. Torimura T, Sata M, Ueno T, Kin M, Tsuji R, Suzaku K, et al. Increased expression of vascular endothelial growth factor is associated with tumor progression in hepatocellular carcinoma. Human Pathol. 1998;29(9):986–91.
46. Kerbel RS. Tumor Angiogenesis. New Eng J Med. 2008;358(19):2039–49.
47. Kim KJ, Li B, Winer J, Armanini M, Gillett N, Phillips HS, et al. Inhibition of vascular endothelial growth factor-induced angiogenesis suppresses tumour growth in vivo. Nature. 1993;362(6423):841.
48. Melnyk O, Shuman MA, Kim KJ. Vascular endothelial growth factor promotes tumor dissemination by a mechanism distinct from its effect on primary tumor growth. Cancer Res. 1996;56(4):921–4.
49. Warren RS, Yuan H, Matli MR, Gillett NA, Ferrara N. Regulation by vascular endothelial growth factor of human colon cancer tumorigenesis in a mouse model of experimental liver metastasis. J Clin Investig. 1995;95(4):1789–97.
50. Ferrara N, Hillan KJ, Gerber H-P, Novotny W. Discovery and development of bevacizumab, an anti-VEGF antibody for treating cancer. Nat Rev Drug Discov. 2004;3(5):391.
51. Cook KM, Figg WD. Angiogenesis inhibitors: current strategies and future prospects. CA Cancer J Clin. 2010;60(4):222–43.

52. Wick W, Gorlia T, Bendszus M, Taphoorn M, Sahm F, Harting I, et al. Lomustine and bevacizumab in progressive glioblastoma. New Eng J Med. 2017;377(20):1954–63.

53. Oza AM, Cook AD, Pfisterer J, Embleton A, Ledermann JA, Pujade-Lauraine E, et al. Standard chemotherapy with or without bevacizumab for women with newly diagnosed ovarian cancer (ICON7): overall survival results of a phase 3 randomised trial. Lancet Oncol. 2015;16(8):928–36.

54. Lamszus K, Lengler U, Schmidt NO, Stavrou D, Ergün S, Westphal M. Vascular endothelial growth factor, hepatocyte growth factor/scatter factor, basic fibroblast growth factor, and placenta growth factor in human meningiomas and their relation to angiogenesis and malignancy. Neurosurgery. 2000;46(4):938–48.

55. Lou E, Sumrall AL, Turner S, Peters KB, Desjardins A, Vredenburgh JJ, et al. Bevacizumab therapy for adults with recurrent/progressive meningioma: a retrospective series. J Neuro-Oncol. 2012;109(1):63–70.

56. Nayak L, Iwamoto FM, Rudnick JD, Norden AD, Lee EQ, Drappatz J, et al. Atypical and anaplastic meningiomas treated with bevacizumab. J Neuro-Oncol. 2012;109(1):187–93.

57. Shih KC, Chowdhary S, Rosenblatt P, Weir AB, Shepard GC, Williams JT, et al. A phase II trial of bevacizumab and everolimus as treatment for patients with refractory, progressive intracranial meningioma. J Neuro-Oncol. 2016;129(2):281–8.

58. Kaley TJ, Wen P, Schiff D, Ligon K, Haidar S, Karimi S, et al. Phase II trial of sunitinib for recurrent and progressive atypical and anaplastic meningioma. Neuro-Oncology. 2014;17(1):116–21.

59. Raizer JJ, Grimm SA, Rademaker A, Chandler JP, Muro K, Helenowski I, et al. A phase II trial of PTK787/ZK 222584 in recurrent or progressive radiation and surgery refractory meningiomas. J Neuro-Oncol. 2014;117(1):93–101.

Emerging Meningioma Therapies I: Precision Medicine, Targeted Therapies, and Mutation-Specific Approaches

Ashley M. Roque and Antonio Omuro

Introduction

Unfortunately, to date, there have been no systemic treatments proven to extend survival in patients with relapsed or refractory meningioma. Chemotherapy agents such as hydroxyurea, temozolomide, ifosfamide, and irinotecan, as well as hormonal agents, interferon alfa 2-beta, EGFR inhibitors (i.e., gefitinib, erlotinib), and angiogenesis inhibitors have all been tried with limited success [1–15], and these therapies are rarely used in the clinical setting (Chap. 13). After radiation and surgical treatments have been exhausted, these tumors continue to progress leading to significant morbidity and mortality. As such, developing new strategies for treatment in relapsed/refractory meningioma is an area of unmet need in neuro-oncology. In today's era of precision medicine, treatment is increasingly becoming individualized, with therapies directed at genetic changes underlying unique phenotypes. Recently, there have been exciting new discoveries leading to a deeper understanding of the genetic and molecular landscape of meningiomas, paving the way to new, more individualized treatment strategies. In this chapter we will review such discoveries and discuss emerging therapies in the treatment of meningioma.

A. M. Roque
Department of Neuro-Oncology, Mount Sinai Hospital, New York, NY, USA
e-mail: ashley.roque@mssm.edu

A. Omuro (✉)
Yale New Haven Hospital and Smilow Cancer Hospital, New Haven, CT, USA

Yale Brain Tumor Center at Smilow Cancer Hospital, New Haven, CT, USA

Department of Neurology, Yale School of Medicine, Yale University, New Haven, CT, USA
e-mail: antonio.omuro@yale.edu

© Springer Nature Switzerland AG 2020
J. Moliterno, A. Omuro (eds.), *Meningiomas*,
https://doi.org/10.1007/978-3-030-59558-6_14

Molecularly Targeted Therapies Directed by Genetic Analyses

To date, treatment choices for meningioma have largely been based on the extent of resection and WHO grade. Meningiomas are divided in WHO Grade I (benign), Grade II (atypical), and Grade III (anaplastic) based on histopathological features including cellularity, number of mitoses, brain invasion, and cytomorphological appearance. Tumors are further classified into 15 distinct variants based on morphological features. While extent of resection and WHO grade are considered the most important predictors of survival, there is significant variability in patient outcomes within these groups. In addition, WHO grading is imprecise as many variables are open to interpretation. Therefore, WHO grade alone cannot reliably predict prognosis and tumor behavior for all patients. Recent knowledge of epigenetic and genetic alterations in meningioma has led to improvement in prognostication at the individual level and prompted investigations into the use of targeted agents.

NF2 Mutations and Deletions

The most commonly altered gene in meningiomas is *NF2*, located on the long arm of chromosome 22 (22q.12.2). Monosomy of chromosome 22 is found in about half of all meningioma cases, including nearly all patients with neurofibromatosis type 2-associated meningiomas and 30–70% of sporadic meningiomas. In most cases this is associated with a focal inactivating mutation in the *NF2* gene in the remaining chromosome, the so-called "double hit" hypothesis [16–20]. *NF2* mutations are found in WHO Grade I, II, and III tumors and are thus felt to be an initial driver in the formation of meningiomas [17, 21]. The *NF2* gene encodes the protein neurofibromin 2 (i.e., merlin or schwanomin) which functions to regulate multiple proliferative pathways such as the hippo, EGFR-Ras-ERK, and PI3K/mTOR/AKT pathways [22–26]. Loss of function of this protein can thus lead to uncontrolled cell growth. As such, meningiomas with *NF2* deletions generally have higher proliferative index, greater recurrence rate, and worse prognosis [18, 20, 27, 28]. Loss of *NF2* function has been shown to increase levels of FAK, a protein tyrosine kinase that is involved in cell migration, proliferation, and invasion [24, 29]. In vitro studies have demonstrated that cell xenograft models of mesothelioma cells with low merlin expression have increased sensitivity to FAK inhibitory agents, making treatment with FAK inhibitors an attractive strategy for meningiomas [30]. Use of a FAK inhibitor (agent GKS2256098) in *NF2*-altered meningiomas is currently being investigated in a national phase II trial.

Neurofibromin regulates multiple pathways, and its tumor suppressive activity is mediated in part by suppression of mTORC1. Prior in vitro work has shown that mTORC1 is constitutively activated in merlin-deficient human meningioma cells [23] and drugs inhibiting mTOR (i.e., rapamycin) inhibit the growth of merlin-deficient arachnoidal and meningioma cells in vitro. Based on these results, several studies have focused on using mTOR inhibition in recurrent/refractory meningiomas both as monotherapy and in combination with other agents. A recently published phase II study evaluated combined treatment with bevacizumab and everolimus (mTOR inhibitor) for patients with recurrent/refractory meningioma. A total of 17 patients with WHO Grade I, II, and III recurrent meningiomas were included in the study and treated with bevacizumab 10 mg/kg on days 1 and 15 and everolimus (10 mg po) in 28-day cycles. No patient had radiographic response, and 15 (88%) had stable disease as their best imaging response. Median PFS in the entire treatment cohort was 22 months, with median PFS of 17.5 months in Grade I tumors and 22 months in Grade II and III tumors. Median overall survival was 23.8 months, and the median duration of disease stabilization was 10 months. This was a small cohort of patients, but results suggest that this combination of therapy may have some activity in higher-grade tumors. It is important to note that patients were enrolled regardless of *NF2* mutation status. The combination of octreotide and everolimus was used in patients with recurrent meningioma, regardless of NF mutation status, in a French phase II study [31]. The study was based on preclinical data demonstrating that the combination of everolimus and octreotide produced a cooperative inhibitory effect on cell proliferation in all tested meningiomas [32]. The study enrolled 20 patients with 37 progressive meningiomas (2 WHO Grade 1, 27 WHO Grade II, and 9 WHO Grade III), 4 of whom had neurofibromatosis type 2. Though the sample size was small, preliminary results were encouraging. 4 patients had a decrease in tumor volume of 10% or greater on volumetric analyses, done 3 months after the initiation of treatment. The 6-month PFS was 58.2% (95% CI 33.5–76.5%), and 12-month PFS was 38% (95% CI 16–60%) [33]. Another in vitro analysis showed that treatment with AZD2014 (vistusertib), a dual mTORC1/mTORC2 inhibitor, inhibited cell proliferation in meningioma cells better than rapamycin and the PAK inhibitor FRAX597 [34]. Two phase II trials of AZD2014 have since been initiated: the first testing the agent in recurrent Grade II/III meningioma and the second in patients with *NF2* and progressive or symptomatic meningiomas.

Non-*NF2*-Deleted Tumors

Until recently, there was limited understanding of the genetic landscape of non-*NF2*-mutated meningiomas. Comprehensive genome analyses of meningiomas have since led to important additional information on driver mutations in these tumors [18, 19, 35]. In an analysis of 50 meningiomas (39 Grade I and 11 Grade II), authors identified frequent mutations in *TRAF7*, *KLF4*, *AKT1*, and *SMO*, which were all mutually exclusive with *NF2* mutations [18]. A total of 79% of tested tumors harbored at least one of these five mutations. There were less frequent mutations in *CREBBP*, *PIK3AC*, *PIK3R1*, *BRCA1*, and *SMARCB1* (which co-occurred with NF2). *TRAF7* was the most commonly found non-*NF2*-associated mutation, seen in 25% of non-*NF2*-mutated tumors. This mutation often co-occurs with *AKT1*, *KLF4*, or *PIK3CA* mutations. Mutations of *TRAF7*, *KLF4*, *AKT1*, *SMO*, and *PIK3AC* are generally found in Grade I meningioma and are associated with benign course and low recurrence rate, except for specific variants of *PIK3CA* (H1047R and E545K) and *SMO* (L412F) which are associated with higher recurrence rates. A study of skull base meningiomas also showed that mutation *AKT1 E17K* was associated with shorter time to recurrence [36]. Mutational profile correlated with histological subtype and tumor location. Most *NF2*-mutated tumors occurred in the convexity and the lateral and posterior skull base, whereas the majority of non-*NF2* meningiomas occurred in the medial skull base. Meningiomas with *SMO* mutations are found near the midline in the medial anterior skull base (near the olfactory groove). A later study of tumors lacking the above known driver genes identified another distinct subset of non-*NF2* meningiomas that harbored recurrent somatic mutations in *POL2RA* [35]. These were found exclusively in Grade I meningiomas, most commonly in the tuberculum sellae.

Based on these sequencing results, new treatments aimed at targeting these driver mutations are being investigated. A multicenter phase II trial, sponsored by the Alliance for Clinical Trials in Oncology group, has been initiated to evaluate the use of several targeted therapies in residual, progressive, and recurrent meningioma. The trial is currently enrolling patients with *AKT1*, *SMO*, and *NF2* mutations to be treated with AKT1, SMO, and FAK inhibitors, respectively. SMO is a key component of the Hedgehog pathway, the activation of which has been shown to increase cell proliferation. Mutations in this pathway have been identified in medulloblastomas and basal cell carcinomas in addition to meningiomas. The use of the SMO inhibitor vismodegib has been approved for use in basal cell carcinoma by the FDA [37]. Its use in medulloblastoma is also an area of active investigation, and small cohorts have shown activity of the drug in *SHH* mutant medulloblastoma [38]. The PI3K/Akt pathway is another important pathway involved in the differentiation, growth, and apoptosis of meningioma cells [17]. Johnson et al. found that PI3K-AKT-p70^{56k} pathway transduced mitogenic signals upon stimulation of PDF-BB in meningioma cells. In the same study, treatment with a PI3K inhibitor resulted in inhibition of meningioma cell growth in association with reduced levels of AKT and p70^{56k} phosphorylation [39]. AKT inhibitors have shown activity in patients harboring AKT mutations in other cancer types, such as breast and gynecological malignancies. In a basket trial including patients with solid cancers and AKT1 mutations treated with AZD5363, 30% of patients with ATK1E17K mutations achieved either stability, partial, or unconfirmed partial response [40]. The agent AZD5363 was used in a single patient with multiple progressive meningiomas (Grades I and III) who demonstrated up to 12.5% reduction in size of their tumors with a durable response of over 1 year [41]. Currently, there are no available drugs for *TRAF7*, *KLF4*, or *POLR2* mutations. However, these mutations can be useful in assessing prognosis as they are generally associated with a low likelihood of recurrence.

Mutations Affecting CDK

While chromosome 22 losses are the most common alterations in meningioma, this likely represents an early event in meningioma development. Progression to atypical and malignant tumor is associated with higher mutation load and more complex karyotype. Higher-grade meningiomas frequently harbor loss of chromosomes 1p, 6q, 10q, 14q, 9p, and 18q and gains of 1q, 9q, 12q, 15q, and 20q [16, 17, 20, 21]. Chromosome 9p alterations are associated with losses of *CDKN2A/p16INKa* (encoding p16), *p14ARF* (encoding p14), and *CDKN2B/p15ARF* (encoding p15) which are all located on 9p21 [16, 21, 42]. These are all important modulators of the p53/pRB pathway which inhibits cell cycle progression and involves Cyclin D, CDK4/6. Loss of these genes is seen in 0% of Grade I, 3% of Grade II, and 38% of Grade III meningiomas [16, 43, 44]. This suggests that this pathway may play a role in malignant progression of meningiomas. A trial of ribociclib, a CDK inhibitor in malignant gliomas and WHO Grade II–III meningiomas (with RB positivity or no RB mutations on next-generation sequencing), is ongoing.

TERT Promoter Mutations

The *TERT* gene encodes for the protein telomerase reverse transcriptase, which leads to the prolonged survival of cancer cells by extending their telomeres. Known mutation hotspots are in the *TERT* promoter region at positions chr5:I, 295,228 (C228T) or chr5:I, 295,250 (C250T) [45, 46]. These mutations are found in several other cancer types including melanoma, glioma, and bladder and thyroid cancer [47]. A recent study identified *TERT* promoter mutations in about 6% of meningiomas, which occurred more frequently in higher-grade tumors (20% of Grade III tumors, 5.7% of Grade II tumors, and 1.7% of Grade I tumors). The mutation was also associated with shorter time to progression, with progression occurring at a median time of 10.1 months in mutated tumors and 179 months in wild-type tumors. In Grade I tumors, *TERT* promoter mutation was associated with progression to a higher tumor grade at recurrence [48]. These results were supported by a meta-analysis of 532 meningioma samples, identifying *TERT* promoter mutations in 8% of tumors. They found statistically significant shortened overall survival and worse prognosis in patients with C228T and C250T mutations in the *TERT* promoter region [49]. These findings suggest that presence of a *TERT* mutation may be a helpful prognostic tool in meningiomas and can be used to help guide treatment decisions. Patients with these mutations may warrant more frequent surveillance and more aggressive treatment paradigms, while development of targeted therapeutics requires more study.

Germline Mutations

Recent work has identified another aggressive subgroup of meningiomas: rhabdoid meningiomas harboring mutations in the breast cancer (BRCA)1-associated protein-1 (i.e., *BAP-1*) tumor suppressor gene. Germline mutations of *BAP-1* underlie the BAP-1 tumor predisposition syndrome which is associated with high risk of uveal and cutaneous melanoma, mesothelioma, renal cell carcinoma, and meningioma. Mutation in *BAP-1* can be seen in sporadic rhabdoid meningiomas as well as those associated with germline mutations and the BAP-1 tumor predisposition syndrome. Shankar et al. evaluated 57 tissue samples from 47 patients with meningiomas with rhabdoid features. Five of these patients showed loss of *BAP-1* protein by immunohistochemical staining and *BAP-1* mutations on gene sequencing studies. They had constitutional DNA available for three of the five patients, and only one of these patients had a germline mutation identified. Compared to patients with WHO Grade II–III *BAP-1* intact meningiomas, BAP-1 tumors were more clinically aggressive. BAP-1-deficient Grade II–II tumors had a median time to progression of 26 months, compared to 116 months in those with BAP-1 intact tumors [50]. There are no currently available therapies directed at BAP-1 mutations. However preclinical studies have suggested that BAP-1 is involved in the DNA damage response and that deficient cells may have increased sensitivity to PARP inhibitors [51, 52]. This information also highlights the importance of testing rhabdoid meningiomas for *BAP-1* mutations and referring those patients for genetic testing and appropriate cancer screening if a germline *BAP-1* mutation is found.

SMARCE1 mutations have recently been implicated in the development of clear cell meningiomas [53, 54]. These tumors are a rare subtype of meningioma, classified as Grade II, and that may occur at a younger age, generally associated with an aggressive clinical course [55]. Germline mutations of *SMARCB1* result in schwannomatosis, and approximately 5% of these individuals develop meningiomas. This mutation has also been identified infrequently in sporadic meningiomas [56]. Lastly, a mutation in *SUFU* was identified as a cause of familial meningioma [57]. *SMARCE1*, *SMARCB1*, and *SUFU* all function in the Sonic Hedgehog signaling pathway, which may have treatment implications for patients with these mutations in the future.

Epigenetic Changes

Recently, DNA methylation status has also been identified as a potentially useful biomarker in meningioma. Sahm et al. studied 497 meningiomas to evaluate the use of genome-wide DNA methylation status as a predictor of tumor recurrence and prognosis. Tumors are segregated into six distinct groups based on methylation status. They found that the degree of methylation was a better predictor of recurrence than WHO grade [58]. These findings represent an exciting discovery that may aid classification of meningiomas in the future. A study by Harmanci et al. [59] compared benign meningiomas to atypical ones. Authors found the majority of primary (de novo) atypical meningiomas display loss of *NF2*, which co-occurs either with genomic instability or recurrent *SMARCB1* mutations. These tumors harbor increased H3K27me3 signal and a hypermethylated phenotype, mainly occupying the polycomb repressive complex 2 (PRC2) binding sites in human embryonic stem cells, thereby phenocopying a more primitive cellular state. Consistent with this observation, atypical meningiomas exhibited upregulation of EZH2, the catalytic subunit of the PRC2 complex, as well as the E2F2 and FOXM1 transcriptional networks. That study established the epigenetic landscape of primary atypical meningiomas and potential therapeutic targets. Clinical trials of epigenetic modulators such as bromodomain inhibitors are being planned.

Conclusions

Discovery of effective systemic treatment options for progressive/recurrent meningiomas is an area of active research in neuro-oncology. Advances in gene sequencing have recently provided further insight into the molecular, genetic, and epigenetic landscape of meningiomas and opened the door for therapeutic advances. Clinical trials using targeted therapies based on mutational profiling are underway, although the rarity of certain phenotypes renders such studies difficult to conduct and accrue. Improving patient referrals for such trials will be key to advance the field. As more follow-up information is collected, genetic and epigenetic data may be used to better predict outcomes and tailor treatment plans for individual patients, perhaps with earlier interventions into the disease course.

References

1. Goodwin JW, Crowley J, Eyre HJ, Stafford B, Jaeckle KA, Townsend JJ. A phase II evaluation of tamoxifen in unresectable or refractory meningiomas: a Southwest Oncology Group study. J Neuro-Oncol. 1993;15(1):75–7.
2. Grunberg SM, Weiss MH, Spitz IM, Ahmadi J, Sadun A, Russell CA, et al. Treatment of unresectable meningiomas with the antiprogesterone agent mifepristone. J Neurosurg. 1991 Jun;74(6):861–6.
3. Hahn BM, Schrell UM, Sauer R, Fahlbusch R, Ganslandt O, Grabenbauer GG. Prolonged oral hydroxyurea and concurrent 3d-conformal radiation in patients with progressive or recurrent meningioma: results of a pilot study. J Neuro-Oncol. 2005;74(2):157–65.
4. Ji Y, Rankin C, Grunberg S, Sherrod AE, Ahmadi J, Townsend JJ, et al. Double-blind phase III randomized trial of the antiprogestin agent mifepristone in the treatment of unresectable meningioma: SWOG S9005. J Clin Oncol. 2015;33(34):4093–8.
5. Johnson DR, Kimmel DW, Burch PA, Cascino TL, Giannini C, Wu W, et al. Phase II study of subcutaneous octreotide in adults with recurrent or progressive meningioma and meningeal hemangiopericytoma. Neuro-Oncology. 2011;13(5):530–5.
6. Kaley TJ, Wen P, Schiff D, Ligon K, Haidar S, Karimi S, et al. Phase II trial of sunitinib for recurrent and progressive atypical and anaplastic meningioma. Neuro-Oncology. 2014;17(1):116–21.
7. Karsy M, Guan J, Cohen A, Colman H, Jensen RL. Medical management of meningiomas: current status, failed treatments, and promising horizons. Neurosurg Clin N Am. 2016;27(2):249–60.
8. Loven D, Hardoff R, Sever ZB, Steinmetz AP, Gornish M, Rappaport ZH, et al. Non-resectable slow-growing meningiomas treated by hydroxyurea. J Neuro-Oncol. 2004;67(1–2):221–6.
9. Nayak L, Iwamoto FM, Rudnick JD, Norden AD, Lee EQ, Drappatz J, et al. Atypical and anaplastic meningiomas treated with bevacizumab. J Neuro-Oncol. 2012;109(1):187–93.
10. Norden AD, Ligon KL, Hammond SN, Muzikansky A, Reardon DA, Kaley TJ, et al. Phase II study of monthly pasireotide LAR (SOM230C) for recurrent or progressive meningioma. Neurology. 2015;84(3):280–6.

11. Norden AD, Raizer JJ, Abrey LE, Lamborn KR, Lassman AB, Chang SM, et al. Phase II trials of erlotinib or gefitinib in patients with recurrent meningioma. J Neuro-Oncol. 2010;96(2):211–7.
12. Reardon DA, Norden AD, Desjardins A, Vredenburgh JJ, Herndon JE 2nd, Coan A, et al. Phase II study of Gleevec® plus hydroxyurea (HU) in adults with progressive or recurrent meningioma. J Neuro-Oncol. 2012;106(2):409–15.
13. Swinnen L, Rankin C, Rushing E, Laura H, Damek D, Barger G. Southwest oncology group s9811: a phase II study of hydroxyurea for unresectable meningioma. J Clin Oncol. 2009;27:15s.
14. Wen PY, Quant E, Drappatz J, Beroukhim R, Norden AD. Medical therapies for meningiomas. J Neuro-Oncol. 2010;99(3):365–78.
15. Wen PY, Yung WA, Lamborn KR, Norden AD, Cloughesy TF, Abrey LE, et al. Phase II study of imatinib mesylate for recurrent meningiomas (North American Brain Tumor Consortium study 01-08). Neuro-Oncology. 2009;11(6):853–60.
16. Choy W, Kim W, Nagasawa D, Stramotas S, Yew A, Gopen Q, et al. The molecular genetics and tumor pathogenesis of meningiomas and the future directions of meningioma treatments. Neurosurg Focus. 2011;30(5):E6.
17. Domingues P, González-Tablas M, Otero Á, Pascual D, Ruiz L, Miranda D, et al. Genetic/molecular alterations of meningiomas and the signaling pathways targeted. Oncotarget. 2015;6(13):10671.
18. Clark VE, Erson-Omay EZ, Serin A, Yin J, Cotney J, Ozduman K, et al. Genomic analysis of non-NF2 meningiomas reveals mutations in TRAF7, KLF4, AKT1, and SMO. Science. 2013;339(6123):1077–80.
19. Brastianos PK, Horowitz PM, Santagata S, Jones RT, McKenna A, Getz G, et al. Genomic sequencing of meningiomas identifies oncogenic SMO and AKT1 mutations. Nat Genet. 2013;45(3):285.
20. Weber RG, Boström J, Wolter M, Baudis M, Collins VP, Reifenberger G, et al. Analysis of genomic alterations in benign, atypical, and anaplastic meningiomas: toward a genetic model of meningioma progression. Proc Natl Acad Sci U S A. 1997;94(26):14719–24.
21. Mawrin C, Perry A. Pathological classification and molecular genetics of meningiomas. J Neuro-Oncol. 2010;99(3):379–91.
22. Curto M, McClatchey A. Nf2/Merlin: a coordinator of receptor signalling and intercellular contact. Br J Cancer. 2008;98(2):256.
23. James MF, Han S, Polizzano C, Plotkin SR, Manning BD, Stemmer-Rachamimov AO, et al. NF2/merlin is a novel negative regulator of mTOR complex 1, and activation of mTORC1 is associated with meningioma and schwannoma growth. Mol Cell Biol. 2009;29(15):4250–61. https://doi.org/10.1128/MCB.01581-08.
24. Suppiah S, Nassiri F, Bi WL, Dunn IF, Hanemann CO, Horbinski CM, et al. Molecular and translational advances in meningiomas. Neuro Oncol. 2019;21(Supplement_1):i4–17.
25. Rong R, Tang X, Gutmann DH, Ye K. Neurofibromatosis 2 (NF2) tumor suppressor merlin inhibits phosphatidylinositol 3-kinase through binding to PIKE-L. Proc Natl Acad Sci. 2004;101(52):18200–5.
26. Cooper J, Giancotti FG. Molecular insights into NF2/Merlin tumor suppressor function. FEBS Lett. 2014;588(16):2743–52.
27. Goutagny S, Yang HW, Zucman-Rossi J, Chan J, Dreyfuss JM, Park PJ, et al. Genomic profiling reveals alternative genetic pathways of meningioma malignant progression dependent on the underlying NF2 status. Clin Cancer Res. 2010;16(16):4155–64.
28. Leuraud P, Dezamis E, Aguirre-Cruz L, Taillibert S, Lejeune J, Robin E, et al. Prognostic value of allelic losses and telomerase activity in meningiomas. J Neurosurg. 2004;100(2):303.
29. Poulikakos P, Xiao G, Gallagher R, Jablonski S, Jhanwar S, Testa J. Re-expression of the tumor suppressor NF2/merlin inhibits invasiveness in mesothelioma cells and negatively regulates FAK. Oncogene. 2006;25(44):5960.
30. Shapiro IM, Kolev VN, Vidal CM, Kadariya Y, Ring JE, Wright Q, et al. Merlin deficiency predicts FAK inhibitor sensitivity: a synthetic lethal relationship. Sci Transl Med. 2014;6(237):237ra68. https://doi.org/10.1126/scitranslmed.3008639.

31. Graillon T, Sanson M, Peyre M, Peyrière H, Autran D, Kalamarides M, et al. A phase II of everolimus and octreotide for patients with refractory and documented progressive meningioma (CEVOREM). J Clin Oncol. 2017;35(15_suppl):2011.
32. Graillon T, Defilles C, Mohamed A, Lisbonis C, Germanetti A-L, Chinot O, et al. Combined treatment by octreotide and everolimus: Octreotide enhances inhibitory effect of everolimus in aggressive meningiomas. J Neuro-Oncol. 2015;124(1):33–43.
33. Graillon T, Sanson M, Peyre M, Peyriere H, Autran D, Kalamarides M, et al. A phase II of everolimus and octreotide for patients with refractory and documented progressive meningioma (CEVOREM). J Clin Oncol. 2017;35(15_suppl):2011.
34. Beauchamp RL, James MF, DeSouza PA, Wagh V, Zhao WN, Jordan JT, et al. A high-throughput kinome screen reveals serum/glucocorticoid-regulated kinase 1 as a therapeutic target for NF2-deficient meningiomas. Oncotarget. 2015;6(19):16981–97.
35. Clark VE, Harmancı AS, Bai H, Youngblood MW, Lee TI, Baranoski JF, et al. Recurrent somatic mutations in POLR2A define a distinct subset of meningiomas. Nat Genet. 2016;48(10):1253.
36. Yesilöz Ü, Kirches E, Hartmann C, Scholz J, Kropf S, Sahm F, et al. Frequent AKT1E17K mutations in skull base meningiomas are associated with mTOR and ERK1/2 activation and reduced time to tumor recurrence. Neuro-Oncology. 2017;19(8):1088–96.
37. Sekulic A, Migden MR, Oro AE, Dirix L, Lewis KD, Hainsworth JD, et al. Efficacy and safety of vismodegib in advanced basal-cell carcinoma. N Engl J Med. 2012;366(23):2171–9.
38. Robinson GW, Orr BA, Wu G, Gururangan S, Lin T, Qaddoumi I, et al. Vismodegib exerts targeted efficacy against recurrent sonic hedgehog–subgroup medulloblastoma: results from phase II pediatric brain tumor consortium studies PBTC-025B and PBTC-032. J Clin Oncol. 2015;33(24):2646.
39. Johnson MD, Okediji E, Woodard A, Toms SA, Allen GS. Evidence for phosphatidylinositol 3-kinase—Akt—p70S6K pathway activation and transduction of mitogenic signals by platelet-derived growth factor in human meningioma cells. J Neurosurg. 2002;97(3):668–75.
40. Hyman DM, Smyth LM, Donoghue MT, Westin SN, Bedard PL, Dean EJ, et al. AKT inhibition in solid tumors with AKT1 mutations. J Clin Oncol. 2017;35(20):2251.
41. Weller M, Roth P, Sahm F, Burghardt I, Schuknecht B, Rushing EJ, et al. Durable control of metastatic AKT1-Mutant WHO Grade 1 meningothelial meningioma by the AKT inhibitor, AZD5363. J Natl Cancer Inst. 2017;109(3):djw320.
42. Banerjee R, Lohse CM, Kleinschmidt-DeMasters BK, Scheithauer BW. A role for chromosome 9p21 deletions in the malignant progression of meningiomas and the prognosis of anaplastic meningiomas. Brain Pathol. 2002;12(2):183–90.
43. Boström J, Meyer-Puttlitz B, Wolter M, Blaschke B, Weber RG, Lichter P, et al. Alterations of the tumor suppressor genes CDKN2A (p16INK4a), p14ARF, CDKN2B (p15INK4b), and CDKN2C (p18INK4c) in atypical and anaplastic meningiomas. Am J Pathol. 2001;159(2):661–9.
44. Lamszus K. Meningioma pathology, genetics, and biology. J Neuropathol Exp Neurol. 2004;63(4):275–86.
45. Huang FW, Hodis E, Xu MJ, Kryukov GV, Chin L, Garraway LA. Highly recurrent TERT promoter mutations in human melanoma. Science. 2013;339(6122):957–9.
46. Horn S, Figl A, Rachakonda PS, Fischer C, Sucker A, Gast A, et al. TERT promoter mutations in familial and sporadic melanoma. Science. 2013;339(6122):959–61.
47. Vinagre J, Almeida A, Pópulo H, Batista R, Lyra J, Pinto V, et al. Frequency of TERT promoter mutations in human cancers. Nat Commun. 2013;4:2185.
48. Sahm F, Schrimpf D, Olar A, Koelsche C, Reuss D, Bissel J, et al. TERT promoter mutations and risk of recurrence in meningioma. J Natl Cancer Inst. 2015;108(5):djv377.
49. Lu VM, Goyal A, Lee A, Jentoft M, Quinones-Hinojosa A, Chaichana KL. The prognostic significance of TERT promoter mutations in meningioma: a systematic review and meta-analysis. J Neuro-Oncol. 2019;142(1):1–10.
50. Shankar GM, Abedalthagafi M, Vaubel RA, Merrill PH, Nayyar N, Gill CM, et al. Germline and somatic BAP1 mutations in high-grade rhabdoid meningiomas. Neuro-Oncology. 2017;19(4):535–45.

51. Shankar GM, Santagata S. BAP1 mutations in high-grade meningioma: implications for patient care. Neuro-Oncology. 2017;19(11):1447–56.
52. Ismail IH, Davidson R, Gagné J-P, Xu ZZ, Poirier GG, Hendzel MJ. Germline mutations in BAP1 impair its function in DNA double-strand break repair. Cancer Res. 2014;74(16):4282–94.
53. Smith MJ, Wallace AJ, Bennett C, Hasselblatt M, Elert-Dobkowska E, Evans LT, et al. Germline SMARCE1 mutations predispose to both spinal and cranial clear cell meningiomas. J Pathol. 2014;234(4):436–40.
54. Smith MJ, Ahn S, Lee JI, Bulman M, Plessis D, Suh YL. SMARCE 1 mutation screening in classification of clear cell meningiomas. Histopathology. 2017;70(5):814–20.
55. Ohba S, Sasaki H, Kimura T, Ikeda E, Kawase T. Clear cell meningiomas: three case reports with genetic characterization and review of the literature. Neurosurgery. 2010;67(3):E870–E1.
56. Smith MJ. Germline and somatic mutations in meningiomas. Cancer Genet. 2015;208(4):107–14.
57. Aavikko M, Li S-P, Saarinen S, Alhopuro P, Kaasinen E, Morgunova E, et al. Loss of SUFU function in familial multiple meningioma. Am J Human Genet. 2012;91(3):520–6.
58. Sahm F, Schrimpf D, Stichel D, Jones DT, Hielscher T, Schefzyk S, et al. DNA methylation-based classification and grading system for meningioma: a multicentre, retrospective analysis. Lancet Oncol. 2017;18(5):682–94.
59. Harmancı AS, Youngblood MW, Clark VE, et al. Integrated genomic analyses of de novo pathways underlying atypical meningiomas. Nat Commun. 2017;8(1):1–14. https://doi.org/10.1038/ncomms16215.

Emerging Meningioma Therapies II: Immunotherapies, Novel Radiotherapy Techniques, and Other Experimental Approaches

15

Corey M. Gill and Priscilla K. Brastianos

Immunotherapy

PD-L1 Expression

PD-L1 expression is strongly associated with immune escape in patients with cancer [1]. Over the last decade, checkpoint inhibitors, which enhance a patient's immune response to cancer, have dramatically changed the treatment landscape for patients with solid tumors [2]. Cancers that have higher mutational burdens, such as melanoma and lung cancer, are associated with improved objective response rates to immunotherapy [3].

In meningiomas, PD-L1 expression is increased with higher grade [4–7], and emerging evidence suggests patients with meningiomas exhibit peripheral immunosuppression [7]. In one study, PD-L1 expression was not independently associated with clinical outcomes, after controlling for clinically relevant characteristics [4]. In a separate study, however, Han et al. reported that higher PD-L1 expression was independently associated with overall survival, when controlling for grade, performance status, extent of resection, and recurrence history [5]. This is an area requiring additional investigation.

There are several open clinical trials evaluating the safety and efficacy of various treatment strategies using checkpoint inhibitors in meningioma patients, including nivolumab (NCT02648997, NCT03604978, NCT03173950), pembrolizumab

C. M. Gill
Icahn School of Medicine at Mount Sinai, New York, NY, USA
e-mail: corey.gill@icahn.mssm.edu

P. K. Brastianos (✉)
Department of Medicine and Neurology, Massachusetts General Hospital/Harvard Medical School, Boston, MA, USA
e-mail: pbrastianos@partners.org

© Springer Nature Switzerland AG 2020
J. Moliterno, A. Omuro (eds.), *Meningiomas*,
https://doi.org/10.1007/978-3-030-59558-6_15

Table 15.1 Active immunotherapy clinical trials for patients with meningioma

NCT number	Title	Phase	Drug
NCT02648997	A Single Arm, Open-Label Phase II Study of Nivolumab in Adult Participants With Recurrent High-Grade Meningioma	2	Nivolumab
NCT03604978	A Phase I/II Study of Nivolumab Plus or Minus Ipilimumab in Combination With Multi-Fraction Stereotactic Radiosurgery for Recurrent High-Grade Radiation-Relapsed Meningioma	1/2	Nivolumab/ipilimumab
NCT03173950	Phase II Trial of the Immune Checkpoint Inhibitor Nivolumab in Patients With Select Rare CNS Cancers	2	Nivolumab
NCT03279692	Phase II Trial of Pembrolizumab in Recurrent or Residual High Grade Meningioma	2	Pembrolizumab
NCT03016091	A Phase II, Open-label, Single Arm Trial of Pembrolizumab for Refractory Atypical and Anaplastic Meningioma	2	Pembrolizumab
NCT03267836	A Phase Ib Study of Neoadjuvant Avelumab and Hypofractionated Proton Radiation Therapy Followed by Surgery for Recurrent Radiation-refractory Meningioma	1	Avelumab
NCT01967823	Phase II Study of Metastatic Cancer That Expresses NY-ESO-1 Using Lymphodepleting Conditioning Followed by Infusion of Anti-NY ESO-1 Murine TCR-Gene Engineered Lymphocytes	2	Anti-NY-ESO-1

(NCT03279692, NCT03016091), and avelumab (NCT03267836) (Table 15.1). Nivolumab and pembrolizumab target PD-1, whereas avelumab targets PD-L1.

Tumor-Infiltrating Lymphocytes

The density and distribution of T-cell and B-cell subpopulations within the tumor microenvironment are emerging biomarkers for clinical outcome and prognosis across various solid tumors [8]. Within meningiomas, Baia et al. performed immunohistochemistry of tumor-infiltrating lymphocytes (TILs) including CD3, CD8, and FOXP3 in 35 meningioma cases [9], finding no association with recurrence status (primary vs recurrence) or tumor grade. Moreover, FOXP3+ lymphocytes were identified in 68% of tumors, and 33% (subset, 4/12) of tumors had CD20+ lymphocytes. Overall, the authors concluded that a subset of meningiomas elicit an immune response, but note that some tumors in fact have heavier infiltrate density than others. While this study did not find an association between TILs and tumor grade, others found that grade III meningiomas are more likely to have CD68+, CD14+, and CD163+ TILs present at the tumor-brain border compared to grade II meningiomas [10].

Additionally, in a separate study, 93 meningioma samples were evaluated for CD4, CD20, CD68, and FOXP3 status using immunohistochemistry [11]. While CD4 and CD68 did not correlate with clinical characteristics, there was a significantly higher density of CD20+ B cells in patients with meningioma recurrence than without recurrence. Importantly, FOXP3+ cells were significantly correlated with increased tumor size, which supports the hypothesis that FOXP3 may play a role in suppressing a sufficient immune response [12, 13]. An observation of increased FOXP3 expression has been reported by others in anaplastic meningiomas compared to lower-grade meningiomas [4]. Thus, this evidence suggests that FOXP3 expression is an important mediator within the tumor microenvironment in meningiomas and may cultivate an environment supportive of oncogenesis.

These findings need validation. In larger cohorts, density and characterization of TILs should be explored to identify and validate a potential biomarker of clinical outcome in patients with meningiomas, especially in the recurrent and high-grade setting.

Beyond associations of TILs with clinical outcomes, in a study of 75 meningioma patients, investigators used cytogenetics and determined that meningiomas with isolated monosomy 22/del(22q) had a higher number of TILs [14]. Given that *NF2* is the most frequent alteration in meningiomas [15] and is associated with chromosome 22 heterozygosity [16], a future study that correlates newer genomic sequencing data and TIL status would help to elucidate how genomic alterations in meningiomas could potentially support, interact with, or predict an immune response.

T-Cell Receptor Engineering

Cancer/testis antigens (CTA) are expressed in certain cancer cells and also in human germ cells, but not by human somatic cells [17, 18]. Identification of CTA that may serve as immunotherapy-based targets is a priority for the National Cancer Institute [19]. One well-characterized antigen is NY-ESO-1, or New York esophageal squamous cell carcinoma 1 [20]. A trial of patients with metastatic synovial cell sarcoma and melanoma who were treated with autologous T cells that were transduced with a T-cell receptor against NY-ESO-1 resulted in an objective clinical response in 52.9% of patients [21].

Within meningiomas, in a discovery cohort of 18 meningiomas, mRNA expression of NY-ESO-1 was appreciated in 27.8% (5/18) of samples [9]. In the expanded validation cohort of 110 cases, 108 or 98.2% of cases expressed NY-ESO-1 using immunohistochemistry. Importantly, intensity of NY-ESO-1 expression was associated with higher tumor grade and decreased disease-free and overall survival. In another study, Syed et al. identified NY-ESO-1 expression in 12% (3/26) of meningioma samples, which were grade I and grade II [22].

Currently, there is an active phase 2 trial, in which patients with recurrent or malignant meningioma are eligible, evaluating the efficacy of anti-NY-ESO-1 murine T-cell receptor gene-engineered lymphocytes (NCT01967823). Notably, patients who have unresectable disease without confirmation of ESO expression are eligible, so long as there is radiographic evidence of meningioma. As more CTA are characterized, future trials may expand the interrogation of such immunotherapy-based vaccines, especially for patients with recurrent and high-grade meningiomas.

Novel Radiotherapy Techniques

Traditionally, meningiomas in the recurrent setting are treated with either photon or proton radiotherapy [23–25]. Beyond these techniques, preclinical and preliminary trial data suggest carbon ion therapy, brachytherapy, peptide receptor radionuclide therapy (PRRT), as well as compounds that may act as radiosensitizers, including protein phosphatase 2A inhibitor and mebendazole, could potentially be added to the treatment armamentarium in the near future (Table 15.2).

Carbon Ion Therapy

Carbon ions are similar to protons but have an increased relative biological effectiveness at the desired tumor depth with a similar low entrance dose profile, which is

Table 15.2 Active novel radiotherapy and other experimental approach clinical trials for patients with meningioma

NCT number	Title	Phase	Class
NCT01795300	Randomized Comparison of Proton and Carbon Ion Radiotherapy With Advanced Photon Radiotherapy in Skull Base Meningiomas: The PINOCCHIO Trial*	N/A	Carbon ion
NCT01166321	Treatment of Patients With Atypical Meningiomas Simpson Grade 4 and 5 With a Carbon Ion Boost in Combination With Postoperative Photon Radiotherapy: A Phase II Trial (MARCIE)	N/A	Carbon ion
NCT03273712	Phase II, Dosimetry Guided, Peptide Receptor Radiotherapy (PRRT) Using 90Y-DOTA tyr3-Octreotide (90Y-DOTATOC) in Children and Adults With Neuroendocrine and Other Somatostatin Receptor Positive Tumors	2	PRRT
NCT03936426	Peptide Receptor Radionuclide Therapy Administered to Participants With Meningioma With 67Cu-SARTATE™: A Single-centre, Open-label, Non-Randomised, Phase I-IIa Theranostic Clinical Trial	1/2	PRRT
NCT02847559	A Phase 2, Single Arm, Multi-center, Open Label Trial Combining Optune With Concurrent Bevacizumab in the Setting of Recurrent or Progressive Meningioma	2	Tumor treatment fields

PRRT peptide receptor radionuclide therapy
ᵃScheduled to begin recruiting May 2019

especially advantageous for radiation-resistant tumors and protection of surrounding eloquent structures, such as the neurovascular structures that are intimately involved with the skull base [26]. Treatment of skull base chondrosarcomas and chordomas with carbon ion radiotherapy resulted in adequate control rates and acceptable toxicity profiles [27, 28].

Combs et al. treated ten meningioma patients with carbon ion radiotherapy, achieving a 5-year survival rate of 75% and 5-year local control rate of 86% [29]. The study included three low-grade meningiomas and seven atypical or anaplastic meningiomas. Other studies have also treated meningioma patients with carbon ion radiotherapy; however, outcomes specific to meningiomas treated with carbon ions were not reported, as cohort level data were reported which included other tumor types or other radiation modalities, such as protons [30–35].

There are currently two active clinical trials evaluating carbon ion radiotherapy in patients with meningiomas. The first study is for patients with atypical meningioma (NCT01166321, MARCIE study) after incomplete resection or biopsy. The second study is scheduled to begin recruiting in May 2019 (NCT01795300, PINOCCHIO study) for patients with skull base meningiomas after incomplete resection or biopsy. The study has four arms: carbon ion radiotherapy, proton therapy, hypofractionated photons, and conventional photons. Notably, patients with higher-grade atypical or anaplastic meningiomas are not eligible for this trial.

Brachytherapy

Treatment of meningiomas with brachytherapy, the placement of radioactive seeds within the resection cavity, has occurred since the 1980s with iodine-125 seeds [36, 37]. Iodine-125 use in a cohort of 21 high-grade meningiomas was associated with a 33% complication rate that required surgical intervention, including 27% of patients developing radiation necrosis [38]. A second study of 42 meningioma patients treated with iodine-125 brachytherapy observed radiation necrosis in 16%, wound breakdown in 12%, hydrocephalus in 8%, as well as infection in 6% and pseudomeningocele in 5%. Such high toxicity rates have therefore limited brachytherapy use in recurrent and high-grade meningiomas.

However, a recent technical report discusses endoscopic endonasal cesium-131 brachytherapy seed placement in a patient with an anaplastic skull base meningioma [39]. No toxicity was reported during a follow-up period of 6.3 months. Moreover, a case series reported resection and cesium-131 brachytherapy seed placement in 19 patients with recurrent, previously irradiated meningiomas [40]. With a median follow-up of 15.4 months, two patients required surgery for complications, and two patients experienced radiation necrosis.

Given that cesium-131 has a half-life of only 9.7 days compared to 60 days for iodine-125 [41], it is possible that cesium-131 brachytherapy use in patients with recurrent or high-grade meningiomas may offer improved biological effectiveness, as compared to patients who have been historically treated with iodine-125 seeds and who experienced markedly high complication rates. A randomized clinical trial in meningioma patients evaluating safety and efficacy of Cesium-131 brachytherapy compared to other radiotherapy methods may be warranted. More data is needed to explore the efficacy of brachytherapy in meningioma patients.

Peptide Receptor Radionuclide Therapy

^{90}Y-DOTATOC and ^{177}Lu-DOTATATE are synthetic somatostatin analogues radio-labeled with a beta-emitting radionuclide that provide targeted radiotherapy to somatostatin-expressing cells. In 39 patients with progressive neuroendocrine tumors, which are classically somatostatin receptor positive, ^{90}Y-DOTATOC administration resulted in an objective response rate of 38% [42].

Similar to neuroendocrine tumors, the majority of meningiomas express the somatostatin receptor [43, 44]. In 29 patients with recurrent or progressive meningiomas treated with ^{90}Y-DOTATOC, 66% of patients had disease stabilization after 3 months of treatment [45]. Median time to progression in grade I meningiomas was 61 months and 13 months in higher-grade II–III meningiomas. In a second study of 34 patients with progressive unresectable meningioma treated with ^{90}Y-DOTATOC and ^{177}Lu-DOTATATE, mean survival from time of recruitment was 8.6 years; stable disease was achieved in 23 patients [46]. Gerster-Gilliéron et al. treated 15 patients with recurrent or progressive meningiomas with ^{90}Y-DOTATOC, reporting a median PFS of at least 24 months [47].

There are currently two clinical trials that are recruiting patients with meningiomas to undergo PRRT: NCT03273712 using 90Y-DOTATOC and NCT03936426 using a newer compound, 67Cu-SARTATE. 67Cu-SARTATE has been shown to have equivalent antitumor activity as ^{177}Lu-DOTATATE in a preclinical model [48].

Protein Phosphatase 2A Inhibitor

Protein phosphatase 2A (PP2A) is a key regulator of the cell cycle and is involved with DNA repair mechanisms, especially those related to repair of chemotherapeutic- and radiotherapy-induced cellular damage [49–51]. LB-100 acts as a small-molecule inhibitor of PP2A; the safety profile has been evaluated in a phase 1 trial [52]. Emerging preclinical evidence also suggests that, when combined with anti-PD-1 blockage, LD-100 promotes an enhanced effector T-cell-mediated response [53].

Ho et al. investigated the use of LB-100 in three human-derived immortalized meningioma cell lines and orthotopic xenograft mouse models [54]. They found that use of LB-100 in irradiated meningioma cells resulted in increased evidence of DNA double-strand breaks, mitotic catastrophic cell death, and G2/M cell cycle arrest. Moreover, in xenograft models, combined LB-100 and radiotherapy prolonged survival when compared to mice treated with radiotherapy alone: median survival 31 days compared to 27 days ($P < 0.05$).

To evaluate whether LB-100 is able to penetrate the blood-brain barrier, NCT03027388 is a phase 2 trial that is currently enrolling patients with glioblastoma. LB-100 will be administered prior to surgery to determine the pharmacokinetics of resected tumor tissue. Given the aforementioned promising in vitro and in vivo preclinical data, further investigation to explore the efficacy of LB-100 in patients with recurrent and high-grade meningiomas is encouraged.

Mebendazole

Mebendazole is an antiparasitic agent with systemic and intracranial activity [55]. Beyond use in parasitic infection, mebendazole inhibited tumor cell growth and facilitated apoptotic cell death in human cancer cell lines and xenograft models [56], including glioblastoma [57] and medulloblastoma [58].

Given that mebendazole acts by disrupting microtubule formation, synergistic use with radiotherapy has recently been investigated in meningioma preclinical models [59]. In a preclinical malignant meningioma mouse model, median survival in radiation treated and combined mebendazole and radiation treated was 33.5 days and 39 days, respectively ($P = 0.0062$). Such improvement in combined therapy supports synergistic effect of mebendazole treatment when combined with radiotherapy. Since mebendazole is a widely used drug with established safety profiles, there is clinical equipoise for a trial to evaluate the safety and efficacy of mebendazole in recurrent and high-grade meningioma when combined with radiotherapy.

Other Experimental Approaches

Tumor Treatment Fields

Tumor treatment fields (Optune™) is a wearable device that emits low-intensity, intermediate-frequency alternating electric fields via transducer arrays applied to the scalp. Such technology has demonstrated efficacy to disrupt microtubules during cell division and leads to eventual cell death in preclinical and animal models [60–63]. In a phase 3 trial evaluating efficacy of tumor treatment fields in patients with recurrent glioblastoma, 237 patients were randomized to tumor treatment fields alone or active chemotherapy control [64]. No improvement in overall survival was seen; however, the trial reported that efficacy was similar to patients who were enrolled in chemotherapy regimens, and patients reported improved toxicity and quality of life.

Recently, 695 patients with newly diagnosed glioblastoma were enrolled and randomized to receive as maintenance therapy either tumor treatment fields with concurrent temozolomide compared to temozolomide monotherapy. Median PFS was 6.7 months in patients who received combined maintenance therapy with

NovoTTF compared to 4.0 months for those who received temozolomide monotherapy. Similarly, median overall survival was 20.9 months compared to 16.0 months [65, 66].

Beyond the recent studies in patients with glioblastoma treated with tumor treatment fields, to date, there are very few meningioma patients who have been treated with this device. Preliminary analysis of a pilot study of six patients with recurrent atypical and anaplastic meningioma who were treated with tumor treatment fields revealed median PFS of 3.3 months (range, 1.0–4.6 months) (NCT01892397) [67]. All six patients failed prior surgical and radiotherapeutic interventions. Best radiographic response was stable disease in four patients, with an additional two patients having progressive disease. The objective response rate was 0%.

Additionally, in a reported case of a patient with newly diagnosed glioblastoma and an incidental meningioma distant from the glioblastoma site, tumor treatment fields therapy was associated with a significant radiographic response of 60% reduction at 20 weeks of the meningioma [68]. Notably, this patient was receiving concurrent temozolomide therapy for the glioblastoma and had received interval radiotherapy to the glioblastoma site.

These limited results have led to a phase 2 trial evaluating the use of tumor treatment fields concurrently with bevacizumab in patients with recurrent or progressive grade II or grade III meningioma (NCT02847559). The study's primary endpoint is PFS at 6 months.

Conclusion

Recurrent meningiomas represent a huge unmet clinical need in neuro-oncology. Historically, traditional chemotherapies have displayed limited efficacy in patients that fail surgery or radiation. With the advent of novel therapies, such as immunotherapy, or newer radiation techniques, there is hope for improved outcomes in this patient population.

References

1. Iwai Y, Ishida M, Tanaka Y, Okazaki T, Honjo T, Minato N. Involvement of PD-L1 on tumor cells in the escape from host immune system and tumor immunotherapy by PD-L1 blockade. Proc Natl Acad Sci. 2002;99(19):12293–7.
2. Larkin J, Chiarion-Sileni V, Gonzalez R, Grob JJ, Cowey CL, Lao CD, et al. Combined nivolumab and ipilimumab or monotherapy in untreated melanoma. N Engl J Med. 2015;373(1):23–34.
3. Yarchoan M, Hopkins A, Jaffee EM. Tumor mutational burden and response rate to PD-1 inhibition. N Engl J Med. 2017;377(25):2500–1.
4. Du Z, Abedalthagafi M, Aizer AA, McHenry AR, Sun HH, Bray M-A, et al. Increased expression of the immune modulatory molecule PD-L1 (CD274) in anaplastic meningioma. Oncotarget. 2015;6(7):4704–16.

5. Han SJ, Reis G, Kohanbash G, Shrivastav S, Magill ST, Molinaro AM, et al. Expression and prognostic impact of immune modulatory molecule PD-L1 in meningioma. J Neuro-Oncol. 2016;130(3):543–52.
6. Everson RG, Hashimoto Y, Freeman JL, Hodges TR, Huse J, Zhou S, et al. Multiplatform profiling of meningioma provides molecular insight and prioritization of drug targets for rational clinical trial design. J Neuro-Oncol. 2018;139(2):469–78.
7. Li YD, Veliceasa D, Lamano JB, Lamano JB, Kaur G, Biyashev D, et al. Systemic and local immunosuppression in patients with high-grade meningiomas. Cancer Immunol Immunother. 2019;68(6):999–1009. https://doi.org/10.1007/s00262-019-02342-8. Epub 2019 Apr 27.
8. Fridman WH, Pagès F, Sautès-Fridman C, Galon J. The immune contexture in human tumours: impact on clinical outcome. Nat Rev Cancer. 2012;12(4):298–306.
9. Baia GS, Caballero OL, Ho JSY, Zhao Q, Cohen T, Binder ZA, et al. NY-ESO-1 expression in meningioma suggests a rationale for new immunotherapeutic approaches. Cancer Immunol Res. 2013;1(5):296–302.
10. Grund S, Schittenhelm J, Roser F, Tatagiba M, Mawrin C, Kim YJ, et al. The microglial/macrophagic response at the tumour-brain border of invasive meningiomas. Neuropathol Appl Neurobiol. 2009;35(1):82–8.
11. Ding Y, Qiu L, Xu Q, Song L, Yang S, Yang T. Relationships between tumor microenvironment and clinicopathological parameters in meningioma. Int J Clin Exp Pathol. 2014;7(10):6973–9.
12. Hori S, Nomura T, Sakaguchi S. Control of regulatory T cell development by the transcription factor Foxp3. Science. 2003;299(5609):1057–61.
13. Fontenot JD, Gavin MA, Rudensky AY. Foxp3 programs the development and function of CD4+CD25+ regulatory T cells. Nat Immunol. 2003;4(4):330–6.
14. Domingues PH, Teodósio C, Otero Á, Sousa P, Ortiz J, Macias M, et al. Association between inflammatory infiltrates and isolated monosomy 22/del(22q) in meningiomas. PloS One. 2013;8(10):e74798.
15. Brastianos PK, Horowitz PM, Santagata S, Jones RT, McKenna A, Getz G, et al. Genomic sequencing of meningiomas identifies oncogenic SMO and AKT1 mutations. Nat Genet. 2013;45(3):285–9.
16. Ruttledge MH, Sarrazin J, Rangaratnam S, Phelan CM, Twist E, Merel P, et al. Evidence for the complete inactivation of the NF2 gene in the majority of sporadic meningiomas. Nat Genet. 1994;6(2):180–4.
17. Simpson AJG, Caballero OL, Jungbluth A, Chen Y-T, Old LJ. Cancer/testis antigens, gametogenesis and cancer. Nat Rev Cancer. 2005;5(8):615–25.
18. Scanlan MJ, Gure AO, Jungbluth AA, Old LJ, Chen Y-T. Cancer/testis antigens: an expanding family of targets for cancer immunotherapy. Immunol Rev. 2002;188(1):22–32.
19. Cheever MA, Allison JP, Ferris AS, Finn OJ, Hastings BM, Hecht TT, et al. The prioritization of cancer antigens: a national cancer institute pilot project for the acceleration of translational research. Clin Cancer Res. 2009;15(17):5323–37.
20. Thomas R, Al-Khadairi G, Roelands J, Hendrickx W, Dermime S, Bedognetti D, et al. NY-ESO-1 based immunotherapy of cancer: current perspectives. Front Immunol. 2018;1:9.
21. Robbins PF, Morgan RA, Feldman SA, Yang JC, Sherry RM, Dudley ME, et al. Tumor regression in patients with metastatic synovial cell sarcoma and melanoma using genetically engineered lymphocytes reactive with NY-ESO-1. J Clin Oncol. 2011;29(7):917–24.
22. Syed ON, Mandigo CE, Killory BD, Canoll P, Bruce JN. Cancer-testis and melanocyte-differentiation antigen expression in malignant glioma and meningioma. J Clin Neurosci. 2012;19(7):1016–21.
23. Goldsmith BJ, Wara WM, Wilson CB, Larson DA. Postoperative irradiation for subtotally resected meningiomas. J Neurosurg. 1994;80(2):195–201.
24. Aghi MK, Carter BS, Cosgrove GR, Ojemann RG, Amin-Hanjani S, Martuza RL, et al. Long-term recurrence rates of atypical meningiomas after gross total resection with or without postoperative adjuvant radiation. Neurosurgery. 2009;64(1):56–60.

25. Wenkel E, Thornton AF, Finkelstein D, Adams J, Lyons S, De La Monte S, et al. Benign meningioma: partially resected, biopsied, and recurrent intracranial tumors treated with combined proton and photon radiotherapy. Int J Radiat Oncol Biol Phys. 2000;48(5):1363–70.
26. Schulz-Ertner D, Tsujii H. Particle radiation therapy using proton and heavier ion beams. J Clin Oncol Off J Am Soc Clin Oncol. 2007;25(8):953–64.
27. Schulz-Ertner D, Nikoghosyan A, Hof H, Didinger B, Combs SE, Jäkel O, et al. Carbon ion radiotherapy of skull base chondrosarcomas. Int J Radiat Oncol Biol Phys. 2007;67(1):171–7.
28. Schulz-Ertner D, Karger CP, Feuerhake A, Nikoghosyan A, Combs SE, Jäkel O, et al. Effectiveness of carbon ion radiotherapy in the treatment of skull-base chordomas. Int J Radiat Oncol Biol Phys. 2007;68(2):449–57.
29. Combs SE, Hartmann C, Nikoghosyan A, Jäkel O, Karger CP, Haberer T, et al. Carbon ion radiation therapy for high-risk meningiomas. Radiother Oncol. 2010;95(1):54–9.
30. Adeberg S, Hartmann C, Welzel T, Rieken S, Habermehl D, von Deimling A, et al. Long-term outcome after radiotherapy in patients with atypical and malignant meningiomas--clinical results in 85 patients treated in a single institution leading to optimized guidelines for early radiation therapy. Int J Radiat Oncol Biol Phys. 2012;83(3):859–64.
31. Rieken S, Habermehl D, Haberer T, Jaekel O, Debus J, Combs SE. Proton and carbon ion radiotherapy for primary brain tumors delivered with active raster scanning at the Heidelberg Ion Therapy Center (HIT): early treatment results and study concepts. Radiat Oncol (London England). 2012;7:41.
32. Combs SE, Welzel T, Habermehl D, Rieken S, Dittmar J-O, Kessel K, et al. Prospective evaluation of early treatment outcome in patients with meningiomas treated with particle therapy based on target volume definition with MRI and 68Ga-DOTATOC-PET. Acta Oncol (Stockholm, Sweden). 2013;52(3):514–20.
33. Mozes P, Dittmar JO, Habermehl D, Tonndorf-Martini E, Hideghety K, Dittmar A, et al. Volumetric response of intracranial meningioma after photon or particle irradiation. Acta Oncol (Stockholm, Sweden). 2017;56(3):431–7.
34. El Shafie RA, Czech M, Kessel KA, Habermehl D, Weber D, Rieken S, et al. Clinical outcome after particle therapy for meningiomas of the skull base: toxicity and local control in patients treated with active rasterscanning. Radiat Oncol (London, England). 2018;13(1):54.
35. El Shafie RA, Czech M, Kessel KA, Habermehl D, Weber D, Rieken S, et al. Evaluation of particle radiotherapy for the re-irradiation of recurrent intracranial meningioma. Radiat Oncol (London, England). 2018;13(1):86.
36. Kumar PP, Good RR, Jones EO, Hahn FJ, McCaul GF, Gallagher TF, et al. A new method for treatment of unresectable, recurrent brain tumors with single permanent high-activity 125iodine brachytherapy. Radiat Med. 1986;4(1):12–20.
37. Gutin PH, Leibel SA, Hosobuchi Y, Crumley RL, Edwards MS, Wilson CB, et al. Brachytherapy of recurrent tumors of the skull base and spine with iodine-125 sources. Neurosurgery. 1987;20(6):938–45.
38. Ware ML, Larson DA, Sneed PK, Wara WW, McDermott MW. Surgical resection and permanent brachytherapy for recurrent atypical and malignant meningioma. Neurosurgery. 2004;54(1):55–63; discussion 63–64.
39. Shafiq AR, Wernicke AG, Riley CA, Morgenstern PF, Nedialkova L, Pannullo SC, et al. Placement of cesium-131 permanent brachytherapy seeds using the endoscopic endonasal approach for recurrent anaplastic skull base meningioma: case report and technical note. J Neurosurg. 2019;1:1–6. https://doi.org/10.3171/2018.11.JNS181943. Online ahead of print.
40. Brachman DG, Youssef E, Dardis CJ, Sanai N, Zabramski JM, Smith KA, et al. Resection and permanent intracranial brachytherapy using modular, biocompatible cesium-131 implants: results in 20 recurrent, previously irradiated meningiomas. J Neurosurg. 2018;131:1819–28.
41. Murphy MK, Piper RK, Greenwood LR, Mitch MG, Lamperti PJ, Seltzer SM, et al. Evaluation of the new cesium-131 seed for use in low-energy x-ray brachytherapy. Med Phys. 2004;31(6):1529–38.

42. Waldherr C, Pless M, Maecke HR, Schumacher T, Crazzolara A, Nitzsche EU, et al. Tumor response and clinical benefit in neuroendocrine tumors after 7.4 GBq (90)Y-DOTATOC. J Nucl Med. 2002;43(5):610–6.
43. Schulz S, Pauli SU, Schulz S, Händel M, Dietzmann K, Firsching R, et al. Immunohistochemical determination of five somatostatin receptors in meningioma reveals frequent overexpression of somatostatin receptor subtype sst2A. Clin Cancer Res. 2000;6(5):1865–74.
44. Reubi JC, Maurer R, Klijn JG, Stefanko SZ, Foekens JA, Blaauw G, et al. High incidence of somatostatin receptors in human meningiomas: biochemical characterization. J Clin Endocrinol Metab. 1986;63(2):433–8.
45. Bartolomei M, Bodei L, De Cicco C, Grana CM, Cremonesi M, Botteri E, et al. Peptide receptor radionuclide therapy with (90)Y-DOTATOC in recurrent meningioma. Eur J Nucl Med Mol Imaging. 2009;36(9):1407–16.
46. Marincek N, Radojewski P, Dumont RA, Brunner P, Müller-Brand J, Maecke HR, et al. Somatostatin receptor-targeted radiopeptide therapy with 90Y-DOTATOC and 177Lu-DOTATOC in progressive meningioma: long-term results of a phase II clinical trial. J Nucl Med. 2015;56(2):171–6.
47. Gerster-Gilliéron K, Forrer F, Maecke H, Mueller-Brand J, Merlo A, Cordier D. 90Y-DOTATOC as a therapeutic option for complex recurrent or progressive meningiomas. J Nucl Med. 2015;56(11):1748–51.
48. Cullinane C, Jeffery C, Walker R, Roselt P, Binns D, van Dam E, et al. Comparing the therapeutic efficacy of 67Cu-SARTATE and 177Lu-DOTA-octreotate in a neuroendocrine tumor model. J Nucl Med. 2018;59(supplement 1):315.
49. Wei D, Parsels LA, Karnak D, Davis MA, Parsels JD, Marsh AC, et al. Inhibition of protein phosphatase 2A radiosensitizes pancreatic cancers by modulating CDC25C/CDK1 and homologous recombination repair. Clin Cancer Res. 2013;19(16):4422–32.
50. Perrotti D, Neviani P. Protein phosphatase 2A: a target for anticancer therapy. Lancet Oncol. 2013;14(6):e229–38.
51. Lee D-H, Chowdhury D. What goes on must come off: phosphatases gate-crash the DNA damage response. Trends Biochem Sci. 2011;36(11):569–77.
52. Chung V, Mansfield AS, Braiteh F, Richards D, Durivage H, Ungerleider RS, et al. Safety, tolerability, and preliminary activity of LB-100, an inhibitor of protein phosphatase 2A, in patients with relapsed solid tumors: an open-label, dose escalation, first-in-human, phase I trial. Clin Cancer Res. 2017;23(13):3277–84.
53. Ho WS, Wang H, Maggio D, Kovach JS, Zhang Q, Song Q, et al. Pharmacologic inhibition of protein phosphatase-2A achieves durable immune-mediated antitumor activity when combined with PD-1 blockade. Nat Commun. 2018;9(1):2126.
54. Ho WS, Sizdahkhani S, Hao S, Song H, Seldomridge A, Tandle A, et al. LB-100, a novel Protein Phosphatase 2A (PP2A) inhibitor, sensitizes malignant meningioma cells to the therapeutic effects of radiation. Cancer Lett. 2018;415:217–26.
55. Keiser J, Utzinger J. Efficacy of current drugs against soil-transmitted helminth infections: systematic review and meta-analysis. JAMA. 2008;299(16):1937–48.
56. Mukhopadhyay T, Sasaki J, Ramesh R, Roth JA. Mebendazole elicits a potent antitumor effect on human cancer cell lines both in vitro and in vivo. Clin Cancer Res. 2002;8(9):2963–9.
57. Bai R-Y, Staedtke V, Aprhys CM, Gallia GL, Riggins GJ. Antiparasitic mebendazole shows survival benefit in 2 preclinical models of glioblastoma multiforme. Neuro-Oncology. 2011;13(9):974–82.
58. Bai R-Y, Staedtke V, Rudin CM, Bunz F, Riggins GJ. Effective treatment of diverse medulloblastoma models with mebendazole and its impact on tumor angiogenesis. Neuro-Oncology. 2015;17(4):545–54.
59. Skibinski CG, Williamson T, Riggins GJ. Mebendazole and radiation in combination increase survival through anticancer mechanisms in an intracranial rodent model of malignant meningioma. J Neuro-Oncol. 2018;140(3):529–38.

60. Kirson ED, Gurvich Z, Schneiderman R, Dekel E, Itzhaki A, Wasserman Y, et al. Disruption of cancer cell replication by alternating electric fields. Cancer Res. 2004;64(9):3288–95.
61. Kirson ED, Dbaly V, Tovarys F, Vymazal J, Soustiel JF, Itzhaki A, et al. Alternating electric fields arrest cell proliferation in animal tumor models and human brain tumors. Proc Natl Acad Sci. 2007;104(24):10152–7.
62. Kirson ED, Schneiderman RS, Dbalý V, Tovaryš F, Vymazal J, Itzhaki A, et al. Chemotherapeutic treatment efficacy and sensitivity are increased by adjuvant alternating electric fields (TTFields). BMC Med Phys. 2009;9:1. https://doi.org/10.1186/1756-6649-9-1.
63. Lee SX, Tunkyi A, Wong E, Swanson KD. Mitosis interference of cancer cells during anaphase by electric field from NovoTTF-100A: an update. J Clin Oncol. 2012;30(15_suppl):e21078.
64. Stupp R, Wong ET, Kanner AA, Steinberg D, Engelhard H, Heidecke V, et al. NovoTTF-100A versus physician's choice chemotherapy in recurrent glioblastoma: a randomised phase III trial of a novel treatment modality. Eur J Cancer. 2012;48(14):2192–202.
65. Stupp R, Taillibert S, Kanner AA, Kesari S, Steinberg DM, Toms SA, et al. Maintenance therapy with tumor-treating fields plus temozolomide vs temozolomide alone for glioblastoma: a randomized clinical trial. JAMA. 2015;314(23):2535.
66. Stupp R, Taillibert S, Kanner A, Read W, Steinberg DM, Lhermitte B, et al. Effect of tumor-treating fields plus maintenance temozolomide vs maintenance temozolomide alone on survival in patients with glioblastoma: a randomized clinical trial. JAMA. 2017;318(23):2306.
67. Wu S, Gavrilovec I, De La Fuente MI, Kreisl T, Kaley T. ACTR-43. Pilot study of optune (novoTTF-100A) for recurrent atypical and anaplastic meningioma. Neuro Oncol. 2016;18(suppl_6):vi11.
68. Schaff L, Armentano F, Harrison C, Lassman A, McKhann G, Iwamoto F. NO-006. Radiographic response of an incidental meningioma in a patient with glioblastoma on novo-TTF therapy. Neuro Oncol. 2013;15(suppl_3):ii99.

Index

© Springer Nature Switzerland AG 2020
J. Moliterno, A. Omuro (eds.), *Meningiomas*,
https://doi.org/10.1007/978-3-030-59558-6